D1760421

Surgical Aspects of Peritoneal Dialysis

Stephen Haggerty

Editor

Surgical Aspects of Peritoneal Dialysis

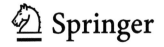

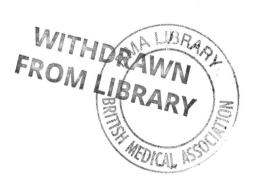

Editor
Stephen Haggerty
Division of Gastrointestinal and
General Surgery
NorthShore University HealthSystem
Evanston, IL
USA

ISBN 978-3-319-52820-5   ISBN 978-3-319-52821-2   (eBook)
DOI 10.1007/978-3-319-52821-2

Library of Congress Control Number: 2017937373

Printed on acid-free paper

This Springer imprint is published by Springer Nature
The registered company is Springer International Publishing AG
The registered company address is: Gewerbestrasse 11, 6330 Cham, Switzerland

I dedicate this book to my lovely wife Pride Turner Haggerty and my three children Peter, Charlie, and Pridie. I appreciate their love and support during this process.

Foreword

Surgeons and Surgical technology have always been an integral part of peritoneal dialysis evolution because infusion of solution into the peritoneal cavity needs a conduit. Christopher Warrick from England in 1740 used the surgical technique to insert a leather pipe in the peritoneal cavity and three years later, Stephen Hale, again from England used two surgical trocars for infusion and drainage of fluids from the peritoneal cavity. Georg Ganter from Germany in 1923 performed peritoneal exchanges in human subjects, using a simple needle to instill and drain one to three liters of specially prepared sterile PD solution that contained appropriate amount of electrolytes and dextrose. He observed that needle allowed free inflow but drainage was very cumbersome. Peritonitis was a frequent complication. To the modern nephrologists involved in peritoneal dialysis, Ganter's observations would be a "loud music"! In the ensuing nearly a century, many innovators including surgeons and nephrologists have worked on designing a dedicated peritoneal dialysis access. In the process, they have used surgical materials like, glass cannulas, trocars, gall bladder trocars, rubber cannulas, Foley catheter, and surgical drains. The disadvantages of these devices were rigidity of the material causing pressure-trauma to the internal organs, air suction and entrapment in the system, fluid leaks and inadequate fixation of devices to the abdominal wall. The result of all these inadequacies was inevitable peritonitis. Innovations in 1950s and 1960s gave us PD catheters that were biocompatible, flexible, less rigid and easily anchored to the abdominal wall. The Tenckhoff catheter, introduced in 1968, was the major breakthrough that saw the peritoneal dialysis become an alternative therapy for ESRD. This catheter has stood the test of time

Based on our 40+ years of clinical experience, I feel the outcome of PD catheters depends upon the experience and technical skills of the operator, including surgeon, interventional nephrologist or radiologist. An ideal catheter insertion would place the catheter tip deep in the pelvis and prevent it from migrating out of pelvis. In order to accomplish this, the operator has to be familiar with the simple but most important component of providing the pelvic tilt to the cuff at the peritoneal entry site. Positioning the catheter terminal segment in the deep pelvis has an additional benefit; keeping the side holes farther away from the omentum. The small amount of intra-peritoneal fluid containing protein bathes the catheter and over-time forms a thin coating outside and inside the catheter. This protein coating of the catheter makes it less likely to be captured by the omentum. It is my observation that omental capture of the terminal segment of the catheter occurs mostly during the first few days after insertion. The second most important step is for the surgeon to ensure that he or she creates an appropriate length of sinus track at the exit site. Too short, too long or too wide a sinus track exposes the higher risk of cuff extrusion or exit site infection. Based on our observations of several hundred cases, Zbylut Twardowski, MD, my respected colleague now retired, concluded that in most human peritoneal dialysis catheter tunnels, during the healing process, the epithelium does not reach to the level of cuff, but grows only for a few millimeters from the exit in the sinus tract. We observed that there are fast healing exits, where the epidermis starts entering into the sinus after 2-3 weeks; and slow healing exits, where the epidermis starts entering into the sinus after 4-6 weeks. The healing process is complete in 4-8 weeks when the epidermis covers approximately half of a visible sinus tract. My goal is to see every sinus tract look like an umbilicus! The third important principle is to preserve the natural shape of the catheter during insertion. The catheter material is a silicone rubber and has its elastic property. When catheter is placed in its unnatural shape, it tends to create opposing forces to get back to its original shape. These forces could cause delayed wound healing, and slowly cause cuff extrusion and catheter tip migration. Lastly and equally important is the care of the catheter by the dialysis nurse, especially during the catheter healing process. The dialysis nurse should ensure at the exit site, the catheter is kept completely immobilized during the entire period of healing. Unintended mobility around the catheter exit site promotes trauma at the site and increase granulation tissue. Consequently, minor bleeding could occur and promote infection. Constricting stitches to immobilize the catheter should be discouraged. When the sinus tract heals completely, the exit site is amazingly resistant to infection. To accomplish excellent results requires a well-coordinated team of surgeons, nephrologists and dialysis nurses. Complications like, catheter tip migration out of pelvis, omental capture, exit infection, cuff extrusion, tunnel infection and ultimately peritonitis can be eliminated or for sure can be minimized. The process of PD catheter placement is an art that has to be seen and cultivated from an expert!

Our PD program is fortunate to have had the expertise of a surgeon, W. Kirt Nichols MD. For over forty years, he collaborated with us both clinically and academically. One of the unique features about our long-term relationship is the open and free communication. In the OR, a Post-op a KUB is performed after every PD catheter placement. Such imaging study provides us a baseline catheter position and a talking point for our discussion for each other's learning. Frequently we discuss whether the surgery met our standards of placement. We have learned a lot from these discussions and have established our own standards. I am sure, during his days at the University of Missouri, Dr. Stephen Haggerty learned from Kirt's experience and long established teamwork approach with nephrology. Not only that Stephen has established a top class PD catheter placement program, it is only fitting that he embarked on writing a book on the surgical aspect of peritoneal dialysis. At the outset, it might raise a question "A book on peritoneal dialysis by a surgeon?" It is my strong conviction that surgeons make or break the functioning and longevity of a PD catheter and the success of the PD program.

Sharing experiences of surgical pioneers like Kirt Nichols, John Crabtree, Stephen Haggerty, and innumerable other surgeons and interventionists through a book is long overdue! The tradition in medical world is to learn from a mentor. A surgeon teaching a colleague surgeon has more impact than any other approach. It is no accident that in this book, 10 of the 15 chapters are dedicated to surgical aspects of peritoneal dialysis. Several world-renowned expert authors have extensively described the pre-op preparation of patients, surgical and laparoscopic insertion technique of different catheter types. Chapters on diagnosis and management of catheter dysfunction and mechanical complications would be well appreciated by all dealing with peritoneal dialysis

There appears to be a resurgence of peritoneal dialysis in the United States and of course, globally its penetration keeps increasing. Training on the surgical aspects of PD should be a part of the overall training related to peritoneal dialysis. Haggerty's book on the Surgical Aspects of Peritoneal Dialysis, a unique treasure. With vast amount of expert knowledge poured in it, would find a niche in the peritoneal dialysis community. As Sir William Osler said "The art of the practice of medicine is to be learned only by experience; 'tis not an inheritance; it cannot be revealed. Learn to see, learn to hear, learn to feel, learn to smell, and know that by practice alone can you become expert." Osler said at other place, "it is harder to acquire the art than the science…. There is still virtue, believe me, in that "long unlovely street", and the old art cannot possibly be replaced by, but must be absorbed in, the new science."

Columbia, MO, USA   Ramesh Khanna, MD
                                                                                                          Karl D. Nolph, MD

Preface

The concept of peritoneal dialysis (PD) has been a work in progress for over a century. The first report of "peritoneal irrigation" as a successful treatment of renal failure was in 1946 by Frank, Seligman, and Fine. Maxwell and colleagues were the first to describe a technique similar to today's form of peritoneal dialysis exchanges in a "closed system" using commercial solutions, disposable tubing, and a nylon catheter in 1959. By 1980, continuous ambulatory peritoneal dialysis (CAPD) had become a proven mode of renal replacement therapy and was being offered in over 116 medical centers in the United States. Its use has steadily grown throughout the world with many countries using it as the primary mode dialysis. Having a functioning intraperitoneal catheter is mandatory in these patients. Across the globe, PD catheters are placed by nephrologists, surgeons, and interventional radiologists based on availability and individual expertise. Peritoneal dialysis catheters may be placed at the bedside, in a fluoroscopic suite, or in an operating room, and it is paramount to minimize complications and maximize longevity of these catheters to have successful PD. To help achieve this, there have been published best available practices and guidelines regarding peritoneal dialysis catheter insertion and care. However, there are no dedicated reference books on the *Surgical Aspects of Peritoneal Dialysis*.

When I started my current practice in 1999 as a general and laparoscopic surgeon, I did not have much interest in placing PD catheters. Like most general surgeons at the time, I was trained in open placement during residency by the transplant surgeons. Soon after starting practice, I was introduced to laparoscopic insertion by my partner Earl Norman, MD, and Mike Carder, NP coordinator of our PD unit. I began placing all PD catheters using a basic laparoscopic technique using a sheath and dilator. I presented and published our initial experience and during my literature review became familiar with the work of John Crabtree of California. He had published several papers on laparoscopic PD catheter insertion and introduced the idea of rectus sheath tunnel and omentopexy. He then began teaching these as "best practices" in PD catheter insertion. To this day, he has published the most papers on peritoneal dialysis access and taught thousands of surgeons on these techniques at the Peritoneal Dialysis University for Surgeons course, sponsored by the International Society of Peritoneal Dialysis. We owe many of the advances in the surgical aspects of peritoneal dialysis to Dr. Crabtree. After learning of these techniques, my practice quickly evolved to advanced laparoscopic insertion, and I became one of the busiest peritoneal dialysis access surgeons in Chicago. I have maintained a scientific interest in PD and related complications through ongoing retrospective and prospective clinical research at our institution. In addition, I have taught several courses to surgeons, published our own institutional data, and been lead author on the SAGES Guideline for Peritoneal Dialysis Access Surgery. Finally, I have had great collaboration with our robust nephrology department and outpatient PD centers to deliver outstanding outcomes to a high volume of patients.

The purpose of *Surgical Aspects of Peritoneal Dialysis* is to provide a reference for physicians, surgeons, and interventionalists who care for renal failure patients who are on or considering peritoneal dialysis as a mode of renal replacement therapy. As the use of PD hopefully grows in the United States as it has done throughout the world, we need experts to care for these patients. Education and attention to detail are important in obtaining good outcomes. This book should provide a foundation of knowledge about the medical and surgical aspects of peritoneal dialysis for surgeons, nephrologists, and interventional radiologists.

Surgical Aspects of Peritoneal Dialysis consists of 15 chapters covering an overview of how peritoneal dialysis works, preoperative considerations, and patient selection, as well as separate chapters on insertion techniques, postoperative care, and complications. I am thrilled that we have had many experts from around the world contributing to this book and hope it helps physicians and surgeons deliver the best care to these challenging patients.

Evanston, IL, USA   Stephen Haggerty, MD, FACS

Contents

Contributors

Ahmed Kamel Abdel Aal, MD, MSc, PhD Department of Radiology, University of Alabama at Birmingham, Birmingham, AL, USA

Fahad Aziz, MD Division of Nephrology, Department of Medicine, University of Missouri-Columbia, Columbia, MO, USA

Nicolas Bonamici, BA Grainger Center for Simulation and Innovation, NorthShore University HealthSystem, Evanston, IL, USA

Edwina A. Brown, MD West London Renal and Transplant Centre, Imperial College Healthcare NHS Trust, Hammersmith Hospital, London, UK

Micah R. Chan, MD, MPH, FACP, FNKF, FASDIN Division of Nephrology, University of Wisconsin School of Medicine and Public Health, Madison, WI, USA

Wael Darwish, MD Department of Radiology, National Cancer Institute, Cairo, Egypt

Pierpaolo Di Cocco, MD West London Renal and Transplant Centre, Imperial College Healthcare NHS Trust, Hammersmith Hospital, London, UK

Frank J.M.F. Dor, MD, PhD West London Renal and Transplant Centre, Imperial College Healthcare NHS Trust, Hammersmith Hospital, London, UK

Amilcar A. Exume, MD Department of General Surgery, Southern California Permanente Medical Group, San Diego, CA, USA

Seth B. Furgeson, MD Division of Renal Diseases and Hypertension, University of Colorado-Anschutz Medical Campus, Denver Health Hospital, Aurora, CO, USA

Stephen Haggerty, MD, FACS Department of Surgery, NorthShore University HealthSystem, Evanston, IL, USA

Ivy N. Haskins, MD Digestive Disease and Surgical Institute, The Cleveland Clinic Foundation, Cleveland, OH, USA

L. Tammy Ho, MD Division of Nephrology and Hypertension, NorthShore University HealthSystem, Evanston, IL, USA

Juaquito M. Jorge, MD Department of Surgery, Northwestern University Feinberg School of Medicine, Chicago, IL, USA

Neenoo Khosla, MD Division of Nephrology and Hypertension, NorthShore University HealthSystem, Evanston, IL, USA

Monika A. Krezalek, MD Department of Surgery, The University of Chicago Pritzker School of Medicine, Chicago, IL, USA

Brendan McCormick, MD, FRCPC Division of Nephrology, Department of Medicine, University of Ottawa and the Ottawa Hospital, Ottawa, ON, Canada

Alan Moreno, MD Division of Nephrology and Hypertension, NorthShore University HealthSystem, Evanston, IL, USA

Amr Soliman Moustafa, MD, MSc Department of Radiology, University of Arkansas for Medical Science, Little Rock, AR, USA

W. Kirt Nichols, MD, MHA Department of Surgery, University of Missouri-Columbia, Columbia, MO, USA

Guner Ogunc, MD Department of General Surgery, University of Akdeniz, Faculty of medicine, Antalya, Turkey

Vassilios E. Papalois, MD West London Renal and Transplant Centre, Imperial College Healthcare NHS Trust, Hammersmith Hospital, London, UK

Steven Rosenblatt, MD, FACS Digestive Disease and Surgical Institute, The Cleveland Clinic Foundation, Cleveland, OH, USA

Nael Saad, MD Department of Radiology, Mallinckrodt Institute of Radiology, Washington University in Saint Louis, St. Louis, MO, USA

Menaka Sarav, MD Division of Nephrology and Hypertension, NorthShore University HealthSystem, Evanston, IL, USA

Isaac Teitelbaum, MD, FACP University of Colorado Hospital, AIP, Aurora, CO, USA

Sana Waheed, MD Division of Nephrology, University of Wisconsin School of Medicine and Public Health, Madison, WI, USA

The Epidemiology of Renal Replacement Therapy

Sana Waheed and Micah R. Chan

Epidemiology of End Stage Renal Disease

Approximately 14% of the US adult population (more than 20 million patients) is affected by chronic kidney disease (CKD) [1]. For an individual, lifetime risk of CKD is high; with more than half of US adults aged 30–64 years old likely to develop CKD (Hoerger et al. 2015). CKD progresses in a substantial proportion of these patients to the point of needing some form of RRT. In 2013 alone, 120,000 patients reached End Stage Renal Disease (ESRD), of which 88% of patients started HD, 9% began PD and 2.6% received a preemptive kidney transplant [1]. (Fig. 1.1) After a year-by-year rise in ESRD incidence over two decades from 1980 through 2000, it has been roughly stable from 2000 to 2013. Regardless, the prevalence of ESRD in the United States has grown in recent years. As of December 31, 2013, there were more than 660,000 prevalent cases of ESRD in the US- an increase of 3.5% since 2012 and an increase of 68% since 2000 [1]. The vast majority of prevalent ESRD population is undergoing in-center hemodialysis (ICHD).

The incidence rates of ESRD increase with age and the majority of patients who develop ESRD have diabetes or hypertension as the underlying cause of their kidney disease. Moreover, there are significant ethnic differences in the prevalence of ESRD. Compared to whites, ESRD prevalence is about 3.7 times higher in African Americans [1]. Recently, this increased risk of kidney disease in this population have been linked to G1 and G2 high-risk alleles for a gene *APOL1* that is located on chromosome 22 [2]. These high-risk alleles provide resistance to disease causing trypanosomiases, which led to their natural selection in the population [3].

Since most symptoms of CKD do not appear till late in the disease process, delay in diagnosis of CKD and referral to nephrology remains a big problem. Based on the USRDS data for patients starting ESRD therapy in 2013, it appears that 25% of patients received no nephrology care and an additional 13% had unknown duration of nephrology care prior to initiation of ESRD therapy. The duration of pre-ESRD care is also associated with age and young patients are most likely to have a longer duration (> 12 months) of pre- ESRD care [1].

The quality of life and the life expectancy of most patients on dialysis are low. Dialysis patients have a much higher mortality rate than the general Medicare population and also compared to Medicare patients with diabetes, acute myocardial infarction, heart failure and cancer. Dialysis patients younger than 80 years old are

S. Waheed, MD • M.R. Chan, MD MPH (✉)
University of Wisconsin School of Medicine and Public Health, Division of Nephrology,
Madison, WI, USA
e-mail: swaheed@medicine.wisc.edu;
mr.chan@hosp.wisc.edu

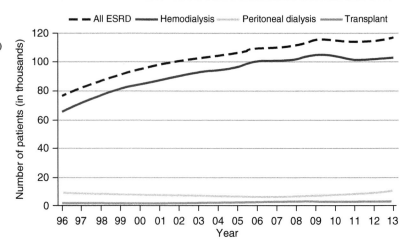

Fig. 1.1 Trends in the annual number of ESRD incident cases (in thousands) by modality, in the U.S. population, 1996–2013-USRDS ADR 2015 (USRDS-ADR [1])

expected to live less than one-third as long as their counterparts without ESRD. The major cause of death in these patients is related to cardiovascular events [1].

Unfortunately, in addition to the increased mortality rate, the quality of life for ESRD patients is adversely affected because of a high symptom burden. Moreover, they are often admitted to hospitals with volume overload, infections and access related complications. On average, ESRD patients are admitted to the hospital nearly twice a year, and about 30% have an unplanned re-hospitalization within the 30 days following discharge [4].

Cost

Chronic maintenance dialysis is an expensive procedure and Centers for Medicare and Medicaid Services extends coverage to all patients with ESRD who require dialysis or transplantation. When this was implemented in 1972, only about 10,000 patients were receiving dialysis, a number that has increased to over 469,000 patients with a cost of 30.9 billion dollars in 2013 [5]. This accounts for 7.1% of the overall Medicare paid claims cost for less than 1% of the total Medicare population [1].

The exact cost per patient per year depends upon the modality used, with HD being the most expensive at approximately $85,000 per patient per year (PPPY), followed by PD, which costs approximately $70,000 PPPY. Transplant is the

most cost effective therapy with an expenditure of approximately $30,000 PPPY [1]. It is significant to point out that the difference in the expenditure of HD and PD in the US is not driven by a lower reimbursement to the dialysis units [6]. The amount paid to the dialysis units is the same for HD and PD but the higher cost for the HD population is mainly attributed to the cost of inpatient care and medication use [7]. Based on these numbers, one can deduce that PD is a financially attractive option for the ever-increasing population of ESRD patients in the US.

Utilization of Peritoneal Dialysis in United States

Although PD has been used as an RRT modality since 1976, the rapid growth of the ESRD population in the early 2000s was mostly due to patients undergoing ICHD [8]. Financial incentives for ICHD and concerns regarding the outcomes on PD were among the major reasons for this disproportionate increase in ICHD and as of 2008, less than 7% of the prevalent ESRD population was on PD [9]. The bundling of dialysis-related services led to a renewed interest in PD nationally with a 50% increase in the prevalent PD population from 2008 to 2013 (45,000 patients were on PD in 2013 compared to 30,000 in 2008) [1].

Despite this increase, the rate of PD utilization in the US is much lower than other countries like Hong Kong, Australia, New Zealand and Canada [10]. This difference cannot be solely attributed to variance in patient characteristics but is rather a result of obstacles impeding the growth of PD in our health care system. Lack of informed decision-making in ESRD patients is the biggest barrier. A quarter of the patients starting dialysis receive no pre-ESRD care but even more worrying is the fact that two-thirds of the patients are not even offered PD as an option despite the fact that 87% of patients would be eligible for it [1, 11, 12]. It is extremely concerning that these numbers challenge the basic principles of autonomy and patient-centered care.

Another important issue is the lack of familiarization with PD in providers since most nephrology training programs focus on HD [13]. Based on the results of a recent survey, 88% of nephrology training program directors felt that PD fellow training was limited and 60% endorsed personal inadequate PD training [14]. As physicians, our practice is limited to what we are most comfortable with. Therefore, these training limitations translate into lower use of PD by providers during independent practice.

In addition to provider related aspects, the most important factor in determining dialysis modality selection is patient choice. Despite being presented with the option of PD, a substantial number of patients choose to undergo HD. Patients report the fear of something catastrophic happening at home without health care provider supervision, lack of space at home and feeling of social isolation as main barriers to selecting PD [15].

In summary, both provider and patient related issues limit the use of PD in the US, which have to be addressed at a national level. Several initiatives like the Home Dialysis University for fellows are addressing the deficiency in provider training. However, most importantly as a team of health care providers, we should emphasize enhancement in patient education and patient empowerment, allowing them to make a decision that suits their lifestyle.

Patient Selection for Peritoneal Dialysis

All ESRD patients should be assessed for PD eligibility. There are very few absolute contraindications to PD, which include lack of residence

Table 1.1 Patient eligibility for peritoneal dialysis

Contraindications	Barriers
Place of residence does not permit PD	Impaired vision or hearing
Active diverticulitis	Insufficient strength or dexterity
Major abdominal surgeries	Immobility
Large unrepaired abdominal wall hernias	Dementia
Increasing abdominal aortic aneurysms	Poor hygiene
Acute psychiatric illness	Non-adherence

Modified from Blake and Quinn [16]

permitting PD, morbid obesity, large unrepaired abdominal wall hernias, expanding abdominal aortic aneurysm and active diverticulitis [16]. Most other factors like impaired vision, hearing, lack of dexterity to make PD connections, immobility and dementia are barriers, and these can potentially be overcome if a patient has assistance at home [16] (Table 1.1).

After evaluation of PD suitability, patients should then be offered a free choice as a part of modality education with written material, websites, videos, group lectures and one-to-one sessions on an as needed basis. The key here is to let the patients decide, as they are more likely to do better with the modality that they are interested in. Most studies show that half of the patients would choose PD if given the right [17].

Comparison of Peritoneal Dialysis to Hemodialysis

Historically, the studies comparing outcomes of PD and HD have focused on mortality and yielded controversial results. An ideal comparison would have been a randomized controlled trial, which has been attempted in the past with very low recruitment rates. Earlier epidemiologic studies based on US renal data system (USRDS) registry showed that PD was associated with a 19% increase in mortality [18]. This became the cornerstone of the argument that PD is somehow an inferior therapy compared to HD. However, there has been a significant improvement in outcomes of PD since then as shown in a study by Mehrotra et al., where the composite outcome of mortality and change in modality over an 8 year period (between 1996 and 2003) showed a 17% improvement in PD outcomes as opposed to HD outcomes where there was no significant improvement [19]. More recent registry data from the USRDS and Denmark shows that there is no significant mortality difference based on the modality for RRT [20, 21]. In the US, the 5-year survival for patients starting RRT between 2002 and 2004 was 33% for PD compared to 35% for HD with no statistical difference.

Residual renal function (RRF) in dialysis patients contributes to small and middle molecular clearance and has effects on mortality with every 0.5 ml/min increase in glomerular filtration rate (GFR) being associated with a 9% lower risk of mortality [22]. HD is associated with a much faster rate of RRF decline (3.7 ml/min compared to 1.4 ml/min for PD at 12 months) which might be related to rapid changes in fluid homeostasis [23]. Moreover, selecting PD as an RRT method prior to transplantation has shown some positive effects on graft function [24].

However, patient outcomes are not only about biomedical outcomes but psychological outcomes are equally important-more so in some cases. PD is associated with more patient satisfaction. Patients receiving PD were much more likely than patients on HD to rate their dialysis care as excellent (86% vs 56% respectively) and including excellent ratings for each specific aspect of clinical care [25]. PD also allows greater flexibility in terms of travel and employment.

To summarize, PD and HD have similar medical outcomes but PD allows more flexibility. Ultimately the choice of RRT modality should be made by patients based on which modality is better suited to their lifestyle as the emphasis for patients is mostly on how they live-rather than how long [26].

Switching from Peritoneal Dialysis to Hemodialysis

The incident rates of PD in the US are lower than expected. Moreover, the probability of patients continuing the initial method of dialysis is much lower on PD compared to HD [27, 28]. A study of approximately 5000 incident PD patients resulted in a technique success of 58% at 5 years [29]. Other studies have shown that the majority of technique failure in PD occurs early (during the first year) and catheter dysfunction and psychosocial problems are more common during this period [30]. Despite the improvement in peritonitis rates in recent years, infections (peritonitis and catheter related) are the main reason for PD patients to transfer to HD overall [31].

Fluid overload likely secondary to ultrafiltration (UF) failure also results in transfer to HD. Loss of RRF and structural changes in the peritoneal membrane with increased lymphatic absorption and small solute transport are contributing to UF failure [32]. Abdominal surgeries, pancreatitis and malnutrition are some of the other reasons implicated in transfer of dialysis modality [33] (Table 1.2).

Risk factors for technique failure include older age, higher peritoneal membrane transport status, diabetes mellitus, lower neighborhood education level and increased body mass index [29, 33–35]. Interestingly, the center size is inversely related to the rate of technique survival. Centers with less than 20 patients have a 1.7 times higher likelihood of transferring to HD compared to centers with a higher number of patients [33]. A possible explanation for this trend is that centers caring for a large PD population are more experienced at dealing with complications and adjusting PD prescriptions to

Table 1.2 Factors involved in switching from PD to HD

Patient factors
Peritonitis
Catheter dysfunction
Ultrafiltration failure
Malnutrition
Patient preference
Abdominal surgeries
Pancreatitis
Patient preference
Provider factors
Center size
Lack of experience managing PD complications

Modified from Huisman and Nieuwenhuizen [33]

increase clearance and improving ultrafiltration without resorting to HD transfer.

It is often difficult to predict which patients will transfer to HD based on baseline characteristics and be able to predict patient success on PD. Therefore, the therapy should be offered to anyone who is interested in the absence of an absolute contraindication [28]. We should also limit the use of the term "technique failure" for transfer to HD as it implies that the patient or providers efforts were futile in some way. Rather, a more encouraging thought process is to consider that with the increased life expectancy of ESRD patients, they will likely need different RRT modalities during their lifetime. Even if someone was successfully able to do PD for 6 months, that's an extra 6 months spent at home instead of traveling to and from a HD unit. Only by this paradigm shift, will we be able to provide excellent care to our ESRD patients in the changing landscape of our healthcare system.

References

1. USRDS-ADR. 2015. USRDS annual data report: epidemiology of kidney disease in the United States. National Institutes of Health, National Institute of Diabetes and Digestive and Kidney Diseases, Bethesda, MD. In.
2. Friedman DJ, Pollak MR. Genetics of kidney failure and the evolving story of APOL1. J Clin Invest. 2011;121:3367–74.
3. Genovese G, Friedman DJ, Ross MD, Lecordier L, Uzureau P, Freedman BI, Bowden DW, Langefeld CD, Oleksyk TK, Uscinski Knob AL, Bernhardy AJ, Hicks PJ, Nelson GW, Vanhollebeke B, Winkler CA, Kopp JB, Pays E, Pollak MR. Association of trypanolytic ApoL1 variants with kidney disease in African Americans. Science. 2010;329:841–5.
4. CMS. 2014. Center for Medicare and Medicaid Services. Report for the standardized readmission ratio. Accessed 25 Mar. https://www.cms.gov/Medicare/Quality-Initiatives-Patient-Assessment-Instruments/ESRDQIP/ Downloads/MeasureMethodologyReport fortheProposed SRRMeasure.pdf.
5. Rettig RA. Special treatment – the story of Medicare's ESRD entitlement. N Engl J Med. 2011;364:596–8.
6. Vanholder R, Davenport A, Hannedouche T, Kooman J, Kribben A, Lameire N, Lonnemann G, Magner P, Mendelssohn D, Saggi SJ, Shaffer RN, Moe SM, Van Biesen W, van der Sande F, Mehrotra R. Reimbursement of dialysis: a comparison of seven countries. J Am Soc Nephrol. 2012;23:1291–8.
7. Berger A, Edelsberg J, Inglese GW, Bhattacharyya SK, Oster G. Cost comparison of peritoneal dialysis versus hemodialysis in end-stage renal disease. Am J Manag Care. 2009;15:509–18.
8. Burkart J. The future of peritoneal dialysis in the United States: optimizing its use. Clin J Am Soc Nephrol. 2009;4(Suppl 1):S125–31.
9. Rivara MB, Mehrotra R. The changing landscape of home dialysis in the United States. Curr Opin Nephrol Hypertens. 2014;23:586–91.
10. Liu FX, Gao X, Inglese G, Chuengsaman P, Pecoits-Filho R, Yu A. A global overview of the impact of peritoneal dialysis first or favored policies: an opinion. Perit Dial Int. 2015;35:406–20.
11. Mendelssohn DC, Mujais SK, Soroka SD, Brouillette J, Takano T, Barre PE, Mittal BV, Singh A, Firanek C, Story K, Finkelstein FO. A prospective evaluation of renal replacement therapy modality eligibility. Nephrol Dial Transplant. 2009;24:555–61.
12. Mehrotra R, Marsh D, Vonesh E, Peters V, Nissenson A. Patient education and access of ESRD patients to renal replacement therapies beyond in-center hemodialysis. Kidney Int. 2005;68:378–90.
13. Mehrotra R, Blake P, Berman N, Nolph KD. An analysis of dialysis training in the United States and Canada. Am J Kidney Dis. 2002;40:152–60.
14. Wadhwa N, Messina C, Hebah N. Does current nephrology fellowship training affect utilization of peritoneal dialysis in the United States? Open J Nephrol. 2013;3:109–14.
15. McLaughlin K, Manns B, Mortis G, Hons R, Taub K. Why patients with ESRD do not select self-care dialysis as a treatment option. Am J Kidney Dis. 2003;41:380–5.
16. Blake PG, Quinn RR, Oliver MJ. Peritoneal dialysis and the process of modality selection. Perit Dial Int. 2013;33:233–41.
17. Manns BJ, Taub K, Vanderstraeten C, Jones H, Mills C, Visser M, McLaughlin K. The impact of education on chronic kidney disease patients' plans to initiate dialysis with self-care dialysis: a randomized trial. Kidney Int. 2005;68:1777–83.
18. Bloembergen WE, Port FK, Mauger EA, Wolfe RA. A comparison of mortality between patients treated with hemodialysis and peritoneal dialysis. J Am Soc Nephrol. 1995;6:177–83.
19. Mehrotra R, Kermah D, Fried L, Kalantar-Zadeh K, Khawar O, Norris K, Nissenson A. Chronic peritoneal dialysis in the United States: declining utilization despite improving outcomes. J Am Soc Nephrol. 2007;18:2781–8.
20. Mehrotra R, Chiu YW, Kalantar-Zadeh K, Bargman J, Vonesh E. Similar outcomes with hemodialysis and peritoneal dialysis in patients with end-stage renal disease. Arch Intern Med. 2011;171:110–8.
21. Heaf JG, Wehberg S. Relative survival of peritoneal dialysis and haemodialysis patients: effect of cohort and mode of dialysis initiation. PLoS One. 2014;9:e90119.

22. Adequacy of dialysis and nutrition in continuous peritoneal dialysis: association with clinical outcomes. Canada-USA (CANUSA) Peritoneal Dialysis Study Group. 1996. J Am Soc Nephrol;7:198–207.

23. Lang SM, Bergner A, Topfer M, Schiffl H. Preservation of residual renal function in dialysis patients: effects of dialysis-technique-related factors. Perit Dial Int. 2001;21:52–7.

24. Van Biesen W, Veys N, Vanholder R, Lameire N. The impact of the pre-transplant renal replacement modality on outcome after cadaveric kidney transplantation: the ghent experience. Contrib Nephrol. 2006;150:254–8.

25. Rubin HR, Fink NE, Plantinga LC, Sadler JH, Kliger AS, Powe NR. Patient ratings of dialysis care with peritoneal dialysis vs hemodialysis. JAMA. 2004;291:697–703.

26. Lee MB, Bargman JM. Survival by dialysis modality-who cares? Clin J Am Soc Nephrol. 2016;6(6):11.

27. Maiorca R, Cancarini GC, Zubani R, Camerini C, Manili L, Brunori G, Movilli E. CAPD viability: a long-term comparison with hemodialysis. Perit Dial Int. 1996;16:276–87.

28. Lan PG, Clayton PA, Saunders J, Polkinghorne KR, Snelling PL. Predictors and outcomes of transfers from peritoneal dialysis to hemodialysis. Perit Dial Int. 2015;35:306–15.

29. Chidambaram M, Bargman JM, Quinn RR, Austin PC, Hux JE, Laupacis A. Patient and physician predictors of peritoneal dialysis technique failure: a population based, retrospective cohort study. Perit Dial Int. 2011;31:565–73.

30. Descoeudres B, Koller MT, Garzoni D, Wolff T, Steiger J, Schaub S, Mayr M. Contribution of early failure to outcome on peritoneal dialysis. Perit Dial Int. 2008;28:259–67.

31. Jaar BG, Plantinga LC, Crews DC, Fink NE, Hebah N, Coresh J, Kliger AS, Powe NR. Timing, causes, predictors and prognosis of switching from peritoneal dialysis to hemodialysis: a prospective study. BMC Nephrol. 2009;10:3.

32. Fusshoeller A. Histomorphological and functional changes of the peritoneal membrane during long-term peritoneal dialysis. Pediatr Nephrol. 2008;23:19–25.

33. Huisman RM, Nieuwenhuizen MG, Th de Charro F. Patient-related and centre-related factors influencing technique survival of peritoneal dialysis in The Netherlands. Nephrol Dial Transplant. 2002;17:1655–60.

34. Snyder JJ, Foley RN, Gilbertson DT, Vonesh EF, Collins AJ. Body size and outcomes on peritoneal dialysis in the United States. Kidney Int. 2003;64:1838–44.

35. Rumpsfeld M, McDonald SP, Johnson DW. Higher peritoneal transport status is associated with higher mortality and technique failure in the Australian and New Zealand peritoneal dialysis patient populations. J Am Soc Nephrol. 2006;17:271–8.

36. Hoerger TJ, Simpson SA, Yarnoff BO, Pavkov ME, Ríos Burrows N, Saydah SH, Williams DE, Zhuo X. The future burden of CKD in the United States: a simulation model for the CDC CKD Initiative. Am J Kidney Dis. 2015;65(3):403–11.

Physiology of Peritoneal Dialysis

2

Alan Moreno and Menaka Sarav

Introduction

The history of peritoneal dialysis is a rich one, and echoes the accumulated knowledge across a multitude of medical specialties and disciplines. The earliest known recorded descriptions of the peritoneal cavity are inscribed in the Ebers Papyrus, an Egyptian medical manuscript dating back to 1550 BC. In ancient Rome, Galen, progenitor to the modern physician, noted its anatomy while treating abdominal injuries to gladiators. Centuries of medical stagnation followed, with renewed interest in the peritoneum blossoming during the Industrial Revolution followed with clinical applications during the twentieth century paving the way for modern peritoneal dialysis. It is now the dominant option in home dialysis therapy, and is the modality of choice in many countries, including Canada, Mexico and Australia, used by about 200,000 patients worldwide [1]. Since its establishment as a viable option for ESRD patients in the 1960s, peritoneal dialysis remains an attractive option for patients and physicians who desire a convenient, flexible and low cost alternative to traditional hemodialysis (HD) [2].

A. Moreno, MD • M. Sarav, MD (✉)
Department of Medicine – Nephrology and Hypertension, North Shore University Health System, Evanston, IL, USA
e-mail: amoreno@northshore.org; msarav@northshore.org

During HD, blood and dialysate interact across a semipermeable membrane, ultimately leading to water removal, solute balance, and toxin clearance. Unlike HD utilizes artificial semi-permeable tubules through which blood passes and is bathed by dialysate, PD harnesses the intrinsic physiologic properties of the peritoneal membrane itself. Additionally, rather than pump-applied pressure gradients in HD, osmotic and solute gradients between dialysate and blood are employed to transport solutes and water via filtration, diffusion and advection in PD.

The Peritoneal Membrane

Central to PD are the properties of the peritoneal membrane – also known as peritoneum – the serous membrane that lines the abdominal cavity. Embryonically derived from layers of mesenchyme, its gross anatomy and cellular constituents were first described in scientific detail in 1862 by the renowned pathologist von Recklinghausen [3].

Anatomy

The peritoneal membrane encompasses a large surface area that roughly, and coincidentally, equals that of the body surface area of an average healthy adult – approximately 1–2 m^2 [4].

S. Haggerty (ed.), *Surgical Aspects of Peritoneal Dialysis*, DOI 10.1007/978-3-319-52821-2_2

Blood flow through the peritoneum is also an important consideration, and can directly affect a patient's dialyzing capabilities. In normal physiologic conditions, estimated blood flow through the peritoneum is 50–100 ml/min, approximately 1% of a person's cardiac output, however this can vary depending on individual anatomy and inflammatory states [4].

The peritoneum is divided into two components:

1. The visceral peritoneum which lines the gut and associated viscera. This comprises 80% of the entire peritoneum, with blood supply coming from the superior mesenteric artery; drainage is through the portal venous system.
2. The parietal peritoneum lines the walls of the abdominal cavity, and comprises the remainder (20%) of the peritoneum. Blood supply of the parietal peritoneum is derived from the abdominal wall vasculature, and drains directly to the inferior vena cava.

Between the parietal and visceral peritoneum is the peritoneal cavity, the site where dialysate "dwells" during exchanges. The cavity is remarkably pliable; while small in healthy persons and housing less than 100 mL of fluid, during peritoneal dialysis upwards of 3 liters of dwell may be tolerated without significant discomfort [4, 5].

The specific extent and proportions of the peritoneum involved during dialysis remain unknown. Although the visceral peritoneum comprises the majority of the membrane surface area, it is largely adhered to fibrous viscera with poorly exposed to dialysate. Consequently it is thought to not contribute significantly to fluid and solute exchange during PD. This lack of contribution has been demonstrated with eviscerated animal studies.

In contrast, despite its limited size, the parietal peritoneum contributes most to the diffusion and ultrafiltration that defines PD primarily due to the availability of usable vasculature to the peritoneal cavity. The concept of "effective peritoneal surface area" is evoked through this discrepancy; simple surface area does not account for the three dimensional differences in capillary distribution, membrane thickness and dialysate – membrane matching. All things being equal, the perfusion of capillaries within the peritoneal membrane can greatly affect the dialyzing capabilities of each individual person.

Histology

Histologically, the peritoneum is a complex, living and dynamic structure that includes and encompasses interstitial matrix, microvasculature, connective tissue and mesothelial cells [4–6]. In general the following landmarks are noted:

(a) Capillary fluid film covering the endothelium of the capillaries
(b) Capillary wall (endothelium)
(c) Endothelium basement membrane
(d) Interstitium
(e) Mesothelium – layer of squamous epithelial cells
(f) Fluid film that overlies the mesothelium

Simplistically, these six landmarks can be thought of as the six layers of resistances to solute transport. There are two popular concept of peritoneal transport; they are complementary rather than mutually exclusive, and will be discussed below.

Models of Transport

The two most popular models of peritoneal transport emphasize the importance of peritoneal vasculature and interstitium. They are the "three pore model" which helped explain how solutes of varying sizes, as well as water are transported and the "distributed model", which has been used to develop the concept of effective peritoneal surface area.

Three Pore Model

This model emphasizes peritoneal capillary endothelium as the critical barrier to the peritoneal transport. Transports of solutes and water movement across these capillaries are mediated by pores of different sizes. The fluid films and the mesothelium – layers a, e and f above are thought to offer only trivial resistance to transport [7, 8].

Ultrapores – the smallest of the pores, these are transcellular with a radius of only 2–5 Å. They also constitute only 2% total pore surface area. These are responsible for the transport of water only and have been experimentally found to correspond to aquaporins (AQP-1) channels, which are known to be the present in the endothelial cell membrane of the peritoneal capillaries. Because of the water selective properties of the ultrapores, sodium is unable to pass through which leads to the initial drop in sodium concentration in dwell fluid (with corresponding increase in sodium concentration in plasma) accounting for the phenomena of "sodium sieving".

Small pores – Pores with radius of 40–50 Å and represent small intercellular defects between endothelial cells. Small pores are large enough to allow transport of both water and solutes, and thus contribute to both diffusion and ultrafiltration. These are the most numerous of the three pore model, comprising over 90% of the total pore surface area and are the dominant site of small solute transportation

Large pores – intercellular pores that constitute radius of 200–300 Å which correspond to large clefts in the endothelium. These are the least abundant and contribute to less than 0.1% of the total effective pore area and macromolecules such as protein are transported by convection through these pores [7–9].

Distributed Model

The distributed model emphasizes the importance of the distribution of capillaries in the peritoneal membrane and the distance water and solutes have to travel from the capillaries across the interstitium to the mesothelium. Transport is dependent on the surface area of the peritoneal capillaries rather than on the total peritoneal surface area [9, 10]. Additionally, the distance of each capillary from the mesothelium determines the relative contribution. The cumulative contribution of all the peritoneal capillaries determines the effective surface area

and the resistance of properties of the membrane. From the distributed model, the concept of "effective peritoneal surface area" has arisen [9–11].

Therefore, two patients with the same peritoneal surface area may have markedly different peritoneal vascularity and so also have different effective peritoneal surface areas. Similarly, a patient's effective peritoneal surface area may vary in different circumstances, for example increasing in peritonitis as the inflammation will increase the vascularity.

Peritoneal Dialysis Transport Physiology

At the heart of PD is transport physiology. It is important to remember that the peritoneal membrane maintains bidirectionality throughout dialysis; however, there is no singular component of the membrane that is the definitive measure for fluid transport (ultrafiltration) or solute transport. Dialysate molecules such as dextrose and water in the peritoneal cavity are subject to the same physiologic principles as are waste products in the blood stream and can cross the membrane into plasma if conditions are favorable.

Ultrafiltration

Ultrafiltration refers to the osmotic flow of water across a dialyzing membrane. It occurs as a consequence of the osmotic gradient between the hypertonic dialysis solution and the relatively hypotonic peritoneal capillary membrane. The movement of fluids across the peritoneal membrane is primarily determined by ultrapores and small pores mechanism and depends on the following:

(a) Concentration gradient for the osmotic agent i.e. glucose. This is maximum at the start of PD dwell and decreases with time due to dilution of the glucose by ultrafiltration and from diffusion of the glucose from the dialysis solution into the blood. The gradient can be maximized by using a higher concentration of the dextrose, or by doing more frequent exchanges [5, 9, 12, 13].

(b) Effective peritoneal surface area, as discussed above under the distributed model.

(c) Reflection coefficient of the osmotic agent (i.e., glucose). This is a measure of how effectively the osmotic agent diffuses out of the dialysis solution into the peritoneal capillaries. It is ranges between 0 and 1. The lower the value the faster the osmotic gradient is lost across a pore and leading to correspondingly less sustained ultrafiltration. Lower numbers are thus not ideal for osmotic agents. Glucose has a reflection coefficient of 0.3 whereas icodextrin is close to 1 [14–16].

(d) Hydrostatic pressure gradient. The hydrostatic pressure is higher in the capillary than the peritoneum and this favors ultrafiltration. This hydrostatic pressure is higher in volume-overloaded ambulatory patients and lower in recumbent or volume depleted patients.

(e) Resorption. Also known as 'fluid loss', and 'wrong way flow', resorption is the reclamation of peritoneal fluid back into circulation. The majority of fluid is resorbed through the membrane itself via hydrostatic convection back through tissue. This occurs among the vasculature in the parietal peritoneum lining the abdominal wall. The remainder is accomplished through the lymphatic system, with the main drainage site being the sub-diaphragmatic lymphatic stomata. Hydrostatic increases in peritoneal cavity pressure, particularly with larger dwell volumes and correspondingly larger pressures, can thus ultimately cause a decrease in net ultrafiltration [4, 17].

(f) Oncotic pressure gradient. A subset of osmotic pressure due to colloids (proteins), this acts to keep fluid in the blood, thereby resisting ultrafiltration [17].

Solute Transportation

Transportation of solutes from the bloodstream to the dialysate fluid depends on two concurrent processes:

(a) Diffusion is the dominant method of small solute transportation in PD, which includes electrolytes, simple sugars and uremic solutes. By definition, diffusion is dependent on concentration gradients of individual solutes between dialysate and blood across the semipermeable peritoneum to facilitate transfer. As in ultrafiltration, the gradient between the dialysate and plasma decreases over time, with the greatest potency occurring in the first hour of a dwell. Numerous other secondary factors will also affect net transport. These include the size of the effective peritoneal surface area, volume of the dialysate, molecular size of the solute, and amount of peritoneal blood flow. Each given solute has its own intrinsic property determining rate of diffusion, and is determined by its molecular weight [4, 5, 9, 13].

(b) Convection – or, more accurately, advection – is clearance of solutes which depends neither on the properties of the solute itself nor the concentration gradient of the solute but, rather, on its relation with the flow of fluid. Solvent drag occurs with the bulk movement of ultrafiltrate across the peritoneum due to osmotic gradients, bringing with it solutes. The amount of solutes carried by the ultrafiltrate is limited by components of peritoneum that allow passage of fluid but not solute. This is seen in with aquaporin channels. This phenomenon is known as 'sieving', and is most commonly observed with sodium when utilizing low molecular weight osmotic molecules for dialysate. In the clinical setting, sodium sieving is an important parameter in assessing the adequacy of free water transport in PD patients, and can become a significant issue during rapid dialysate cycling [14].

Dialysis Solutions

In 1923, Gantar injected normal saline into the peritoneal cavity of uremic guinea pigs, thereby performing the first known attempt at peritoneal dialysis in animals. A failed attempt in PD on a uremic woman soon followed, again using normal saline. The importance of PD fluid hyperosmolarity in inducing fluid removal became apparent, with Heusser first adding dextrose to PD solutions in 1927 [3].

Modern PD solutions are varied, however they share important distinguishing features: a primary osmotic agent, electrolytes and buffers. Given that the average PD patient uses 7–10 *tons* per year of dialysate, certain considerations are important in determining an ideal solution, namely expense, safety and efficacy.

Osmotic Agents

As mentioned earlier, hydrostatic gradients are the primary engine of ultrafiltration in hemodialysis. Due to inherent limitations of anatomy, however, utilizing pressure gradients in PD is close to impossible. Fluid transport in PD is thus reliant on osmotic differences between dialysate and plasma to move water.

(a) Low Molecular Weight Agents – Inexpensive, easy to produce, and relatively safe, sugar based agents are the dominant osmotic agents even today, though their structural components may differ. Dextrose (D-glucose) remains the most commonly used agent, with solutions containing variable concentrations standardized into 1.5%, 2.5% and 4.5%. Fluid osmolality ranges between 346 and 485 mOsm/kg; higher concentrations lead to greater ultrafiltration. Due to their low reflection coefficients, they are readily diffusible through the peritoneal membrane into plasma [14, 18]. With their passage several phenomena can be noted. First, the osmotic potency of the dialysate diminishes overtime, reducing ultrafiltration. Second, unsurprisingly hyperglycemia and hyperinsulinemia can ensue. With diabetes being the leading cause of end stage renal disease worldwide this can become a significant issue. A consideration when using small molecular weight sugar based osmotic agents is their susceptibility to forming cytotoxic glucose degradation products (GDP) during fluid sterilization processes. These can further react with native proteins forming advanced glycation end products (AGE) [19]. Long term exposure to these components leads to superoxide radicals, mesothelial necrosis and fibrosis which raises concern for association with PD failure [5, 6, 19–21].

(b) High Molecular Weight Agents – High molecular weight agents such as glucose polymers, dextran polypeptides and the like, range in weight from 10 k to 350 k Daltons. The most commonly utilized polymer is icodextrin at 7.5%, a glucagon isomer that averages roughly 16 k Daltons. Icodextrin circumvents many of the issues that plague lower molecular weight sugars. Due to its high reflection coefficient, it remains in dialysate much longer – its diffusion into the bloodstream is limited to lymphatic resorption and consequently maintains ultrafiltration capabilities for a longer time period. They are removed from dialysate either through lymphatic absorption or through endothelial large pores. This property allows icodextrin solutions to also have much less osmolarity than dextrose-based solutions – 282 mOsm/kg compared to 346 mOsm/kg for a 1.5% dextrose solution. The smaller osmolarity of icodextrin solutions are supplemented by osmotic pull of electrolytes that have diffused from plasma to the dialysate [16, 18, 22].

Electrolytes

Electrolyte additives in PD dialysate generally run low to better facilitate diffusion, clearance, and ultimately removal during exchanges. Potassium, for example, is usually not added to dialysate, and any deficiencies can easily be corrected with oral supplementation. Sodium sieving can cause an abrupt hypernatremia within the first hour of PD exchanges whilst using dextrose based dialysate due to increased isolated ultrafiltration of water. Due to the tendency of PD patients towards hypernatremia, sodium in dialysate tend to run lower than plasma levels to encourage diffusion of sodium out of plasma. Commercial solutions range between 130 and 137 mmol/L internationally.

Calcium levels have a tendency to be low in renal patients due to failure to synthesize calcitriol. Supplementation can be added to solutions, though with caution as patients tend to be on calcium containing phosphate binders or vitamin D supplementation.

Buffers

Buffering components mixed into dialysis fluids have been used control acidosis in PD since Dr. Boen used bicarbonate in the 1960s [3]. However its propensity to precipitate calcium and magnesium led to its replacement with lactate and similar containing solutions.

Today, lactate is the most commonly used buffer due to its efficacy, and compatibility. Lactate is metabolized to bicarbonate in the liver though its acidic nature is thought to possibly contribute to cellular death. Lactate based solutions also have an unfortunate tendency to cause inflow pain as well as abdominal discomfort. Bicarbonate solutions have stubbornly continued to be a suitable alternative for buffering; it is particularly useful for patients wishing to avoid infusion pain provided that they are separated from calcium or magnesium solutions [18]. Realistically this can be a cumbersome experience for patients and caregivers alike.

Assessment of Membrane Transport Status

Measurements of membrane transport status is critical in both predicting an individual patient's physiologic response to dialysis as well as assessing and evaluating their current status to adjust needed prescriptions.

Peritoneal Equilibration Test (PET)

Described in 1987 by Twardowski and colleagues, this was the first and still most utilized standardized evaluation of patient response to peritoneal dialysis [23, 24]. By checking the levels of a given solute in the dialysate and plasma, nephrologists can determine the dialyzing capabilities of a patient and estimate adequacy. The initial body of work emphasized categorizing peritoneal membrane solute transport characteristics amongst four distinct patient types: high, high-average, low-average, and low depending on their rate of solute transport. The test is

Table 2.1 An example of D/P ratio categorization for creatinine levels

$D/P_{creatinine}$ ratio at 4 h	Transporter type
$D/P_{creatinine}$ 0.81–1.03	High
$D/P_{creatinine}$ 0.65–0.81	High average
$D/P_{creatinine}$ 0.50–0.65	Low average
$D/P_{creatinine}$ 0.34–0.5	Low

Modified from Twardowski [23]

typically performed as an in-office visit four to 6 weeks after initiation of PD to allow for membrane stabilization. The test requires complete drainage of the overnight dwell, with reinfusion of a standardized fluid (2 L of 2.5% dextrose).

The dialysate is sampled as soon as infusion is completed, and repeated at 2 and 4 h intervals. Dwell urea, creatinine, sodium, and glucose levels are checked. A concurrent blood (plasma) sample is checked at the same intervals, and compared with dialysate characteristics. These are presented as D/P (D for dwell, P for plasma) and are termed equilibration ratios. The equilibration ratios between the urea, creatinine, sodium and glucose should be compared with each other to ensure concordance of measurement (Table 2.1).

Higher transporters achieve the most rapid and complete equilibrium for solutes creatinine and urea because they have a relatively large effective peritoneal surface area or low membrane resistance. However high transporters rapidly lose their osmotic gradient for ultrafiltration because the dialysate glucose diffuses into the blood through the highly permeable membrane. They also have higher dialysate protein losses and so tend to have lower serum albumin levels.

Conversely, despite the slow movement of solutes in low transporters and need for longer dwell times, lack of ultrafiltration is rarely an issue due to longer maintenance of the osmotic gradient. High average and low average transporters have intermediate values for these ratios and for ultrafiltration and protein losses (Fig. 2.1). In practice, high transporters do best on PD regimens that involve frequent short duration dwells, so that ultrafiltration is optimized while the low transporters do best on regimens based on long high volume dwell times so that diffusion is maximized.

Fig. 2.1 Dialysate to plasma ratio for creatinine (Adapted from Zbylut et al. [24])

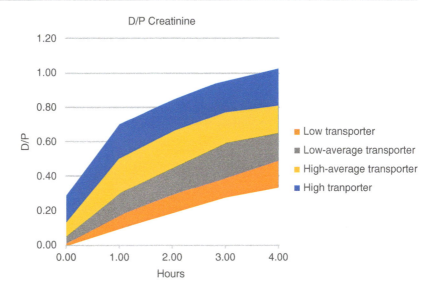

Other testing modalities include the Fast PET, an abbreviated test which only samples dwell and plasma creatinine and glucose at the 5 h mark and the Modified PET, which evaluates ultrafiltration failure using an osmotic challenge by utilizing a more concentrated dextrose solution (4.25% 2 L dextrose). Ultrafiltration less than 400 mL during a Modified PET is diagnostic for peritoneal membrane failure [4, 23, 24].

Adequacy of Dialysis

In the broadest sense, adequacy is the overall assessment of the efficacy of dialysis and is an expression of the overall gestalt of a patient's well-being [25, 26]. Ultimately the goal of dialysis is to maintain a patient's subjective quality of life. In practice this is difficult to quantify.

While being secondary goals, outcomes such as solute clearance, acid base maintenance, maintenance of electrolyte equilibrium, and mineral bone disease prevention, are objective and easier to quantify. Urea and its clearance became the most commonly used markers for adequacy after 1981, when a study performed by the National Cooperative Dialysis Study noted that significantly better outcomes were noted in patients with lower BUN levels for patients undergoing hemodialysis [27].

In the clinical setting, urea clearance is normalized to body water levels (Kt/V_{urea}) and is measured at 1 month after starting PD concurrently with the PET then subsequently every 4 months thereafter [23, 24]. Urea clearance is comprised of clearance from peritoneal dialysis itself and clearance from any residual kidney function and have to be individually calculated, and then added together.

The components of Kt/V_{urea} are as follows:

K – This is the *daily* clearance of urea, and can be obtained by the D/P_{urea} ratio multiplied by the total volume of dialysate (dwell plus ultrafiltrate) for the PD portion. For assessing urea clearance of the kidneys, D (dialysate) is substituted by U (urine). Correspondingly this is multiplied by the volume of urine produced rather than dialysate volume.

t – This is time, in days. Standard measurements of Kt/V_{urea} is expressed as a weekly value, so this number is typically 7.

V – This is the volume of distribution of urea, and can be obtained by the Watson formula which is available online. It is roughly 60% of a patient's ideal body weight.

Survival on PD has documented associations with maintaining higher Kt/V levels. Initial studies recommended maintaining weekly Kt/V levels of greater than 2.0 though this has since relaxed. The most recent guidelines from KDOQI committee recommends maintaining the total Kt/V_{urea} (peritoneal and urinary clearance) above 1.7 [25].

Peritoneal Dialysis Modalities

Peritoneal dialysis is divided into two main modalities: continuous ambulatory peritoneal dialysis (CAPD) and automated peritoneal dialysis (APD). The choice of peritoneal dialysis to use depends on numerous factors including transport phenotype; however, by and large patient and caregiver preference is the main determinant. There is no difference in survival outcomes between CAPD and APD.

Continuous Ambulatory Peritoneal Dialysis (CAPD)

Developed and refined by Drs. Popovich, Moncrief and Nolph in the 1970s, CAPD was the dominant modality worldwide for a number of years though automated peritoneal dialysis (APD) has since caught up [1, 15, 28]. CAPD requires a continued dwell throughout the day, with exchanges between used dialysate and fresh solutions performed four times per day. Fluid volume per exchange is 2 L. Residual kidney function, patient size, and transport characteristics of the patient will influence subsequent fluid volumes, exchange frequency as well as solution types though these changes are typically made after formal PET and adequacy measurements are performed a month after PD has started.

CAPD offers the advantage of portability, and longer dwell times to facilitate better solute clearance and ultrafiltration. In patients whose residual kidney function is terminal or are low transporters with poor ultrafiltration, CAPD may be the only feasible peritoneal dialysis option. The main disadvantages is the inconvenience of performing exchanges throughout the day, as well as higher rates of peritonitis due to persistent fluid in the peritoneal cavity.

Automatic Peritoneal Dialysis (APD)

The use of cyclers became more mainstream in the early 1980s. APD is now the most common form of PD in the United States. The cycler attempts to compress a patient's dialysis during their least active part of the day – during sleep. This is an especially attractive option in patients who have active schedules, or who require help from persons whose time is limited.

Unsurprisingly, exchanges are performed more frequently and more rapidly compared to CAPD, and the dwell is completely drained once the patient detaches from the cycler in the morning. While high transporters benefit from faster exchanges to limit excessive ultrafiltration, in low transporters this can be problematic and lead to inadequate fluid removal and solute clearance. Using icodextrin in APD is difficult as well, as it typically requires longer dwell periods to realize its full effects.

Fortunately, automated peritoneal dialysis itself is flexible enough to be subdivided into distinct modalities which can help circumvent the problems described above; however, they all share the same characteristic of using a cycler overnight. Several of the more common variables are described below.

(a) Nightly intermittent peritoneal dialysis (NIPD) – "Dry APD", this is the purest form of automated peritoneal dialysis as there are no exchanges performed during the day. The only time a patient undergoes dialysis is when they are asleep.

(b) Continuous cycling peritoneal dialysis (CCPD) – also known as "wet" APD, an additional exchange (or two) is performed during the day in addition to nightly cycling.

(c) Tidal peritoneal dialysis – a common modality in Europe, TPD addresses the problem of reduced dwell time with serial exchanges by instead maintaining a constant dwell throughout the night to allow for more UF and diffusion. Overfilling can be a problem with these patients.

(d) Intermittent peritoneal dialysis – infrequent dialysis over the course of several days [4, 15, 28].

References

1. Jain AK, Blake P, Cordy P, Garg AX. Global trends in rates of peritoneal dialysis. J Am Soc Nephrol JASN. 2012;23(3):533–44.
2. Chaudhary K, Sangha H, Khanna R. Peritoneal dialysis first: rationale. Clin J Am Soc Nephrol. 2011;6(2): 447–56.
3. Palmer RA. As it was in the beginning: a history of peritoneal dialysis. Perit Dial Int. 1982;2(1): 16–22.
4. Peter G, Blake JTD, editors. Physiology of peritoneal dialysis. In: Daugirdas JT, Blake PG, Ing TS, editors. Handbook of dialysis. 7th ed. Philadelphia: Wolters Kluwer; 2015.
5. Devuyst O, Margetts PJ, Topley N. The pathophysiology of the peritoneal membrane. J Am Soc Nephrol. 2010;21(7):1077–85.
6. Rippe B. Pathophysiological description of the ultrastructural changes of the peritoneal membrane during long-term continuous ambulatory peritoneal dialysis. Blood Purif. 1994;12(4–5):211–20.
7. Rippe B, Simonsen O, Stelin G. Clinical implications of a three-pore model of peritoneal transport. Adv Perit Dial. 1991;7:3–9. Toronto.
8. Rippe B. Free water transport, small pore transport and the osmotic pressure gradient three-pore model of peritoneal transport. Nephrol Dial Transplant. 2008;23(7):2147–53.
9. Flessner MF, Fenstermacher JD, Dedrick RL, Blasberg RG. A distributed model of peritoneal plasma transport: tissue concentration gradients. Am J Physiol. 1985;248(3):F425–35.
10. Flessner MF. Distributed model of peritoneal transport: implications of the endothelial glycocalyx. Nephrol Dial Transplant. 2008;23(7): 2142–6.
11. Flessner MF. Small solute transport across specific peritoneal tissue surfaces in the rat. J Am Soc Nephrol. 1996;7(2):225–32.
12. Rippe B, Stelin G. Simulations of peritoneal solute transport during CAPD. Application of two-pore formalism. Kidney Int. 1989;35(5):1234–44.
13. Ronco C. The "nearest capillary" hypothesis: a novel approach to peritoneal transport physiology. Perit Dial Int. 1996;16(2):121–5.
14. Chen TW, Khanna R, Moore H, Twardowski ZJ, Nolph KD. Sieving and reflection coefficients for sodium salts and glucose during peritoneal dialysis in rats. J Am Soc Nephrol. 1991;2(6):1092–100.
15. Ronco C, Kliger A, Amici G, Virga G. Automated peritoneal dialysis: clinical prescription and technology. Perit Dial Int. 2000;20(Suppl 2):S70–6.
16. Davies SJ, Woodrow G, Donovan K, Plum J, Williams P, Johansson AC, Bosselmann HP, Heimbürger O, Simonsen O, Davenport A, Tranaeus A, Divino Filho JC. Icodextrin improves the fluid status of peritoneal dialysis patients: results of a double-blind randomized controlled trial. J Am Soc Nephrol. 2003;14(9): 2338–44.
17. Durand PY, Chanliau J, Gamberoni J, Hestin D, Kessler M. Intraperitoneal pressure, peritoneal permeability and volume of ultrafiltration in CAPD. Adv Perit Dial. 1992;8:22–5.
18. García-López E, Lindholm B, Davies S. An update on peritoneal dialysis solutions. Nat Rev Nephrol. 2012;8:10.
19. Witowski J, Jörres A, Korybalska K, Ksiazek K, Wisniewska-Elnur J, Bender TO, Passlick-Deetjen J, Breborowicz A. Glucose degradation products in peritoneal dialysis fluids: do they harm? Kidney Int Suppl. 2003;84:S148–51.
20. Rippe B, Simonsen O, Heimbürger O, Christensson A, Haraldsson B, Stelin G, Weiss L, Nielsen FD, Bro S, Friedberg M, Wieslander A. Long-term clinical effects of a peritoneal dialysis fluid with less glucose degradation products. Kidney Int. 2001;59(1):10.
21. Erixon M, Wieslander A, Lindén T, Carlsson O, Forsbäck G, Svensson E, Jönsson JA, Kjellstrand P. How to avoid glucose degradation products in peritoneal dialysis fluids. Perit Dial Int. 2006;26(4):497.
22. Mujais S, Vonesh E. Profiling of peritoneal ultrafiltration. Kidney Int. 2002;62:S17–22.
23. Twardowski ZJ. The fast peritoneal equilibration test. Semin Dial. 1990;3(3):141–2.
24. Zbylut J, Twardowski KON, Khanna R, Prowant BF, Ryan LP, Moore HL, Nielsen MP. Peritoneal equilibration test. Perit Dial Int. 1987;7(3):138–48.
25. Clinical practice guidelines for peritoneal adequacy, update 2006. Am J Kidney Dis. 2006;48(Suppl 1):8.
26. Blake PG. Adequacy of dialysis revisited. Kidney Int. 2003;63(4):1587–99.
27. Lowrie EG, Laird NM, Parker TF, Sargent JA. Effect of the hemodialysis prescription on patient morbidity. N Engl J Med. 1981;305(20):1176–81.
28. Michels WM, Verduijn M, Boeschoten EW, Dekker FW, Krediet RT. Similar survival on automated peritoneal dialysis and continuous ambulatory peritoneal dialysis in a large prospective cohort. Clin J Am Soc Nephrol. 2009;4(5):943–9.

Patient Selection for Peritoneal Dialysis

Neenoo Khosla

Introduction

Despite apparent cost benefits, improved quality-of-life indicators, and initiatives to increase selection of the modality, the utilization of peritoneal dialysis (PD) remains low in many industrialized countries. Although many nephrology groups strive to provide patients an equal opportunity to choose PD versus hemodialysis (HD), utilization of PD varies greatly from practice to practice. One reason is a lack of understanding of which patients are eligible for PD. In addition, there is a lack of understanding of the difference between contraindications to PD as opposed to barriers to choosing the modality. Contraindications to PD are those that cannot be overcome despite the physician and/or patient choice. There are clear surgical contraindications to PD such as active intra-abdominal infection, loss of domain/unrepairable hernia and dense abdominal adhesions which are not amenable to laparoscopic lysis [1]. In addition, there are medical contraindications such as documented loss of peritoneal function/ultrafiltration failure of the peritoneal membrane, and severe protein malnutrition and or proteinuria >10 g/day [2, 3]. Much of the time, medical contraindications to PD are actually barriers that could be overcome with careful effort and institution of proper support systems. This chapter will clarify all patients that should be considered eligible for PD. Also medical contraindications versus barriers to PD will be contrasted. Lastly, possible solutions to overcome these barriers will be discussed.

Surgical Contraindications to Peritoneal Dialysis

Decreased Capacity of Peritoneal Cavity

The peritoneal cavity must allow up to 2 liters of fluid to dwell at any time for peritoneal dialysis to be effective. In pediatric patients, an exchange volume of 1,000–1,100 mL/m^2 BSA is recommended, though in infants and toddlers less than 2 years of age, this may be decreased to 800 mL/m^2 BSA [3, 4]. Women starting third trimester of pregnancy or patients with extensive abdominal adhesions that are not amenable to surgical correction do not have appropriate capacity of the peritoneal cavity for dialysate [3]. However, it is difficult to predict the degree of adhesions preoperatively. After abdominal surgery adhesions between the omentum and abdominal wall occur in over 80% of patients and involve the small intestine up to 20% of the time [5]. In a sample of 436 patients who underwent PD catheter placement, Crabtree et al. reported the need for

N. Khosla, MD
Division of Nephrology, Department of Internal
Medicine, Northshore University Healthsystem,
Evanston, IL, USA
e-mail: nkhosla@northshore.org

adhesiolysis in 32% of those who had prior abdominal surgery (58%), but only 3.3% in those without prior abdominal surgery. It is not surprising that they found adhesiolysis was needed more commonly based on the number of prior operations, ranging from 22.7% after one operation to 52% if the patient had a history of four or more operations [6]. However, the severity of adhesive disease may only be evident after attempted lysis of adhesions and catheter placement as shown in his study where the incidence of catheter failure from extensive adhesions was only 1.8%. In a similar study of 217 catheter insertions, Keshvari found a 42.8% incidence of previous abdominal surgery and 27% incidence of adhesions. Extensive laparoscopic adhesiolysis was required in only three patients. When comparing the patients who had adhesions and those without, he found no difference in the incidence of mechanical complications or need for revision [7]. Catheters have also been placed in a suprahepatic location in patients with a hostile pelvis precluding low placement of a catheter, and in infants undergoing open heart surgery with successful dialysis [8]. Therefore, history of prior abdominal surgery is not a contraindication to trying peritoneal dialysis if surgeons with experience in advanced laparoscopy can attempt lysis of adhesions and catheter placement in these patients.

Lack of Integrity of the Abdominal Wall

Uncorrected mechanical defects that prevent effective PD such as surgically irreparable hernia, omphalocele, gastroschisis, diaphragmatic hernia, pericardial window into the abdominal cavity, and bladder extrophy are also contraindications, although rare exceptions to this rule have been described [9]. The volume of dialysate must dwell in the abdomen where the peritoneum is well vascularized. Therefore these conditions prevent proper peritoneal dialysis and may lead to fluid leak into the pleural space or soft tissues. Because of the increased intraabdominal pressure with peritoneal dialysis, the incidence of abdominal wall hernia is almost 30% in adults and up to 40% in children [10, 11]. Literature regarding giant abdominal wall hernia repair before or during peritoneal dialysis is lacking. However, ventral and inguinal hernia repair may be performed preoperatively or concomitantly with PD catheter insertion and may allow effective PD [12]. More details on hernia repair in PD patients are found in a subsequent chapter. If adequate hernia repair is not successful, there tends to be rapid enlargement and dialysate leak [13, 14], thus these patients may no longer be candidates for PD.

Eligible Patients for Peritoneal Dialysis

Most patients are medically eligible for PD. Peritoneal dialysis has few absolute medical contraindications. One large Dutch study demonstrated that only 17% of end-stage kidney disease (ESKD) patients had a medical contraindication to PD [15]. The most common was previous major abdominal surgery. Many patients in this study had a social contraindication to PD. That is, there was an inability to perform PD exchanges by themselves. In a US study, only 23% of eligible patients had a medical contraindication to PD, consistent with 17–21% seen in studies from other countries [16].

Thus, medical eligibility for PD must remain broad. Specifically, the scope of patients eligible for PD should not be limited to those who have progressive chronic kidney disease (CKD) who are followed in outpatient clinics for a period of time. Certainly, pre- ESKD care allows for modality education and optimal patient choice [17]. Patients who are urgent starts or require unplanned dialysis are often only considered for HD via a central venous catheter (CVC). Nephrologists often delay or even inadvertently deny modality education in such patients. This is more often the case if there is uncertainty of renal recovery. Urgent start with acute PD catheter placement has been shown to be safe and feasible. It may be associated with increased risk of mechanical complications but, unlike with HD via CVC catheter, is not associated with increased risk of infections complications [18]. Patients who require unplanned dialysis should be evaluated for barriers and contraindications to PD and offered this modality if appropriate. Urgent start PD should be considered and a transitioning outpatient Nurse- assist PD program should be established until such patients can be educated to perform independent home care.

As mentioned, another at risk group, who is denied modality education, is patients who start dialysis for acute kidney injury. These patients are most often started on HD via a CVC catheter with the thought of imminent renal recovery. However, a number of these patients at 30–60 days show no signs of renal recovery. These patients for multiple reasons, including comorbid debilitating illnesses, forgotten modality education and/or a perception that the patient is "doing well on HD", are never offered PD. They are often directly referred for arteriovenous access placement without consideration of PD eligibility.

Another unique opportunity to transition patients to PD is HD transfers from outside dialysis units that may be stable but who have not been offered modality education at previous centers. Lastly, patients who have failed multiple arteriovenous accesses for HD require reevaluation of PD eligibility and concerted efforts to overcome barriers to transitioning to PD must be made.

Beyond proper eligibility, there are true medical contraindications to PD. Psychiatric illness that prevents safe and hygienic self care is a clear contraindication. Additionally, patients who demonstrate a consistent lack of medical compliance and follow up are not able to be offered PD. Patients who have significant lung disease with poor lung compliance often cannot tolerate PD secondary to restriction of ventilation from dialysate fill volumes. Lastly, patients with severe neurologic disease, movement disorder, or severe arthritis preventing self care whom have no caregivers cannot perform PD.

Barriers to Peritoneal Dialysis

The Elderly

There are patient groups that nephrologists often overlook as appropriate for PD. Firstly, the geriatric population is a population of patients often overlooked for PD. In 2004, a Dutch study showed that older age was associated with more contraindications to PD therapy and stronger likelihood to be directed to HD therapy [15]. This group of patients often has barriers to rather than contraindications to PD. In the elderly, the goal of care shifts more from quantity of life the quality of life. PD is well- suited for this goal of care. The modality avoids hospitalizations and complications of HD. Careful efforts to evaluate eligibility and overcome barriers are critical in this patient population [19].

They are several potential advantages of PD in the elderly. Most importantly is increased cardiovascular stability with PD. The potential for cardiovascular disease and related complications increases with age. Elderly can most benefit from the hemodynamic stabilities of PD. Additionally, vascular access surgeries are avoided with PD. Elderly often have poor target veins and require repeated vascular procedures. This modality also avoids chronic venous catheter when arteriovenous access cannot be created. Lastly, PD does not require anti-coagulation and lowering the risk of G.I. bleeding.

Conversely, there are potential problems in the elderly. There are an increased number of and complex co- morbidities in older patients that may prevent them from actually performing the dialysis exchanges. These include depression, dementia, impaired vision, decrease physical and mental abilities that impair self-performance of dialysis procedure. These limitations are real but can be overcome. Manual dexterity problems can be partly overcome with connection assistant devices and certainly use of the cycler is important. There are other adaptive CAPD systems such as the rotary disc system. Home care assistance from family, friends, and home nurses allows more patients to receive PD at home. Some patients can start with assisted PD with a RN and then graduate to self-care. Family or friends can be trained as an assistant and models can be developed with two daily nursing visits. Employment and training of a dedicated care giver can be considered and finally more assisted living centers or skilled nurse facilities should be available to elderly patients to perform PD. Healthcare policies supporting assisted PD can increase utilization and this has been shown in a number of countries, including Canada and France [20]. Assisted PD does not cost more than in- center HD even when the cost of home care provider is taken into account [21]. In conclusion PD is not contraindicated in the elderly and offers advantages over in center HD. Homecare assistance can allow more elderly patients to receive PD. PD mortality is affected by the increased risk of co morbidities at this age but not due to the modality per se.

Obesity

Obesity is often considered medical contraindications to PD. Obese patients with ESKD are less likely to initiate PD in the United States [22]. There are several reasons for this. Obese patients are often not offered PD as a modality. Clinicians are inexperienced and thus less comfortable with the management of PD in obese patients. Also, there are misconceptions about the outcomes of PD in obese patients. The relationship between body mass index (BMI) and mortality in dialysis patients is opposite of the relationship in the non-CKD population. A low BMI (<22) is associated with an increased risk of death, regardless of modality of dialysis. Obesity (BMI > 30) seems to confirm a survival advantage in patients with ESKD. This benefit seems to be more pronounced in HD as compared to PD. However, there is no clear evidence that the mortality significantly differs between obese patients on PD versus on HD [23–25].

There are mechanical and technical reasons obesity can pose problems in performing PD. These include higher risks of catheter leak, exit site infections and peritonitis. Also, there are concerns that patients with high BMI may have difficulty achieving solute clearance and adequate ultrafiltration. Early catheter placement and proper positioning of PD catheter by the surgeon using an upper abdominal or presternal exit site can help reduce catheter leaks, exit site

infections and peritonitis. Achieving adequate clearance in the obese patient can be achieved with larger dwell volumes and use of CCPD. Careful monitoring of residual kidney function is paramount in the obese patient as the loss of this function may require transition to HD. In conclusion, obesity is not an absolute contraindication a PD. Careful planning on catheter placement and diligence to achieve adequacy of dialysis can allow the obese patient to successfully undergo PD.

Polycystic Kidney Disease

Patients with polycystic kidney disease (PKD) are one last patient population group that is often not considered for PD. It is often felt that the risk of complications and technique failure due to the limited intraabdominal space is higher in patients with PKD. There are clear considerations that must be made as this patient population. There is a theoretical higher likelihood to develop hernia, cyst rupture and increased pain when adding PD fluid to an abdomen with enlarged kidneys. However, in a number of retrospective and observational studies the technical survival, quality of dialysis, duration in therapy and rates of complications in PD are comparable in patients with cystic or noncystic kidney disease. Therefor PKD should not be considered a medical contraindication to PD [26].

In conclusion, in industrialized countries PD is underutilized partly from poor assessment of eligibility and contraindications. There are very few medical contraindications to PD. There are several things that need to occur to promote increased utilization of this modality. Certainly efforts to promote pre ESKD care are is essential. In addition, patients that start dialysis without predialysis care should be considered eligible for PD. Efforts to overcome barriers to PD by offering support, such as assist devices and home care takers, should be employed. Challenging patient populations, such as elderly and the obese, must not be excluded from PD.

References

1. Haggerty SP, Roth S, Walsh D, Stefanidis D, Price R, Fanelli R, Penner T, Richardson W. Guidelines for laparoscopic peritoneal dialysis access surgery. Surg Endosc. 2014;11:3016–45.
2. Foundation NK. K/DPQI Clinical practice guidelines for peritoneal dialysis adequacy: update 2000. Am J Kidney Dis. 2001;37:S65–136.
3. Foundation NK. KDOQI Clinical Practice Guidelines and Clinical Practice Recommendations for 2006 updates: hemodialysis adequacy, peritoneal dialysis adequacy and vascular access. Am J Kidney Dis. 2006;48:S1–S322.
4. Fischbach M, Stefanidis CJ, Watson AR. Guidelines by an ad hoc European committee on adequacy of the paediatric peritoneal dialysis prescription. Nephrol Dial Transplant. 2002;17:380–5.
5. Menzies D, Ellis H. Intestinal obstruction from adhesions–how big is the problem? Ann R Coll Surg Engl. 1990;72:60–3.
6. Crabtree JH, Burchette RJ. Effect of prior abdominal surgery, peritonitis, and adhesions on catheter function and long-term outcome on peritoneal dialysis. Am Surg. 2009;75:140–7.
7. Keshvari A, Fazeli MS, Meysamie A, Seifi S, Taromloo MK. The effects of previous abdominal operations and intraperitoneal adhesions on the outcome of peritoneal dialysis catheters. Perit Dial Int. 2008;30:41–5.
8. Murala JS, Singappuli K, Provenzano Jr SC, Nunn G. Techniques of inserting peritoneal dialysis catheters in neonates and infants undergoing open heart surgery. J Thorac Cardiovasc Surg. 139:503–5.
9. Yildiz N, Memisoglu A, Benzer M, Altuntas U, Alpay H. Can peritoneal dialysis be used in preterm infants with congenital diaphragmatic hernia? J Matern Fetal Neonatal Med. 2013;26:943–5.
10. Del Peso G, Bajo MA, Costero O, Hevia C, Gil F, Diaz C, Aguilera A, Selgas R. Risk factors for abdominal wall complications in peritoneal dialysis patients. Perit Dial Int. 2003;23:249–54.
11. von Lilien T, Salusky IB, Yap HK, Fonkalsrud EW, Fine RN. Hernias: a frequent complication in children treated with continuous peritoneal dialysis. Am J Kidney Dis. 1987;10:356–60.
12. Garcia-Urena MA, Rodriguez CR, Vega Ruiz V, Carnero Hernandez FJ, Fernandez-Ruiz E, Vazquez Gallego JM, Velasco Garcia M. Prevalence and management of hernias in peritoneal dialysis patients. Perit Dial Int. 2006;26:198–202.
13. Leblanc M, Ouimet D, Pichette V. Dialysate leaks in peritoneal dialysis. Semin Dial. 2001;14:50–4.
14. Tzamaloukas AH, Gibel LJ, Eisenberg B, Goldman RS, Kanig SP, Zager PG, Elledge L, Wood B, Simon D. Early and late peritoneal dialysate leaks in patients on CAPD. Adv Perit Dial. 1990;6:64–71.
15. Jager KJ, Korevaar JC, Dekker FW, Krediet RT, Boeschoten EW, Netherlands Cooperative Study on Adequacy of Dialysis Study Group. The effect of contraindications and patient preference on dialysis modality selection in ESRD patients in the Netherlands. Am J Kidney Dis. 2004;43:891–9.
16. Mehrotra R, Marsh D, Vonesh E, et al. Patient education and access of ESRD patients to renal replacement therapies: beyond in-center hemodialysis. Kidney Int. 2005;68:378–90.
17. Goovaerts T, Jadoul M, Goffin E. Influence of a pre-dialysis education programme (PDEP) on the mode of renal replacement therapy. Nephrol Dial Transplant. 2005;20:1842–7.
18. Alkatheeri AMA, Blake PG, Gray D, Jain AK. Success of urgent-start peritoneal dialysis in a large Canadian Renal Program. Perit Dial Int. 2015;36:171–6.
19. Li PK, Law MC, Chow KM, Leung CB, Kwan BC, Chung KY, Szeto CC. Good patient and technique survival in elderly patients on continuous ambulatory peritoneal dialysis. Perit Dial Int. 2007;27(Suppl 2):S196–201.
20. Oliver MJ, Quinn RR, Richardson EP, Kiss AJ, Lamping DL, Manns BJ. Home care assistance and the utilization of peritoneal dialysis. Kidney Int. 2007;71(7):673–8.
21. Dratwa M. Costs of home assistance for peritoneal dialysis: a European survey. Kidney Int. 2008;73(Suppl 108):S72–5.
22. Snyder JJ, Foley RN, Gilbertson DT, Vonesh EF, Collins AJ. Body size and outcomes on peritoneal dialysis in the United States. Kidney Int. 2003;64:1838–44.
23. Abbott KC, Glanton CW, Trespalacios F, Oliver D, et al. Body mass index, dialysis modality, and survival: analysis of the United States Renal Data System Dialysis Morbidity and Mortality Wave II Study. Kidney Int. 2004;65:597–605.
24. Johnson DW, Herzig KA, Purdie DM, et al. Is obesity a favorable prognostic factor in peritoneal dialysis patients? Perit Dial Int. 2000;20:715–21.
25. Aslam N, Bernardini J, Fried L, et al. Large body mass index does not predict short-term survival in peritoneal dialysis patients. Perit Dial Int. 2002;22:191–6.
26. Lobbedez T, Touam M, Evans D, Ryckelynck JP, Knebelman B, Verger C. Peritoneal dialysis in polycystic kidney disease patients. Report from the French peritoneal dialysis registry (RDPLF). Nephrol Dial Transplant. 2011;26(7):2332–9.

Perioperative Planning Assessment and Preparation

Amilcar A. Exume

Introduction

Peritoneal Dialysis Access Surgery can be fraught with post procedural technique failure and complications. The five key premises of this chapter advise a method of proper risk identification and mitigation, preoperative training, PD team coordination, precise mapping, and perioperative care. Difficulties to be addressed with best perioperative practices are ubiquitous and pertinent.

Early PD technique failure rates range up to 35% in adults [1]. Pediatric early PD technique failure rates of 30% within 2 months are common, with median catheter life less than 19 months [2–4].

The predominant etiology of early technique failure is infectious. This patient demographic beset with uremia, and prevalent diabetes mellitus, malnutrition, heart failure, have impaired host defenses with increased risk of infection [5]. In a large Australian series PD catheter related infection was the cause of 48% of conversions from PD to hemodialysis [6]. Very wide divergence of peritonitis rates are noted between as well as within industrialized countries. Registry reports of 0.06 episodes per year in Taiwan up to 1.66 episode peritonitis per year in Israel. Regions within the same country have 20 fold variations in peritonitis rates. eg Austria [7].

Mechanical complications are frequent as well. A 10% early postoperative mechanical catheter failure rate is common [8], and >25% rates in pediatric series [3, 4, 9]. Wide variations in observed rates of infectious and mechanical complications and improved outcomes with implementation of best practices are the impetus for the information offered here [10]. The preoperative office assessment, history and physical exam, as well as laboratory and other testing identify risks and suggest appropriate adaptive plans. As Christian N. Bovee said: "The method of the enterprising is to plan with audacity and execute with vigor".

History and Physical Exam

History of Present Illness

Elderly age per se is not a contraindication to peritoneal dialysis catheter implantation surgery. Adequate dexterity, visual acuity, cognition and home support are key areas to confirm preoperatively in these patients [11, 12].

For patients on hemodialysis, several historic aspects are very helpful in the preoperative period. Surgery can be arranged a day following a regular scheduled dialysis date, or an additional dialysis session can be arranged the day before catheter implantation. This helps to optimize fluid and electrolyte balance and perioperative consequences of uremia. Knowledge of the patient's

A.A. Exume, MD
Department of General Surgery, Southern California Permanente Medical Group,
4647 Zion Avenue, San Diego, CA 92120, USA
e-mail: amilcar.a.exume@kp.org

© Springer International Publishing AG 2017
S. Haggerty (ed.), *Surgical Aspects of Peritoneal Dialysis*, DOI 10.1007/978-3-319-52821-2_4

dry weight (usual weight immediately following dialysis) may be used to calculate volume status based on immediate preoperative measured weight. Awareness of the preoperative baseline daily urine output can assist with decisions on perioperative fluid therapy planning [13].

In autosomal dominant polycystic kidney disease there is a generally reported association of hernia and diverticulosis. The postoperative PD insertion outcomes are similar to unaffected patients. Preoperative awareness of polycystic kidney disease is useful in planning peritoneal entry, careful scrutiny of the abdominal wall and preoperative catheter site mapping [14].

A history of paraesophageal or Morgagni hernia may be associated with symptomatic enlargement or recurrence following peritoneal dialysis institution. Sliding hiatal hernias identified preoperatively are not reported to be problematic [15, 16].

Review of Systems

Symptoms of orthopnea or PND may suggest evaluation for fluid overload that can be optimized prior to supine positioning for surgery. Palpitations may suggest hypokalemia, hyperkalemia or other electrolyte disturbance all common in this patient subset [17].

A history of excessive snoring, somnolent respiratory pauses, or diurnal drowsiness may indicate obstructive sleep apnea syndrome. Awareness by the Anesthesiologist is especially valuable for PD insertion under local anesthetic and sedation where excessive abdominal wall motion in the oversedated sleep apneic can impair intraperitoneal visibility.

Past Surgical History

If patient has received a renal transplant, information on recent or ongoing immunosuppressive therapy can be useful in perioperative management, particularly in identification of need for perioperative stress dose steroids.

A ventriculo-peritoneal shunt still permits safe dialysis catheter peritoneal access surgery. Concerns for increased meningitis risk are not supported in reported cases. Tactical preoperative mapping to avoid injury to the existing shunt is sufficient [18–20].

Recent fundoplication may predispose to peritoneal dialysate transdiaphragmatic leak and herniation [21].

A history of breast implants still in situ is a relative contraindication to presternal peritoneal dialysis catheter implantation. The risk of implant injury during presternal tunneling of the extended catheter and subsequent secondary infection of the implant in case of a tunnel infection are the concerns [22].

A history of prior peritonitis, visceral perforation, intraabdominal or pelvic surgery all raise concerns for intraperitoneal adhesion. Peritoneal adhesions are reported in up to 90% of patients with a history of major abdominal surgery [23]. This rate is thought to be lower for patients with only a history of laparoscopic surgery. Lunderdorff prospectively randomized 105 patients with tubal pregnancy to laparoscopy versus laparotomy surgery. In followup 73 of these patients selected a second look operation for assessment of tubal anatomy. At operation there were significantly more adhesions in the group randomized to laparotomy $p < 0.001$ [24]. Keshvari et al. noted at exploratory laparoscopy in 217 consecutive peritoneal access procedures a 27% rate of intraperitoneal adhesions among patients with prior abdominal surgery versus a 2.8% rate seen in those without prior abdominal surgery [25]. Increased complication rates are noted for fluoroscopic, blind percutaneous, and open surgery peritoneal dialysis catheter placement in patients with intraabdominal adhesions. The increased problems of catheter tip migration, catheter malposition, kinking, and tube blockage are largely averted with application of a laparoscopic approach in such cases [25, 26, 55]. Crabtree in a prospective series of 244 patients with prior abdominal surgery, only 3.3% could not be implanted laparoscopically due to adhesions [27]. Therefore, laparoscopic peritoneal dialysis access can be safely attempted in patients with prior abdominal surgery or history of peritonitis. Ongoing peritonitis, inflammatory bowel disease, carcinomatosis, astroschisis, omphalocele, bladder extrophy, and diaphragmatic hernia, irreparable abdominal wall defects remain contraindications to peritoneal dialysis catheter placement in the pediatric and adult populations [28, 29].

Past Medical History

The preoperative renal failure patient typically suffers from medical comorbidities, some being etiologic to their renal disease. These must be identified preoperatively and the condition must be optimized for anesthesia and surgery. Hypertension and diabetes mellitus represent the two most frequent comorbidities.

The prevalence of hypertension in the end stage renal disease population is 50–60% [30]. Hypervolemia and increased sympathoadrenal tone are the main drivers of secondary hypertension in chronic renal failure patients [31]. Davenport et al. in a multicenter retrospective analysis of 183,609 general and vascular surgical patients found a 1.29% incidence of perioperative adverse cardiac events. Multivariate analysis indicated no independent association of preoperative hypertension with these adverse cardiac events [32]. Ajaimy in a retrospective cohort review of 209 adult preoperative renal transplant patients noted 53% presenting to the preoperative area with severe hypertension(diastolic bp >110 or systolic bp >180). The preoperatively severe hypertensives had similar one year outcomes to those without severe hypertension [30]. Charlson studied 278 elective noncardiac surgery patients with hypertension and/or diabetes in a prospective observational trial. Preoperative hypertension (mean arterial pressure ≥ 110) was associated with intraoperative hypotension defined as >1 h with ≥20 mm Hg drop in mean arterial pressure (p < 0.0001) [33]. There is no evidence that improved cardiac risk is achieved by postponing surgery to a subsequent date for better preoperative blood pressure control [17, 34].

Routine antihypertensive therapy should be continued in the perioperative period [31]. Some authors have advised holding angiotensin converting enzyme (ACE) inhibitors and angiotensin receptor blockers (ARBs) the morning of surgery [35]. The American College of Cardiology and American Heart Association (ACC/AHA) guidelines find continuation of ACE inhibitors and ARB's perioperatively is reasonable as no outcome difference is demonstrated despite more frequent transient intraoperative hypotension [36]. Avoidance of perioperative hypotension to preserve residual renal function may be the appropriate priority in renal failure patients. It is reasonable to hold these agents in the immediate preoperative period. Avoidance of perioperative hypotension may better preserve residual renal function [33]. Good blood pressure control with close monitoring facilitates this goal. The perioperative management of hypertension consists in continuation of baseline preoperative therapy, limiting the use of hypertension inducing drugs, and acute control with short acting agents as needed. Rescheduling of surgery for preoperative hypertension should be rare.

Platinga in a review of 8188 US patients found a 40% incidence of chronic kidney disease in diabetic patients and a 17% incidence in prediabetics [37]. The 2013 European Renal Association–European Dialysis and Transplant Association (ERA-EDTA) Registry identified diabetes as the primary cause in 24% of incident end stage renal disease patients. Goodenough et al. in a prospective review of 438 colon and bariatric surgery patients demonstrated a twofold increased rate of major complications with an elevated preoperative Hba1c ≥6.5%. Although hba1c preoperative reduction is achievable, there is lack of evidence that delay of surgery to achieve this goal improves postoperative outcomes [38, 39]. Kwon et al. performed a multicenter retrospective review of 11,633 patients undergoing elective colorectal and bariatric surgery. Patients with perioperative hyperglycemia glc > 180 mg/dl had significant 2 fold increased rate of infection, as well as increased risk of reoperation, and a 2.7 fold increased in hospital mortality. Most importantly this risk was reversed by using perioperative insulin for glycemic control [40]. The authors find that conventional glycemic management should suffice [39, 41]. Delay of PD access surgery in type II diabetics for optimization of glycemic control is rarely indicated as long as adequate sliding scale insulin therapy is used perioperatively [191].

Family History

Response of the patient or family to anesthesia and any prior sensitivities or adverse reactions is elicited. A personal or family history of poor susceptibility to local anesthetics is best identified prior to scheduling a catheter insertion under local anesthesia [42, 43].

Social History

Pet ownership history is useful due to the risk of biting or clawing of PD catheter tubing and resultant peritonitis risk. The patient's ability to exclude cats and other domesticated animals from the room while dialysis exchanges are performed is required [44].

Smoking if present should be discontinued 6–8 weeks prior to surgery.

Patients with active drug or alcohol abuse should be preoperatively carefully screened to assure ability with available home support to comply with therapy, otherwise catheter placement for home therapy is contraindicated [45].

Allergy

Antibiotic allergies particularly to cephalosporins or vancomycin and allergies to topical adhesives may help with selection of perioperative prophylaxis and postoperative surgical site dressings [43]. A history of iodinated contrast allergy should be identified if fluoroscopic PD access is being considered [17].

Medications

Nephrotoxic drugs should be avoided to the extent possible even in patients with end stage renal disease. Nongnuch et al. in a large observational prospective international trial correlated a 35–47% reduced mortality risk with every 1 ml/min of preserved residual renal function [46]. In children with end stage kidney failure superior growth velocity, decreased left ventricular hypertrophy, and decreased rates of PD associated peritonitis are noted protective effects of residual renal function [18, 47, 48].

Physical Examination

A comprehensive physical exam is necessary for potential peritoneal dialysis to help assess the candidacy of the patient and help minimize risk. Below is a summary of pertinent components of the exam.

Skin

Careful screening for cutaneous infection is beneficial [43]. In a retrospective review of 164 patients by Tiong et al. 3 patients developed peritonitis within a month of PD catheter insertion. All three of these patients had ongoing cutaneous infection, these included 1 groin abscess, 1 forearm abscess, 1 above knee amputation site wound infection [26]. Torso intertriginous or any dermatitis should be addressed prior to surgery if possible, and planned incision and catheter exit sites should be marked to avoid these areas.

Cardiac

Cardiac auscultation for pericardial rub may indicate uremic pericarditis that might benefit from preoperative optimization. A gallop may indicate preoperative heart failure to be addressed.

Lungs

A respiratory finding of rales may indicate fluid overload. Diminished breath sounds may indicated pleural effusion. Tachypnea and Kausmal's breathing can occur in respiratory compensation for metabolic acidosis of renal failure.

Abdomen

The abdominal exam is probably the most important in planning for peritoneal dialysis catheter insertion. Inspection may reveal obesity, pannus, skin infections and scars which may affect tunnel and exit site mapping. Scars may signify prior surgery and need to be confirmed by the surgical history. The presence of a pannus is notable and site planning is needed to avoid emergence of the dialysis catheter tunnel within this fatty fold and the associated deleterious excess catheter mobility. The abdominal shape must be carefully considered to select an optimal convex, patient visible and nondependent catheter exit. In the very obese this will usually be upper abdominal or presternal. The presence of an ostomy, a chronic tube drain such as gastrostomy, long term drain, or percutaneous cystostomy all necessitate siting the catheter exit and tunnel at a distance away.

A careful and thorough exam for ventral, umbilical and inguinal hernias is crucial since abdominal wall hernia is reported in 5–20% of patients for peritoneal dialysis catheter placement. Half of these are noted preoperatively and half are noted intraoperatively. Peritoneal dialysis candidates with prior abdominal surgery have higher prevalent rates of hernia [49, 50]. Autosomal dominant polycystic kidney disease patients have prevalence rates of abdominal wall hernia as high as 45% [51]. Increased intraabdominal pressure and weakening of the abdominal wall may play a role not only in polycystic kidney disease patients but also in chronic PD patients [51, 52].

The prevalence of clinically apparent abdominal wall hernia in chronic PD patients is reported at 10–25% due to the increase in resting intraperitoneal pressure up to five times normal [53, 54]. Garcia Ureña in a prospective observational study of 122 incident PD patients diagnosed 17% with hernias. Of these hernias 1/3 were identified postoperatively during a mean 24 month followup [52]. De Ugarte et al. in a pediatric single institution retrospective review with 72 month median surveillance found a 14% reoperation rate for hernia after PD catheter insertion [3]. Hernias in adults and children frequently increase in size with dialysis and are a significant source of dialysate leak. Therefore all hernias should be repaired prior to initiation of PD. Hernia repair can usually be undertaken at the same time as insertion making pre or intraoperative diagnosis very important. Unfortunately, If a patient has an irreparable abdominal wall hernia, this absolutely precludes successful peritoneal dialysis [55].

Neurologic

Neurologic evaluation should confirm basic visual acuity, dexterity, cognitive ability, and coordination. The patient will need to perform site care directly if an abdominal exit or using a mirror if a presternal exit site is selected [22]. Blindness is not a contraindication for assisted peritoneal dialysis.

Extemity

Extremity evaluation of any arteriovenous fistula or graft and its patency, identification of hand dominance, and future plans for dialysis can inform preoperative intravenous line site selection. Excess peripheral edema may indicate the need for preoperative diuresis [13].

Recommended Screening Labs

Urinanalysis

Urinanalysis is recommended as any identified urinary tract infections should be treated prior to peritoneal access placement.

Basic Metabolic Profile

Baseline Electrolytes Blood Urea Nitrogen, and Creatinine are recommended. A preoperative serum potassium is helpful as preoperative end stage renal failure patients are often hyperkalemic [31, 56]. Pinson et al. noted a 19% rate of perioperative hyperkalemia in chronic renal failure patients [57]. A complete blood count is indicated as anemia is routinely present in this patient population. Leukocytosis may lead to identification of unsuspected infection. Thrombocytopenia is not uncommon in renal failure patients and may necessitate withdrawal of causative medication preoperatively or perioperative precautionary monitoring and intervention.

Complete Blood Count

Although platelet transfusion is typically favored for preoperative patients with a platelet count below 50,000/mm^3, hemolytic uremic syndrome have relative contraindication to platelet transfusion. In a retrospective review by Weil et al. 26 patients were identified with a mean platelet count of 37,100/mm^3. These patients underwent surgical peritoneal dialysis access placement and no bleeding complications were noted. The authors suggest that most thrombocytopenic children with hemolytic uremic syndrome requiring peritoneal dialysis can have their catheters placed without the need for platelet transfusion [58].

Pregnancy Test

Preoperative pregnancy testing is recommended in potentially fertile women. Although fertility rates are decreased in end stage renal disease pregnancy during dialysis is increasingly being reported. In women on dialysis results may be difficult to interpret as serum hcg levels may be elevated in the absence of pregnancy [59–61].

Coagulation Studies

Coagulopathy is ubiquitous in end stage renal disease. Platelet adhesion and aggregation are deficient in chronic kidney disease [62]. Bleeding occurs in up to 50% of prevalent renal failure outpatients. This most commonly presents with excessive bruising, bleeding at venipuncture sites, menorrhagia, gastrointestinal bleeding, and in the retroperitoneum. Chronic kidney disease patients have a fivefold increased risk of intracranial hemorrhage than the general population [63]. An observational review of 1503 venous thromboembolism patients demonstrated a twofold increased short and long term major bleeding risk

for patients with stage IV and V chronic kidney disease [64]. Prothrombin Time (INR) and Partial Thromboplastin Time (PTT) may detect coagulation disorders that might result in excessive procedural blood loss. These are recommended for screening by some authors [13, 65]. Without suggestion of bleeding tendency by history, medication list, and physical findings the INR and PTT were not tested in most peritoneal access case series [17]. Template Bleeding Time is not routinely useful in the preoperative screening of renal failure patients. There is poor correlation of bleeding time and the occurrence of perioperative bleeding [66].

Electrocardiogram

In the general population preoperative ECG for noncardiac surgery is rarely helpful in the asymptomatic general population without known cardiovascular disease (2014 ACA/AHA and ESC and ESA guidelines) [36]. In the renal failure population given the high frequency of cardiovascular disease and arrhythmias, a baseline preoperative ECG is useful.

Chest X-Ray

A chest radiograph is not routinely indicated preoperatively unless a specific clinical indication presents [13, 17].

Other Imaging

Imaging for hernia may be considered due to the clinical significance of even small hernias. A 15% rate of peritoneal dialysis technique loss has been noted with the repair of hernias detected after peritoneal dialysis has been initiated [43, 50, 67]. Additionally up to a third of hernias are diagnosed postoperatively [52]. Many of these clinically missed hernias can be detected intraoperatively during catheter insertion with laparoscopy [49]. Abdominal wall hernias in peritoneal dialysis preoperative patients in order of incidence are umbilical, inguinal, incisional, then ventral. Reported higher risk subsets among renal failure patients include elderly males, nulliparous females, patients with autosomal dominant polycystic kidney disease, mitral valve prolapse, systemic lupus erythematosus, low body weight, history of prior laparotomy, and history of prior herniorraphy [67].

Peritoneoscintigraphy is known to be a sensitive imaging test for hernia. Kopecky et al. conducted a prospective observational trial of 48 patients without clinical suggestion of hernia shortly after initiation of CAPD. During a mean 11.5 month followup, although 14 patients had scintigraphically detected abdominal wall defects, only 4 of these (29%) had progression to clinical evidence. This is therefore not a useful screening preoperative test [68].

Preoperative imaging is suggested in patients with symptoms or history suggestive of abdominal wall hernia unconfirmed by a thorough physical examination. This is particularly applicable when an open surgical, Y-TEC peritoneoscopic, percutaneous fluoroscopic or blind percutaneous insertion is planned, since laparoscopy allows visual inspection for hernias intraoperatively. The favored noninvasive testing modality in order of decreasing sensitivity include noncontrast MRI, non intravenous contrast CT, and abdominal wall musculoskeletal ultrasound [69–71].

Patient Risk Stratification

Perioperative risk stratification guides patient selection, informed consent, preoperative preparation of the patient, periprocedural monitoring, and optimal deployment of the multidisciplinary team.

The most widely utilized risk evaluative tool is the American Society of Anesthesiologist physical status classification (ASA) Table 4.1.

The majority of peritoneal access surgery patients will be categories ASA III or IV [73, 74]. In patient's deemed at prohibitive risk for general anesthetic alternative options can be planned. These options include laparoscopic catheter placement under local anesthetic, open surgical insertion under local anesthetic, open surgical insertion under TAPP (transverses abdominis plane block), open surgical insertion under spinal anesthethetic, Y tec peritoneoscopic or percutaneous methods under local anesthetic [75–77].

Pulmonary

Pulmonary patient risk stratification depends on identification of risk factors, use of a pulmonary stratification tool when there is concern, and liberal utilization of perioperative risk mitigative strategies.

Table 4.1 ASA classification

ASA class	Definition	Examples
ASA I	A normal healthy patient	Healthy nonsmoker
ASA II	Mild systemic disease	Mild diseases, smoker, controlled DM(diabetes mellitus or Htn (hypertension) BMI(body mass index) >30 up to 40
ASA III	Severe systemic disease	Moderate to severe diseases ESRD (end stage renal disease) on regular dialysis, COPD, BMI > 40 Poorly controlled Htn or DM
ASA IV	Systemic disease that is a constant threat to life	ESRD not on regular dialysis, recent myocardial infarction, recent cerebrovascular accident, recent transient ischemic attack, coronary artery stent placement less than 3 months prior, ongoing cardiac ischemia
ASA V	Moribund patient not expected to survive without operation	Ruptured abdominal or thoracic aneurysm, ischemic bowel with cardiac or multiorgan system dysfunction
ASA VI	Brain dead organ removal for donor purposes	

Source: (Adapted ASA web site) [72]

The preoperative history and physical can screen for the following pulmonary risk factors. Further more specific testing ordered on basis of elicited findings.

Risk factors for periprocedural pulmonary complication include:

1. Chronic obstructive pulmonary disease (COPD)
2. Age > 60
3. Cigarette smoking
4. Congestive heart failure (CHF)
5. ASA class ≥ II
6. Functional Dependence (need for device or human assistance with activities of daily living)
7. Obstructive Sleep Apnea Syndrome
8. Pulmonary hypertension (correlates with increased perioperative chf, hemodynamic instability, and respiratory failure)
9. Use of general anesthetic for planned peritoneal access catheter surgery
10. Serum albumin less than 3.5 g/dL
11. Emergency Surgery
12. BUN ≥ 21 mg/dL or Cr > 1.5 mg/dL

Risk Stratification when indicated may utilize 2 accessible pulmonary patient risk indices. The NSQIP (National Surgical Quality Improvement) Surgical Risk Calculator for postoperative pneumonia risk, and ARISCAT (Assess Respiratory Risk in Surgical Patients in Catalonia). Both tools are extensively validated. The NSQIP Surgical Risk Calculator is demonstrated to have a very high predictive discriminatory correlation for postoperative pulmonary complication [78].

Canet et al. developed the ARISCAT in 2010, an externally validated major perioperative pulmonary risk index. This prognosticator utilizes seven weighted clinical factors. These risk factors are age, history of respiratory infection with a month before surgery, the anatomic site of planned surgery, the duration of the procedure, the operative urgency, and the preoperative oxygen saturation. In a multicenter validation trial 5099 consecutive nonobstetric patients had inpatient surgery under general, neuraxial, or plexus block anesthesia. Patients were followed in this study throughout their postoperative hospital stay for up to 5 weeks. A C statistic of 0.80 was realized, demonstrating a high predictive discrimination for patients having or not having postoperative pulmonary adverse outcome [79, 80].

Pulmonary Risk Mitigative Strategies

1. Smoking cessation for at least 8 weeks prior to surgery. Some data suggest that preoperative smoking cessation for less than 6 weeks may increase perioperative pulmonary risk [81]. 2. Excellent preoperative control of asthma reverses the perioperative asthmatic risk of general anesthesia [82]. Perioperative bronchodilator therapy can be useful in COPD, asthma, and pulmonary hypertension. Inhaled corticosteroid therapy can optimize perioperative asthma and COPD.

Cardiovascular

Cardiac risk: A 28–41% adult prevalence of ischemic heart disease at initial dialysis is internationally reported [83]. The hemodialysis population has been reported to have a 35 fold higher annual cardiovascular mortality compared to the general population [83]. Left ventricular hypertrophy, diastolic dysfunction, coronary artery disease, and hypertension are very common in end stage renal disease patients. Perioperative cardiac risk markers are categorized as active cardiac conditions or as clinical cardiac risk factors. Active cardiac conditions require cardiovascular investigation, and treatment prior to surgery. These are listed in Table 4.2 below. Clinical cardiac risk factors such as compensated heart failure and diabetes mellitus do not require routine preoperative noninvasive cardiac testing for peritoneal dialysis access surgery [84].

Surgical procedures can be classified in terms of their inherent cardiac risk level. The American College of Cardiology and the American Heart Association guidelines stratify noncardiac surgery into low <1%, and high >1% risk levels for

Table 4.2 Preoperative cardiac risk factors

American College of Cardiology/American Heart Association Perioperative Cardiac Risks
Active Cardiac Conditions
Unstable coronary syndromes
Myocardial infarction (≤30 days)
Unstable or severe angina (Canadian class III or IV)
Decompensated heart failure
Significant arrhythmias
High-grade atrioventricular block
Symptomatic ventricular arrhythmias with uncontrolled ventricular rate
Supraventricular arrhythmias with uncontrolled ventricular rate
Severe valvular disease
Clinical Cardiac Risk Factors
Compensated or prior heart failure
Renal Insufficiency
History of ischemic heart disease
Diabetes Mellitus
History of cerebrovascular disease

Adapted (Cardiac Risk Stratification for Noncardiac Surgery Grasso and Wael [84])

30 day major adverse cardiac events. Major adverse cardiac events being defined to include myocardial infarction, pulmonary edema, ventricular fibrillation, primary cardiac arrest, and complete heart block. Germane factors that influence this stratification include anticipated perioperative blood loss, operative fluid shifts, and duration of surgery. By these criteria peritoneal dialysis access procedures have an inherently low cardiac risk [36].

The overall cardiac risk stratification must not only consider the inherent procedural risk, but also consider the procedural timing urgency, and the cardiac comorbidities of the patient [17, 36]. Any of three preoperative cardiac risk stratification models are recommended by the ACC. These are the RCRI revised cardiac risk index, NSQIP derived MICA myocardial infarction and cardiac arrest calculator, and the NSQIP national surgical quality improvement program broad surgical risk calculator [85].

The Revised Cardiac Risk Index (or Lee Index) counts the preoperative presence of six equally weighted factors: coronary artery disease, heart failure, cerebrovascular disease, diabetes mellitus requiring insulin, high risk noncardiac surgery, and renal insufficiency

(Cr > 2 mg/dl). Elevated risk (major adverse perioperative cardiac event >1%) is predicted if two or more risk factors are present [141]. This method overestimates the risk of peritoneal dialysis access surgery.

The NSQIP derived MICA risk model assesses risk of myocardial infarction or cardiac arrest in the 30 day perioperative period. The independent patient variables for this model are ASA (American Society of Anesthesiologist) class, functional status, age, Cr >1.5 g/dl, and type of surgery. This model is derived from data on >400,000 patients [32].

This third risk model applies to cardiac, pulmonary and a broad array of perioperative risk. The American College of Surgeons NSQIP online risk calculator tool uses 20 patient variables built on a database of 2.7 million operations. It predicts perioperative mortality and morbidity modeled for 11 outcomes. As of 2016 this tool includes procedure specific outcome prognostication for laparoscopic, percutaneous, open peritoneal dialysis catheter insertion and catheter removal. The predictions of this calculator correlate very closely with clinically observed patient complication rates [188, 189]. This broad prognosticator is available for pediatric peritoneal dialysis access patients as well [86].

Bleeding

Bleeding risk at time of surgery and postoperatively are a concern given the known platelet dysfunction and common anticoagulant use in chronic kidney disease patients (Table 4.3). Mital et al. retrospectively reviewed 263 consecutive patients after surgically placed Tenckhoff catheters. They evaluated the incidence of perioperative major bleeding complications. Major bleeding was defined as ≥3% decline in hematocrit, or the need for surgical intervention or blood transfusion within 2 weeks of insertion. A 2% rate of major bleeding was identified. A third of the patients with major bleeding were thrombocytopenic preoperatively. Half of the major bleeds were in patients on preoperative warfarin or postoperative heparin [65].

Table 4.3 Reported bleeding rate as complication of PD catheter insertion [3, 4, 9, 10, 25, 65, 77, 87–107]

Case series authors	Reported bleeding rate	Comments
Case series	Bleeding episodes/total patients	Description
Fluoroscopic Percutaneous		
Vaux et al. (2008)	0/209	No clinically significant bleeding
Medani et al. (2012)	0/151	No clinically significant bleeding
Moon et al. (2008)	1/134	
Ozener et al. (2001)	5/133	
Perakis et al. (2009)	5/86	
Reddy et al. (2010)	4/64	
Voss et al. (2012)	0/51	
Jacobs et al. (1992)	3/45	
Zaman et al. (2005)	1/36	
Maya et al. (2007)	0/32	No clinically significant bleeding
Trung et al. (2013)	2/30	
Chula et al. (2013)	2/26	
Open Surgical Placement		
Rinaldi et al. (2004)	6/503	Hemoperitoneum
Mital et al. (2004)	6/292	Minor pericannular bleeds
Li et al. (2012)	20/244	Pediatric series
Phan et al. (2012)	0/214	Pediatric series
Robison et al. (1984)	3/173	Pediatric series
Carpenter et al. (2016)	0/173	Pediatric series
Medani et al. (2012)	0/162	Pediatric series five of the 7 were
Stone et al. (2013)	0/134	minor bleeds
Yeh et al. (1992)	4/115	
Ozener et al. (2001)	0/82	
Park et al. (2014)	0/78	
Perakis et al. (2009)	2/75	
Gadallah et al. (1999)	0/72	
Radtke et al. (2015)	0/70	
Kim et al. (2015)	7/60	
Blind Percutaneous		
Medani et al. (2012)	0/151	Pericannular bleeding
Park et al. (2014)	2/89	Minor bleeding
Chula et al. (2013)	3/53	
Peritoneoscopic		
Asif et al. (2004)	4/82	Blood tinged dialysate
Gadallah et al. (1999)	0/76	
Laparoscopic		
Crabtree et al. (2009)	1/428	Port site abdominal wall bleeding
Attaluri et al. (2010)	1/197	Reoperatively controlled
Keshvari et al. (2010)	1/175	Delayed mild bleeding
Penner et al. (2015)	1/87	
Voss et al. (2012)	0/51	

Bleeding Risk Table

Early preoperative interdiction can be initiated at time of consultation when an elevated bleeding complication risk level is prospectively identified. These measures include amelioration of anemia, and a short course of estrogen therapy.

Anemia associated with chronic kidney disease is frequent. Improvement of anemia reduces uremic surgical bleeding through platelet function effects including increased platelet endothelial interaction. Recombinant erythropoietin is a useful agent for optimizing hemostasis. A hematocrit level of 30% is recommended. The benefit of further correction above 30% must be weighed against the increased thrombotic risk [63].

Estrogen administration safely and effectively improves procedural hemostasis in male and female patients with azotemia. Conjugated estrogen can be administered at a dose of 0.6 mg/kg intravenously over 30 min once daily for 5 days. This achieves a procoagulant effect on circulating factor VIII, von Willebrands factor, protein S, endothelial nitric oxide, and platelet ADP and thromboxane A2 levels. A 5–7 day preprocedural course provides maximal effect. Postoperative dosing is not necessary [63, 108–110].

Anti-platelet Therapy

Cardiovascular risk is prevalent among end stage renal disease patients. Among pediatric renal failure patients left ventricular hypertrophy is noted in >80% at initiation of dialysis. Cardiovascular disease is causative in 20–40% of deaths in pediatric end stage kidney failure [47]. Adults with end stage kidney disease have a 20–50 fold increased risk for premature cardiovascular disease compared to the general population [83, 111, 112]. Cerebrovascular risk is also elevated in renal failure patients. A 2015 meta-analysis by Masson et al. included over 30,000 strokes identified a linear relation of GFR and stroke risk. A 7% increased stroke risk was noted for every 10 ml/min/1.73 m^2 decrease in GFR [113].

As a result of the prevalence of cardiovascular disease, atrial fibrillation, and cerebrovascular disease among renal disease patients long term antiplatelet and anticoagulation therapy are a frequent issue in preoperative planning. The surgeon or interventionalist in collaboration with consultants must balance the relative perioperative risk of bleeding and the risk of thromboembolism to develop a patient specific optimal strategy. This includes timing of withholding anticoagulants, approaches of coagulopathic reversal, bridging protocols, and timing the resumption of maintenance therapy.

Let us start with the component best known to the surgeon or interventionalist. According to the ACC/AHA (American College of Cardiology and the American Heart Association) operative bleeding risk is now stratified as:

Low <2% 2 day risk of major periprocedural bleed and
High > 2% 2 day risk of major periprocedural bleed.

Low risk procedures include pacemaker or cardiac defibrillator insertion, abdominal hernia repair, axillary node dissection, dental extraction, or cholecystectomy [114]. Peritoneal dialysis access insertion based on broad historical experience has a low operative bleeding risk.

Chronic Oral Anticoagulation

Oral anticoagulant therapy is often encountered in the severe or end stage renal disease patient (gfr < 30). The prevalence of atrial fibrillation in this group has been noted in up to 20% [116]. Preoperative warfarin or novel oral anticoagulants require thoughtful decisions on the need for interruption of therapy, use of parenteral bridging, and postoperative resumption of oral therapy. Interdisciplinary consultation is advisable as there are no large randomized trials that assess the risk benefit of full anticoagulation in severe renal failure patients. Cataract, dermatologic, implantable cardiac device insertion, and dental extractive surgery are safely conducted under full oral anticoagulation [121, 177, 190]. Although PD access surgery is also a low bleeding risk procedure, the potential for hidden intraperitoneal bleeding favors a conservative approach. In the absence of specific studies of PD access surgery on full oral anticoagulant therapy the table below summarizes pharmacologic guidance from available data in renal disease patients with gfr 15–30 (Table 4.4). The nature of the anticoagulant, its antidote, the elimination half life in renal impairment, and options of management based on a patient's thromboembolic risk. Bridging therapy is discouraged when avoidable due to increased

Table 4.4 Half-life of various oral anticoagulant drugs [178–187]

Oral anticoagulant Therapy alone[a]	T½ elimination gfr 15–30 ml/min	Low thrombotic risk patient Time from last anticoagulant dose to incision 4–5 t½	Moderate thrombotic risk patient Time from last anticoagulation dose to incision 2–3 t½	High thrombotic risk patient Time from last anticoagulation dose to incision
Warfarin Vitamin K antagonist Reversal vitamin k FFP, PCC[b]	35 h	Hold 5–7 days	Hold 3–4 days	Uninterrupted warfarin versus 5–7 day warfarin hold with heparin bridge
Dabigatran (Pradaxa) Direct thrombin Inhibitor Reversal hemodialysis, or idarucizumab	27.5 h	5–6 days	2–3.5 days	Uninterrupted dabigatran versus 5 day hold with heparin bridge
Rivaroxaban (Xarelto) Direct factor Xa inhibitor Reversal PCC[b] Adexanet alfa[c]	9.5 h	2 days	1 day	Bridge usually unnecessary due to rapid onset offset of effect
Apixaban (Eliquis) Direct factor Xa inhibitor Reversal PCC[b] Adexanet alfa[c]	17.3 h	3 days	2 days	Uninterrupted dabigatran versus 3 day hold with heparin bridge
Edoxaban (Savaysa) Direct factor Xa inhibitor Reversal PCC[b] Adexanet alfa[c]	17.5 h	3 days	2 days	Uninterrupted edoxaban versus 3 day hold with heparin bridge

FFP fresh frozen plasma
[a]Not combined with antiplatelet therapy
[b]*PCC* prothrombin complex concentrate
[c]Adexanet alpha undergoing premarket clinical trials

bleeding risk compared to uninterrupted therapeutic anticoagulation.

Chronic antiplatelet therapy is frequently encountered in preoperative peritoneal access patients. Colette et al. in a multicenter regional study of 502 incident hemodialysis patients found a 61.3% prevalence of chronic antiplatelet therapy [115]. Agents commonly used for antiplatelet therapy include aspirin, P2Y12 receptor inhibitors such as clopidogrel (Plavix) prasugrel (Effient) and ticagrelor (Brilinta) [116].

Aspirin therapy that is indicated for cardiac or vascular indications may be continued perioperatively without interruption for low bleeding risk procedures (2014 American College of Cardiology/American Heart Association Guidelines, 2014 European Society of Cardiology/European Society of Aneaesthesiology Guidelines) [36, 120].

The POISE-2 trial randomly assigned 10,010 noncardiac preoperative patients at risk for vascular complications to low dose perioperative aspirin or placebo. The 30 day death or nonfatal MI rate was statistically not different at 7% for both groups. The major bleeding rate in the aspirin treated group was higher (4.6% versus 3.8%, p = 0.04, [117].

Shpitz et al. prospectively evaluated the effect of low dose aspirin (mostly 100 mg daily) on postoperative bleeding in end-stage renal disease patients. These patients underwent 52 consecutive open surgical peritoneal dialysis catheter placements or removals. Twenty-nine patients were on aspirin and this was continued perioperatively without interruption 23 control patients were not on chronic aspirin therapy. There was a 17.2% minor bleeding rate in the aspiring group and a

13% bleeding rate in the control group. Only one major bleed occurred and this was in the control group. 2/3 of the bleeding observed occurred with catheter removal. From this data the authors conclude that PD catheter insertion or removal can be safely performed with uninterrupted conventional low-dose aspirin therapy [118].

Large trials on perioperative aspirin use in renal failure patients are lacking. In Summary, the cardiology society guidelines, POISE 2 trial results, Shpitz data, and the low bleeding risk of peritoneal dialysis access surgery suggest safety in perioperative continuation of chronic aspirin therapy when medically indicated [36, 117, 119–121].

Surgeons and Interventionalists have been even more reticent to continue P2Y12 platelet aggregation inhibition therapy periprocedurally. Among end stage renal disease patients clopidogrel (Plavix) tends to have less bleeding risk than prasugrel or ticagrelor [122–124] Combined aspirin clopidogrel use without perioperative interruption demonstrated a 6.8 fold increased pocket hematoma risk in meta-analyzed cardiac implantable electronic device insertions [119].

In the largest retrospective trial of major noncardiac surgery involving 2154 patients, Strosberg et al. demonstrated no increased periprocedural bleeding with clopidogrel alone continued within 5 days prior to incision [125]. Furthermore, Chu et al. performed the largest prospective randomized controlled trial of noncardiac surgical patients, and administered single agent clopidogrel perioperatively. In 39 patients they observed no difference in perioperative bleeding with uninterrupted versus a 7 day preoperatively held clopidogrel [126]. A 5–7 day preoperative hold of clopidogrel is historically recommended. There is now sufficient data to suggest that low bleeding risk procedures such peritoneal dialysis access can safely be performed without interruption of single agent clopidogrel. Dual agent aspirin and clopidogrel perioperative use still requires careful consideration of thromboembolic proclivity, duration of need for dual antiplatelet therapy, bleeding risk, and alternative options for dialysis access.

Office Preoperative Preparation

Preoperative Mapping and Planning of Insertion and Exit Site

PD catheter mapping is the most important preoperative step unique to peritoneal access placement by the surgeon or interventionalist. Omission of adequate mapping predisposes to a litany of demonstrated complications including: Drain or infusion pain, catheter dysfunction, peritonitis, catheter tip migration, superficial cuff extrusion, injury during subsequent operations. Increased risk of tunnel infection and exit site infection, as well as catheter kinking and patient discomfort at the exit site.

The primary objectives of mapping are to establish optimal catheter tip position, optimal catheter tunnel, and optimal exit site positioning. The catheter tip should be positioned in the pelvis sufficiently deeply to allow good dependent drainage, and decreased omental wrapping, as outflow dysfunction is a most common cause of catheter failure [103]. Drain pain is most commonly observed when the catheter tip is too deeply positioned in the pelvis. Clinically significant drain pain occurs in 13–25% of patients. This estimate does not include patients who tolerate the pain, convert to manual exchanges, or convert to hemodialysis because of the pain [127]. Drain pain occurs by a siphoning effect against deep cul de sac fenestrated catheter tip apposition to sensitive parietal pelvic peritoneum [128–131].

The key to an optimal catheter tip placement is distal cuff abdominal wall mapping. Historically a number of landmarks have been used for deep cuff mapping. The anterior superior iliac spine, specified distance superior to planned exit site [6], some distance relative to umbilicus [43, 100, 132–134], and pubic symphysis [43, 107]. An anthropometric anatomic study by Crabtree et al. found a 21 cm variation in the distance of the umbilicus to the symphysis pubis in 200 adult patients. There was wide variation in the distance of the anterior superior iliac spine to the symphysis pubis making it an unreliable anatomic marker also. The pubic symphysis has been confirmed laparoscopically to be a consistent externally identifiable landmark to catheter tip placement in the true pelvis [135].

Mapping of the deep cuff location is performed in the office with the patient supine. A sample straight tip catheter can be used by positioning the first side hole of a straight catheter on the upper border of the symphysis pubis. If a curled tip catheter insertion is planned, the upper or proximal border of the coil can be placed over the pubic symphysis. The deep cuff location is then marked on the skin as the catheter is extended along the planned tunnel course. Some catheter manufacturers provide plastic marking stencils designed for this purpose also [1, 128, 135, 136]. The deep cuff position should be moved more laterally to coincide with the rectus muscle position in patients with diastasis. Bilateral mapping may be considered in patients anticipated to have extensive lower abdominal adhesions [25].

The patient's clothing or work tool belt line, nonvisible or inaccessible areas of the abdominal skin, cutaneous intertriginous, inframammary, or surgical scar folds, chronic dermatitis, incontinence susceptible skin, planned sites of postoperative bath tub or whirlpool water exposure, bra lines, thicker portions of breast, gastrostomy or ostomy placement areas should be identified with the patient seated and supine. The belt line is best identified with patient dressed. Once these hazard zones are marked, a catheter configuration and exit site is selected that best avoids them. The catheter tunnel should eschew contact with existing or planned prosthetic abdominal wall mesh, a ventriculoperitoneal shunt, breast implants, midline abdomen or midline sternum(risk of laparotomy or sternotomy operative catheter damage) [8, 22, 29, 55, 128, 137–140, 142–146].

Informed consent in peritoneal access procedures includes good doctor patient communication in review of indications, risks, benefits, and alternatives. Setting rational expectations of outcome, and explaining adjunctive procedures that may become indicated at laparoscopic exploration is valuable. These include selective omentopexy, abdominal wall herniorraphy, adhesiolysis, epiploic appendage resection, ovariopexy, and fallopian tubopexy [8, 49, 165].

Infection Prevention

Infection is a common early postoperative peritoneal dialysis access complication. It is an overwhelming and often avertable cause of catheter loss and peritoneal dialysis interruption. Tunnel, exit site, and peritoneal infection early after peritoneal dialysis procedures are usually caused from endogenous microbes [5, 147, 148]. Staphylococci are the most frequently cultured organism. Selective preoperative nasal *Staphylococcus aureus* decolonization in peritoneal dialysis access may be prudent.

The close correlation between endonasal S. aureus colonization and exit site infection has been known for greater than 20 years [43]. Lye et al. in a 4 year trial with 146 chronic PD patients found higher rates of exit site infection, peritonitis, and catheter loss in nasal *S. aureus* carriers ($p < 0.01$) [149].

In prevalent peritoneal dialysis patients a broad genomic heterogeneity of *S. aureus* nasal colonization is consistently demonstrated. Clinical *S. aureus* infections during a 6 month trial by Aktas et al. found a 90% genomic concordance with identified endonasal *S. aureus* [150]. Many earlier studies also confirm autologous origin of PD related peritonitis and exit site infections [151–153].

Two large studies in broad populations demonstrate reduction in clinical early postoperative infection when nasal and cutaneous staphylococcal decolonization is administered. Bode et al. in a randomized double blind placebo controlled trial, PCR rapidly screened general hospital admissions for nasal *S. aureus* colonization. 808 nasal *S. aureus* colonized patients had surgical procedures acutely after admission. The nasal mupirocin and chlorhexidine bath treatment group had a 79% reduced risk of deep surgical site infection compared to placebo [154].

Schweitzer et al. conducted the pragmatic STOP SSI multicenter trial with 38,000 cardiac, knee and hip arthroplasty surgical patients. Despite a low (39%) protocol full compliance for nasal and cutaneous decolonization, treated subjects demonstrated a 40%

reduction in staphylococcal complex surgical site infections [155].

There is evidence to suggest decreased infection rates with the institution of maintenance antistaphyloccal prophylaxis among prevalent PD patients. A 2004 Cochrane review found nasal mupirocin reduced exit site and tunnel infections in patients being dialyzed peritoneally [156]. Blowey et al. in a randomized controlled trial demonstrated a higher incidence of dialysis related infection among pediatric nasal *S. aureus* carriers. This was rendered equivalent to noncarriers during the month following decolonization therapy [157]. In a multicenter double blind randomized placebo controlled trial the Mupirocin Study Group demonstrated a significant reduction in staphyloccal exit site infections with nasal mupirocin nasal decolonization in nasal carrier adult PD patients. Crabtree et al. carried out a 2 year surveillance and nasal mupirocin treatment of *S. aureus* carriers. The rates of peritonitis ($p = 0.0002$) and catheter loss ($p = 0.01$) were reduced in the treatment group compared to historic controls [158]. The nasal carriage rate of *S. aureus* is 20% in the general population and higher among dialysis patients [154, 155]. *S. aureus* nasal carriage confers a five to tenfold increased risk of staphylococcal surgical site infection [148]. The Italian Society of Nephrology Peritoneal Dialysis Study Group recommends bid nasal mupirocin prophylaxis for 3 days preoperatively and 3 days postoperatively. The International Society of Peritoneal Dialysis is ambivalent about the need for preoperative nasal decolonization due to lack of data on this specific indication. Preoperative nasal *S. aureus* screening and preoperative prophylactic treatment of carriers can be recommended on the basis of the information so far reviewed [8].

The benefit of preoperative chlorhexidine whole-body showering or bathing has not been adequately studied in preoperative peritoneal dialysis patients. The use of this low cost low risk potentially beneficial intervention is left to individual practitioner preference [159, 160].

Preoperative Training

Preoperative training helps optimize outcomes following PD access insertion. Hall et al. in a longitudinal multicenter trial, assigned 620 incident patients to conventional versus enhanced peritoneal dialysis training. The enhanced training patients demonstrated significantly improve procedural compliance ($p < .0001$), lower exit site infection rates 18.5/1000 patient months vs 31.8/1000 patient months ($p = .00349$), and lower infection related drop out rates from peritoneal dialysis 1.6% vs 5.6% ($p = .0069$) [161].

In an International Society of Peritoneal Dialysis 76 center survey, longer pre-dialysis training times for families were associated with the lowest pediatric peritoneal dialysis related infection rates ($p < 0.05$) [162].

Bordin et al. in a retrospective analysis of peritonitis rates at 120 dialysis centers found a strong correlation of improved peritoneal infection free duration with pre-dialysis education. A rate of 1 peritonitis episode/26 months improved to 1 peritonitis episode/32 months with pre-dialysis education ($p < 0.05$) [163].

Pre-dialysis PD training time was noted to vary from 6 to 96 h in an international multicenter survey [164]. ISPD guidelines advise thorough training of patients and participating family members. Motor skills, concepts, procedures and problem solving in peritoneal dialysis home care must be assured through a standardized teaching plan [29, 161].

PD Team Coordination

Collaboration within a team facilitates successful timing, fulfilling social supportive needs, and optimal delivery of care. The Renal Association UK, and the International Society for Peritoneal Dialysis recommend that each center establish a dedicated team involved in the implantation and care of peritoneal catheters [8, 166]. In addition, care coordination for optimal timing of PD catheter placement improves the rate of successful peritoneal dialysis start [167]. The team consists of Nephrologist, Primary care physician, medical specialists, nurses, social workers, perioperative staff, dialysis unit team, and interventionalist or surgeon. Nephrologists are the primary drivers of this team. When the decision is made a patient will begin PD, Education is begun at the dialysis unit, either by nurse or nurse practitioner and the patient is referred to surgeon or interventionalist. If the patient is to have surgical placement, an expedited process must take place of pre-op risk stratification and optimization. This is in combination with surgeon, primary care physician and appropriate medical specialist. Finally, the procedure is accomplished with carful coordination with outpatient nephrology and the operating room team. Postoperatively the nephrologist and dialysis unit continue support for the patient, with the surgeon on standby in case there are complications. It should be noted that a surgeon and operating room team with interest, experience and skill in dealing with these complex patients is paramount to a successful process [168].

Team coordination of nursing assessment and social supportive needs can be critical to successful post implantation outcomes. For instance, impaired visual acuity is a barrier that can be overcome with well coordinated assisted PD in adults and children [169, 170]. If a presternal catheter placement is planned, a nursing evaluation prior to surgery can assure that the patient can perform exit site care using a mirror. If not, then home assistance must be assured prior to catheter insertion in this position [22]. In addition, cognitive impairment is twofold more prevalent in elderly end stage renal disease patients than age matched cohort. With increasing age beyond 60 the pivotal value of reliable, trainable, home assistance enhances successful results. Developmental cognitive disability among younger patients also requires assurance of adequate home support for successful PD [170–172]. Confirmation of this support can avert postoperative technique failure [173]. Finally, preoperative psychosocial screening team communication is essential to optimal outcomes because socioeconomic adversity, poor home conditions, poor hygiene,

lack of space for storage of supplies, drug abuse, poor motivation to self care are all competitive risks factors to successful reliable peritoneal access [169, 170, 174].

Advanced coordination with the Nephrologist, dialysis unit, and procedural scheduling is important. For patients with hemodialysis access, a dialysis session the day before catheter insertion reduces uremic platelet dysfunction. It also allows optimization of electrolyte and fluid volume status at the time of catheter insertion. Postoperative catheter care, training, and initiation of peritoneal dialysis can be optimally sequenced in this way [34, 175–178].

Summary

A plethora of variables impact the establishment of functional, reliable, sustained peritoneal access for dialysis. Preoperatively the Interventionalist or Surgeon must identify the anatomic, physiologic, social, and medical risks. Once the patient's candidacy is confirmed, a detailed strategy is elaborated to overcome any barriers to success by medical optimization, thorough patient training, and detailed catheter mapping. This strategy is best realized by a collaborative team of nephrologist, medical specialists, nurses, social workers, perioperative staff, dialysis unit team, and interventionalist or surgeon.

> The method of the enterprising is to plan with audacity and execute with vigor. (Christian N. Bovee)

Bibliography

1. Hagen SM, Lafranca JA, Ijzermans JNM, Dor FJMF. A systematic review and meta-analysis of the influence of peritoneal dialysis catheter type on complication rate and catheter survival. Kidney Int. 2014;85(4):920–32. Web
2. Cribbs RK, Greenbaum LA, Heiss KF. Risk factors for early peritoneal dialysis catheter failure in children. J Pediatr Surg. 2010;45:585–9.

3. Phan J, Stanford S, Joshua ZJ, Daniel DA. Risk factors for morbidity and mortality in pediatric patients with peritoneal dialysis catheters. J Pediatr Surg. 2013;48(1):197–202.

4. Carpenter JL, Sara FC, Sarah SJ, Paul MK, Darrell CL, Jed NG, Ashwin PP, Mary BL. Outcomes after peritoneal dialysis catheter placement. J Pediatr Surg. 2016;51(5):730–3.

5. Wikdahl A, Engman U, Stegmayr B, Sorenssen J. One-dose cefuroxime I.v. and I.p. reduces microbial growth in PD patients after catheter insertion. Nephrol Dial Transplant. 1997;12(1):157–60.

6. Johnson DW, Wong J, Kathryn WJ, Kirwan R, Griffin A, Preston J, Wall D, Scott CB, Nicole IM, David MW, Carmel HM, David NL. A randomized controlled trial of coiled versus straight swan-neck Tenckhoff catheters in peritoneal dialysis patients. Am J Kidney Dis. 2006;48(5):812–21.

7. Zhang L, Carmel Hawley M, David Johnson W. Focus on peritoneal dialysis training: working to decrease peritonitis rates. Nephrol Dial Transplant. 2016;31:214–22.

8. Frost JH, Bagul A. A brief recap of tips and surgical manoeuvres to enhance optimal outcome of surgically placed peritoneal dialysis catheters. Int J Nephrol. 2012;2012:1–7.

9. Stone ML, Damien LJ, John BP, Victoria NF, Daniel MP, Eugene MD, Bradley RM, Bartholomew KJ. Surgical outcomes analysis of pediatric peritoneal dialysis catheter function in a rural region. J Pediatr Surg. 2013;48(7):1520–7.

10. Attaluri V, Lebeis C, Brethauer S, Rosenblatt S. Advanced laparoscopic techniques significantly improve function of peritoneal dialysis catheters. J Am Coll Surg. 2010;211(6):699–704.

11. Castrale C, Evans D, Verger C, Fabre E, Aguilera D, Ryckelynck J-P, Lobbedez T. Peritoneal dialysis in elderly patients: report from the French Peritoneal Dialysis Registry (RDPLF). Nephrol Dial Transplant. 2009;25:255–62.

12. Koc YA. Is peritoneal dialysis a therapeutic option for polycystic kidney disease? 15 years' experience in a single center. Nephrol Therapeut. 2016;12:215–20.

13. Forrington S, Bannard-Smith J. Preoperative assessment of the patient with kidney disease. Anaesth Intensive Care Med. 2015;16(6):253–6.

14. Yang J-Y, Chen L, Chao C-T, Peng Y-S, Chiang C-K, Kao T-W, Chien K-L, Wu H-Y, Huang J-W, Hung K-Y. Outcome comparisons between patients on peritoneal dialysis with and without polycystic kidney disease. Medicine. 2015;94(48):e2166.

15. Hughes GC, Ketchersid TL, Lenzen JM, Lowe JE. Thoracic complications of peritoneal dialysis. Ann Thorac Surg. 1999;67(5):1518–22.

16. Lew SQ. Hydrothorax: pleural effusion associated with peritoneal dialysis. Perit Dial Int. 2010;30(1):13–8.

17. Buffington M, Abreo K. Preoperative evaluation of a patient for peritoneal dialysis catheter. Intervent Nephrol. 2013:281–91.

18. Bakkaloglu SA, Saygili A, Sever L, Noyan A, Akman S, Ekim M, Aksu N, Doganay B, Yildiz N, Duzova A, Soylu A, Alpay H, Sonmez F, Civilibal M, Erdem S, Kardelen F. Assessment of cardiovascular risk in paediatric peritoneal dialysis patients: a Turkish Pediatric Peritoneal Dialysis Study Group (TUPEPD) Report. Nephrol Dial Transplant. 2009;24(11):3525–32.

19. Ram Prabahar M, Sivakumar M, Chandrasekaran V, Indhumathi E, Soundararajan P. Peritoneal dialysis in a patient with neurogenic bladder and chronic kidney disease with ventriculoperitoneal shunt. Blood Purif. 2008;26:274–8.

20. Grünberg J, Verocay MC, Rébori A, Pouso J. Comparison of chronic peritoneal dialysis outcomes in children with and without spina bifida. Pediatr Nephrol. 2007;22:573–7.

21. Clarke D, Hall C, Shaw D. Transdiaphragmatic herniation of peritoneal dialysis fluid post Nissen's operation: an unusual cause for a mass on the chest radiograph. Pediatr Radiol. 1997;27:813–4.

22. Crabtree JH, Burchette RJ. Comparative analysis of two-piece extended peritoneal dialysis catheters with remote exit-site locations and conventional abdominal catheters. Perit Dial Int. 2010;30(1):46–55.

23. Liakakos T, Thomakos N, Paul FM, Dervenis C, Ronald YL. Peritoneal adhesions: etiology, pathophysiology, and clinical significance. Digest Surg Dig Surg. 2001;18(4):260–73.

24. Lundorff P, Hahlin M, Källfelt B, Thorburn J, Lindblom B. Adhesion formation after laparoscopic surgery in tubal pregnancy: a randomized trial versus laparotomy**supported by grant 8683 from The Swedish Medical Research Council, Sweden, and by the Göteborg Medical Society, Göteborg, Sweden. Fertil Steril. 1991;55(5):911–5.

25. Keshvari A, Fazeli MS, Meysamie A, Seifi S, Taromloo MK. The effects of previous abdominal operations and intraperitoneal adhesions on the outcome of peritoneal dialysis catheters. Perit Dial Int. 2010;30(1):41–5.

26. Tiong HY, Poh J, Sunderaraj K, Wu YJ, Consigliere DT. Surgical complications of Tenckhoff catheters used in continuous ambulatory peritoneal dialysis. Singap Med J. 2006;47(8):707–11.

27. Crabtree JH, Raoul BJ. Effective use of laparoscopy for long-term peritoneal dialysis access. Am J Surg. 2009;198(1):135–41.

28. Dolan NM, Borzych-Duzalka D, Suarez A, Principi I, Hernandez O, Al-Akash S, Alconchar L, Breen C, Fischbach M, Flynn J, Pape L, Piantanida JJ, Printza N, Wong W, Zaritsky J, Schaefer F, Warady BA, White CT. Ventriculoperitoneal shunts in children on peritoneal dialysis: a survey of the international pediatric peritoneal dialysis network. Pediatr Nephrol Pediatr Nephrol. 2012;28(2):315–9.

29. Warady BA, Bakkaloglu S, Newland J, Cantwell M, Verrina E, Neu A, Chadha V, Yap H-K, Schaefer F. Consensus guidelines for the prevention and treat-

ment of catheter-related infections and peritonitis in pediatric patients receiving peritoneal dialysis: 2012 update. Perit Dial Int. 2012;32(Suppl_2):S32–86.

30. Ajaimy M, Lubetzky M, Kamal L, Gupta A, Dunn C, De GB, Akalin E, Kayler L. Kidney transplantation in patients with severe preoperative hypertension. Clin Transplant. 2015;29(9):781–5.

31. Yee J, Parasuraman R, Narins RG. Selective review of key perioperative renal-electrolyte disturbances in chronic renal failure patients. Chest. 1999;115(5):149S–57S.

32. Davenport DL, Ferraris VA, Hosokawa P, Henderson WG, Khuri SF, Mentzer RM. Multivariable predictors of postoperative cardiac adverse events after general and vascular surgery: results from the patient safety in surgery study. J Am Coll Surg. 2007;204(6):1199–210.

33. Charlson ME, Mackenzie RC, Gold PJ, Ales KL, Topkins M, Shires GT. Preoperative characteristics predicting intraoperative hypotension and hypertension among hypertensives and diabetics undergoing noncardiac surgery. Ann Surg. 1990;212(1):66–81.

34. Jones DR, Lee HT. Surgery in the patient with renal dysfunction. Med Clin N Am. 2009;93(5):1083–93.

35. Mythen M. Anesthetic implications of concurrent diseases. In: Fleisher LA, editor. Millers anesthesia. 8th ed. München: Elsevier Health Sciences; 2015. p. 1156–225.

36. Fleisher LA, Fleischmann KE, Auerbach AD, Barnason SA, Beckman JA, Bozkurt B, Davila-Roman VG, Gerhard-Herman MD, Holly TA, Kane GC, Marine JE, Nelson MT, Spencer CC, Thompson A, Ting HH, Uretsky BF, Wijeysundera DN. 2014 ACC/AHA guideline on perioperative cardiovascular evaluation and management of patients undergoing noncardiac surgery. J Am Coll Cardiol. 2014;64(22).

37. Plantinga LC, Crews DC, Coresh J, Miller ER, Saran R, Yee J, Hedgeman E, Pavkov M, Eberhardt MS, Williams DE, Powe NR. Prevalence of chronic kidney disease in US adults with undiagnosed diabetes or prediabetes. Clin J Am Soc Nephrol. 2010;5(4):673–82.

38. Goodenough CJ, Liang MK, Nguyen MT, Nguyen DH, Holihan JL, Alawadi ZM, Roth JS, Wray CJ, Ko TC, Kao LS. Preoperative glycosylated hemoglobin and postoperative glucose together predict major complications after abdominal surgery. J Am Coll Surg. 2015;221(4):854–61.e1.

39. Duggan EW, Klopman MA, Berry AJ, Umpierrez G. The Emory University Perioperative Algorithm for the Management of Hyperglycemia and Diabetes in Non-cardiac Surgery Patients. Curr Diab Rep. 2016;16(3):34.

40. Kwon S, Thompson RE, Dellinger P, Rogers T, Flum D. Importance of perioperative glycemic control in general surgery: a report from the surgical care and outcomes assessment program. J Surg Res. 2012;172(2):274.

41. Kao LS, Meeks D, Moyer VA, Lally KP. Perioperative glycaemic control regimens for preventing surgical site infections in adults. Cochrane Database Syst Rev. 2009;(3):CD006806.

42. Trescot A. Local anesthetic resistance. Pain Physician. 2003;6:291–3. Web.

43. Santarelli S, Amici G, Bernacooni T, Bonforte G, Ceraudo E, Zeiler M. Best practice: the peritoneal dialysis catheter. J Nephrol. 2013;26(21):S4–S75.

44. Piraino B, Bernardini J, Brown E, Figueiredo A, Johnson DW, Lye W-C, Price V, Ramalakshmi S, Szeto C-C. ISPD position statement on reducing the risks of peritoneal dialysis-related infections. Perit Dial Int. 2011;31(6):614–30.

45. Crabtree JH, Penner T, Armstrong SW, Burkart J. Peritoneal dialysis university for surgeons: a peritoneal access training program. Perit Dial Int. 2015;36:177–81.

46. Nongnuch A, Assanatham M, Panorchan K, Davenport A. Strategies for preserving residual renal function in peritoneal dialysis patients. Clin Kidney J. 2015;8(2):202–11.

47. Cadnapaphornchai MA, Teitelbaum I. Strategies for the preservation of residual renal function in pediatric dialysis patients. Pediatr Nephrol. 2014;29:825–36.

48. Boehm M, Vécsei A, Aufricht C, Mueller T, Csaicsich D, Arbeiter K. Risk factors for peritonitis in pediatric peritoneal dialysis: a single-center study. Pediatr Nephrol. 2005;20(10):1478–83.

49. Crabtree JH, Burchette RJ. Peritoneal dialysis catheter embedment: surgical considerations, expectations, and complications. Am J Surg. 2013;206:464–71.

50. Balda S, Power A, Papalois V, Brown E. Impact of hernias on peritoneal dialysis technique survival and residual renal function. Perit Dial Int. 2013;33(6):629–34.

51. Morris-Stiff G, Coles G, Moore R, Jurewicz A, Lord R. Abdominal wall hernia in autosomal dominant polycystic kidney disease. Br J Surg. 1997;84(5):615–7.

52. Garcia-Urena MA, Rodriguez CR, Vega Ruiz V, Carnero Hernandez FJ, Fernandez-Ruiz E, Vazquez Gallego JM, Velasco Garcia M. Prevalence and management of hernias in peritoneal dialysis patients. Perit Dial Int. 2006;26:198–202.

53. Mahale AS, Katyal A, Khanna R. Complications of per ito-neal dialysis related to increased intra-abdominal pressure. Adv Perit Dial. 2003;19:130–5.

54. Gotloib L. Hemodynamic effects of increasing intra-abdominal pressure in peritoneal dialysis. Peritoneal Dial Bull. 1981;1:41–3.

55. Haggerty S, Roth S, Walsh D, Stefanidis D, Price R, Fanelli RD, Penner T, Richardson W. Guidelines for laparoscopic peritoneal dialysis access surgery. Surg Endosc. 2014;28(11):3016–45.

56. Ayach T, Nappo RW, Paugh-Miller JL, Ross EA. Postoperative hyperkalemia. Eur J Intern Med. 2015;26(2):106–11.

57. Pinson CW, Schuman ES, Gross GF, Schuman TA, Hayes JF. Surgery in long-term dialysis patients. Am J Surg. 1986;151(5):567–71.

58. Weil BR, Andreoli SP, Billmire DF. Bleeding risk for surgical dialysis procedures in children with hemolytic uremic syndrome. Pediatr Nephrol. 2010;25(9):1693–8. Print

59. Cabiddu G, Castellino S, Gernone G, Santoro D, Giacchino F, Credendino O, Daidone G, Gregorini G, Moroni G, Attini R, Minelli F, Manisco G, Todros T, Piccoli GB. Best practices on pregnancy on dialysis: The Italian Study Group on Kidney and Pregnancy. J Nephrol. 2015;28(3):279–88.

60. Jesudason S, Grace BS, Mcdonald SP. Pregnancy outcomes according to dialysis commencing before or after conception in women with ESRD. Clin J Am Soc Nephrol. 2013;9(1):143–9.

61. Vazquez-Rodriguez JG. Dialisis peritoneal Y embarazo. Cir Cir. 2010;78(2):181–7. Web; Vijt D, Castro MJ, Endall G, Lindley E, Elseviers M. Post insertion catheter care in peritoneal dialysis (Pd) centres across Europe. Part 2: complication rates and individual patient outcomes. EDTNA-ERCA J. 2004;30(2):91–6.

62. Lutz J, Menke J, Sollinger D, Schinzel H, Thurmel K. Haemostasis in chronic kidney disease. Nephrol Dial Transplant. 2014;29(1):29–40.

63. Pavord S, Myers B. Bleeding and thrombotic complications of kidney disease. Blood Rev. 2011;25(6):271–8.

64. Parikh AM, Spencer FA, Lessard D, Emery C, Baylin A, Linkletter C, Goldberg RJ. Venous thromboembolism in patients with reduced estimated GFR: a population-based perspective. Am J Kidney Dis. 2011;58(5):746–55. Web

65. Mital S, Fried LF, Piraino B. Bleeding complications associated with peritoneal dialysis catheter insertion. Perit Dial Int. 2004;24(5):478–80.

66. Lind SE. The bleeding time does not predict surgical bleeding. Blood. 1991;77:2547–52.

67. Yang S-F, Liu C-J, Yang W-C, Chang C-F, Yang C-Y, Li S-Y, Lin C-C. The risk factors and the impact of hernia development on technique survival in peritoneal dialysis patients: a population-based cohort study. Perit Dial Int. 2014;35(3):351–9.

68. Kopecky RT, Frymoyer PA, Witanowski LS, Thomas FD, Wojtaszek J, Reinitz ER. Prospective peritoneal scintigraphy in patients beginning continuous ambulatory peritoneal dialysis. Am J Kidney Dis. 1990;15(3):228–36.

69. Imam TH, Tucker JD, Taur AS, Yamanishi FJ, Aka PK. Preoperative peritoneal scintigraphy. Perit Dial Int. 2012;32(3):357–60.

70. Miller J, Cho J, Michael MJ, Saouaf R, Towfigh S. Role of imaging in the diagnosis of occult hernias. JAMA Surg. 2014;149(10):1077.

71. Rydahl C, Thomsen HS, Marckmann P. High prevalence of nephrogenic systemic fibrosis in chronic renal failure patients exposed to gadodiamide, a gadolinium-containing magnetic resonance contrast agent. Investig Radiol. 2008;43(2):141–4.

72. ASA House of Delegates. American society of anesthesiologists – ASA physical status classification system. American Society of Anesthesiologists – ASA Physical Status Classification System. American Society of Anesthesiologists, 15 Oct 2014. Web. 23 May 2016.

73. Tiret L, Hatton F, Desmonts JM, Vourc'h G. Prediction of outcome of anaesthesia in patients over 40 years: a multifactorial risk index. Statist Med. 1988;7(9):947–54.

74. Goldstein A, Keats AS. The risk of anesthesia. Anesthesiology. 1970;33:130–43.

75. Keshvari A, Najafi I, Jafari-Javid M, Yunesian M, Chaman R, Taromlou MN. Laparoscopic peritoneal dialysis catheter implantation using a Tenckhoff trocar under local anesthesia with nitrous oxide gas insufflation. Am J Surg. 2009;197:8–13.

76. Henshaw DS, Baker ML, Weller RS, Reynolds JW, Jaffe JD. Transversus abdominis plane block as the primary anesthetic for peritoneal dialysis catheter surgery. J Clin Anesth. 2016;31:182–8.

77. Wu R, Okrainec A, Penner T. Laparoscopic peritoneal dialysis catheter insertion using nitrous oxide under procedural sedation. World J Surg. 2014;39(1):128–32.

78. Mutter TC, Chateau D, Moffatt M, Ramsey C, Roos LL, Kryger M. A matched cohort study of postoperative outcomes in obstructive sleep apnea. Anesthesiology. 2014;121:707–18.

79. Dutta S, Cohn SL, Pfeifer KJ, Slawski BA, Smetana GW, Jaffer AK. Updates in perioperative medicine. J Hosp Med. 2015;11(3):231–6.

80. Mazo V, Sabaté S, Canet J, Gallart L, de Abreu MG, Belda J, Langeron O, Hoeft A, Pelosi P. Prospective external validation of a predictive score for postoperative pulmonary complications. Anesthesiology. 2014;121(2):219–31.

81. Yamashita S, Yamaguchi H, Sakaguchi M, Yamamoto S, Aoki K, Shiga Y, Yu H. Effect of smoking on intraoperative sputum and postoperative pulmonary complication in minor surgical patients. Respir Med. 2004;98(8):760–6.

82. Smetana GW. Preoperative pulmonary risk stratification for noncardiothoracic surgery: systematic review for the American College of Physicians. Ann Intern Med. 2006;144(8):581.

83. Parfrey PS, Foley RN. The clinical epidemiology of cardiac disease in chronic renal failure. J Am Soc Nephrol. 1999;10:1606–15.

84. Grasso AW, Wael Jaber A. Cardiac risk stratification for noncardiac surgery. Cardiac Risk Stratification for Noncardiac Surgery. Cleveland Clinic; 2014. Web. 12 Aug 2016.

85. Ford MK. Systematic review: prediction of perioperative cardiac complications and mortality by the revised cardiac risk index. Ann Intern Med. 2010;152(1):26.

86. American College of Surgeons, and American Pediatric Surgical Association. American College of Surgeons National Surgical Quality Improvement Program Pediatric. ACS NSQIP Pediatr. ACS APSA. http://riskcalculator.facs.org/peds/

87. Vaux EC, Torrie PH, Barker LC, Naik RB, Gibson MR. Percutaneous fluoroscopically guided placement of peritoneal dialysis catheters-a 10-year experience. Semin Dial. 2008;21(5):459–65.

88. Medani S, Shantier M, Hussein W, Wall C, Mellotte G. A comparative analysis of percutaneous and open surgical techniques for peritoneal catheter placement. Perit Dial Int. 2012;32(6):628–35.

89. Moon JY. Fluoroscopically guided peritoneal dialysis catheter placement: long-term results from a single center. Perit Dial Int. 2008;28(2):163–9.

90. Ozener C. Technical survival of CAPD catheters: comparison between percutaneous and conventional surgical placement techniques. Nephrol Dial Transplant. 2001;16(9):1893–9.

91. Perakis KE, Stylianou KG, Kyriazis JP, Mavroeidi VN, Katsipi IG, Vardaki EA, Petrakis IG, Stratigis S, Kroustalakis NG, Alegakis AK, Daphnis EK. Long-term complication rates and survival of peritoneal dialysis catheters: the role of percutaneous versus surgical placement. Semin Dial. 2009;22(5):569–75.

92. Reddy C, Dybbro PE, Guest S. Fluoroscopically guided percutaneous peritoneal dialysis catheter placement: single center experience and review of the literature. Ren Fail. 2010;32(3):294–9.

93. Voss D, Hawkins S, Poole G, Marshall M. Radiological versus surgical implantation of first catheter for peritoneal dialysis: a randomized non-inferiority trial. Nephrol Dial Transplant. 2012;27(11):4196–204.

94. Jacobs IG, Gray RR, Elliott DS, Grosman H. Radiologic placement of peritoneal dialysis catheters: preliminary experience. Radiology. 1992;182(1):251–5.

95. Zaman F, Pervez A, Atray NK, Murphy S, Work J, Abreo KD. Fluoroscopy-assisted placement of peritoneal dialysis catheters by nephrologists. Semin Dial. 2005;18(3):247–51.

96. Maya ID. Ultrasound/fluoroscopy-assisted placement of peritoneal dialysis catheters. Semin Dial. 2007;20(6):611–5.

97. Quach T, Tregaskis P, Menahem S, Koukounaras J, Mott N, Walker RG. Radiological insertion of Tenckhoff catheters for peritoneal dialysis: a 1-year single-centre experience. Clin Kidney J. 2013;7(1): 23–6.

98. Chula DC, Campos RP, de Alcântara MT, Riella MC, do Nascimento MM. Percutaneous and surgical insertion of peritoneal catheter in patients starting in chronic dialysis therapy: a comparative study. Semin Dial. 2013;27(3):E32–7.

99. Verrina E, Edefonti A, Gianoglio B, Rinaldi S, Sorino P, Zacchello G, Lavoratti G, Maringhini S, Pecoraro C, Calevo MG, Turrini Dertenois L, Perfumo F. A multicenter experience on patient and technique survival in children on chronic dialysis. Pediatr Nephrol. 2004;19(1):82–90.

100. Li CL, Cui TG, Gan HR. A randomized trial comparing conventional swan-neck straight-tip catheters to straight-tip catheters with an artificial subcutaneous swan neck. Perit Dial Int. 2009;29:278–84.

101. Robison RJ. Surgical considerations of continuous ambulatory peritoneal dialysis. Surgery. 1984;96: 723–30.

102. Yeh T. Catheter-related complications of continuous ambulatory peritoneal dialysis. Eur J Surg. 1992;158:277–9.

103. Kim JE, Park SJ, Oh JY, Kim JH, Lee JS, Kim PK, Shin JI. Noninfectious complications of peritoneal dialysis in Korean children: a 26-year single-center study. Yonsei Med J. 2015;56(5):1359.

104. Gadallah MF, Pervez A, El-Shahawy MA, Sorrells D, Zibari G, Mcdonald J, Work J. Peritoneoscopic versus surgical placement of peritoneal dialysis catheters: a prospective randomized study on outcome. Am J Kidney Dis. 1999;33(1):118–22.

105. Radtke J, Lemke A, Kemper MJ, Nashan B, Koch M. Surgical complications after peritoneal dialysis catheter implantation depend on children's weight. J Pediatr Surg. 2016;51(8):1317–20.

106. Asif A, Tawakol J, Khan T, Vieira CF, Byers P, Gadalean F, Hogan R, Merrill D, Roth D. American Society of Diagnostic and Interventional Nephrology: modification of the peritoneoscopic technique of peritoneal dialysis catheter insertion: experience of an interventional nephrology program. Semin Dial. 2004;17(2):171–3.

107. Crabtree JH, Burchette R. Effect of prior abdominal surgery, peritonitis, and adhesions on catheter function and long-term outcome on peritoneal dialysis. Am Surg. 2009;75(2):140–8.

108. Kalman RS, Pedrosa MC. Evidence-based review of gastrointestinal bleeding in the chronic kidney disease patient. Semin Dial. 2014;28(1):68–74.

109. Livio M, Mannucci PM, Viganò G, Mingardi G, Lombardi R, Mecca G, Remuzzi G. Conjugated estrogens for the management of bleeding associated with renal failure. N Engl J Med. 1986;315(12): 731–5.

110. Hedges SJ, Dehoney SB, Hooper JS, Amanzadeh J, Busti AJ. Evidence-based treatment recommendations for uremic bleeding. Nat Clin Pract Nephrol. 2007;3(3):138–53.

111. Lees JS, Mark PB, Jardine AG. Cardiovascular complications of chronic kidney disease. Medicine. 2015;43(8):469–73.

112. de Jager DJ. Cardiovascular and noncardiovascular mortality among patients starting dialysis. JAMA. 2009;302(16):1782.

113. Masson P, Webster AC, Hong M, Turner R, RichardI L, Craig JC. Chronic kidney disease and the risk of stroke: a systematic review and meta-analysis. Nephrol Dial Transplant. 2015;30(7):1162–9.

114. Spyropoulos AC, Douketis JD. How I treat anticoagulated patients undergoing an elective procedure or surgery. Blood. 2012;120(15):2954–62.

115. Collette C, Clerc-Urmès I, Laborde-Castérot H, Frimat L, Ayav C, Peters N, Martin A, Agrinier N, Thilly N. Antiplatelet and oral anticoagulant therapies in chronic hemodialysis patients: prescribing practices and bleeding risk. Pharmacoepidemiol Drug Saf. 2016;25:935–43.

116. Schwartzenberg S, Eli LI, Sagie A, Korzets A, Kornowski R. The quandary of oral anticoagulation in patients with atrial fibrillation and chronic kidney disease. Am J Cardiol. 2016;117(3):477–82.

117. Devereaux P, Mrkobrada M, Sessler DI, et al. Aspirin in patients undergoing noncardiac surgery. N Engl J Med. 2014;370:1494–503.

118. Shpitz B, Plotkin E, Spindel Z, Buklan G, Klein E, Bernheim J, Korzets Z. Should aspirin therapy be with held before insertion and/or removal of a permanent peritoneal dialysis catheter? Am Surg. 2002;68(9):762–4.

119. Yang X, Wang Z, Zhang Y, Yin X, Hou Y. The safety and efficacy of antithrombotic therapy in patients undergoing cardiac rhythm device implantation: a meta-analysis. Europace. 2015;17(7):1076–84.

120. 2014 ESC/ESA guidelines on non-cardiac surgery: cardiovascular assessment and management. Eur Heart J. 2014;35(35):2383–431.

121. Douketis JD, Spyropoulos AC, Spencer FA, Mayr M, Jaffer AK, Eckman MH, Dunn AS, Kunz R. Perioperative management of antithrombotic therapy. Chest. 2012;141(2 Suppl):e326S–50S.

122. Samama C-M. Gestion péri-opératoire des antiplaquettaires. Arch Cardiovasc Dis Suppl. 2012;4: 236–9.

123. Jeong KH, Cho JH, Woo JS, Kim JB, Kim W-S, Lee TW, Kim KS, Ihm CG, Kim W. Platelet reactivity after receiving clopidogrel compared with ticagrelor in patients with kidney failure treated with hemodialysis: a randomized crossover study. Am J Kidney Dis. 2015;65:916–24.

124. Bouatou Y, Samer C, Fontana P, Daali Y, Desmeules J. Evidence-based choice of P2Y12 inhibitors in end stage renal disease patients: a mini-review. CDM Curr Drug Metab. 2015;16:97–104.

125. Strosberg DS, Corbey T, Henry JC, Starr JE. Preoperative antiplatelet use does not increase incidence of bleeding after major operations. Surgery. 2016;160:968–76.

126. Chu EW, Chernoguz A, Divino CM. The evaluation of clopidogrel use in perioperative general surgery patients: a prospective randomized controlled trial. Am J Surg. 2016;211:1019–25.

127. Blake P. Drain pain, overfill, and how they are connected. Perit Dial Int. 2014;34(4):342–4.

128. Crabtree JH. Peritoneal dialysis catheter implantation: avoiding problems and optimizing outcomes. Semin Dial. 2014;28(1):12–5.

129. Crabtree JH. Development of surgical guidelines for laparoscopic peritoneal dialysis access: down a long and winding road. Perit Dial Int. 2015;35(3): 241–4.

130. Twardowski ZJ, Nolph K, Khanna R. The need for a "swan neck" permanently bent, arcuate peritoneal dialysis catheter. Perit Dial Int. 1985;5: 219–23.

131. Juergensen PH, Rizvi H, Vicente CJ, Alan KS, Fredric FO. Value of scintigraphy in chronic peritoneal dialysis patients. Kidney Int. 1999;55(3): 1111–9.

132. Xie J, Kiryluk K, Ren H, Zhu P, Huang X, Shen P, Xu T, Chen X, Chen N. Coiled versus straight peritoneal dialysis catheters: a randomized controlled trial and meta-analysis. Am J Kidney Dis. 2011;58: 946–55.

133. Rubin J, Didlake R, Raju S, Hsu H. A prospective randomized evaluation of chronic peritoneal catheters. Insertion site and intraperitoneal segment. ASAIO Trans. 1990;36(3):M497–500.

134. Stegmayr BG, Wikdahl AM, Bergstrom M. A randomized clinical trial comparing the function of straight and coiled Tenckhoff catheters for peritoneal dialysis. Perit Dial Int. 2005;25:85–8.

135. Crabtree JH, Fishman A. A laparoscopic method for optimal peritoneal dialysis access. Am Surg. 2005;71:135–43.

136. Crabtree JH. Construction and use of stencils in planning for peritoneal dialysis catheter implantation. Perit Dial Int. 2003;23:395–402.

137. Imvrios G, Tsakiris D, Gakis D, Takoudas D, Koukoudis P. Prosthetic mesh repair of multiple recurrent and large abdominal hernias in continuous ambulatory peritoneal dialysis patients. Perit Dial Int. 1994;14:338–43.

138. Zaritsky J, Warady BA. Peritoneal dialysis in infants and young children. Semin Nephrol. 2011;31: 213–24.

139. Dolan NM, Borzych-Duzalka D, Suarez A, Principi I, Hernandez O, Al-Akash S, Alconchar L, Breen C, Fischbach M, Flynn J, Pape L, Piantanida JJ, Printza N, Wong W, Zaritsky J, Schaefer F, Warady BA, White CT. Ventriculoperitoneal shunts in children on peritoneal dialysis: a survey of the international pediatric peritoneal dialysis network. Pediatr Nephrol. 2012;28(2):315–9.

140. Crabtree JH, Burchette RJ, Siddiqi NA. Optimal peritoneal dialysis catheter type and exit site location: an anthropometric analysis. ASAIO J. 2005; 51(6):743–7.

141. Mooney JF, Hillis GS, Lee VW, Halliwell R, Vicaretti M, Moncrieff C, Chow CK. Cardiac assessment prior to non-cardiac surgery. Intern Med J. 2016;46(8):932–41.

142. Hansson JH, Watnick S. Update on peritoneal dialysis: core curriculum 2016. Am J Kidney Dis. 2016;67(1):151–64.

143. Warchol S, Roszkowska-Blaim M, Latoszynska J, Jarmolinski T, Zachwieja J. Experience using presternal catheter for peritoneal dialysis in Poland: a multicenter pediatric survey. Perit Dial Int. n.d.;23:242–8.

144. Stringel G, Mcbride W, Weiss R. Laparoscopic placement of peritoneal dialysis catheters in children. J Pediatr Surg. 2008;43(5):857–60.

145. Flanigan M, Gokal R. Peritoneal catheters and exit-site practices toward optimum peritoneal access: a review of current developments. Perit Dial Int. 2005;25:132–9.

146. Banshodani M, Kawanishi H, Moriishi M, Shintaku S, Ago R, Hashimoto S, Nishihara M, Tsuchiya S. Umbilical hernia in peritoneal dialysis patients:

surgical treatment and risk factors. Ther Apher Dial. 2015;19(6):606–10.

147. Lefebvre A, Saliou P, Lucet JC, Mimoz O, Keita-Perse O, Grandbastien B, Bruyère F, Boisrenoult P, Lepelletier D, Aho-Glélé LS. Preoperative hair removal and surgical site infections: network meta-analysis of randomized controlled trials. J Hosp Infect. 2015;91(2):100–8.

148. Hetem DJ, Bootsma MC, Bonten MJ. Prevention of surgical site infections: decontamination with mupirocin based on preoperative screening for *Staphylococcus aureus* carriers or universal decontamination? Clin Infect Dis. 2015;62(5):631–6.

149. Lye WC, Leung SO, Van Der Straaten J, Lee EJ. Staphyloccus aureus CAPD-related infections are associated with nasal carriage. Adv Perit Dial. 1994;10:163–5.

150. Aktas E, Pazarli O, Külah C, Cömert F, Külah E, Sümbüloğlu V. Determination of *Staphylococcus aureus* carriage in hemodialysis and peritoneal dialysis patients and evaluation of the clonal relationship between carriage and clinical isolates. Am J Infect Control. 2011;39(5):421–5.

151. Sewell CM. Staphylococcal nasal carriage and subsequent infection in peritoneal dialysis patients. J Am Med Assoc. 1982;248(12):1493.

152. Sesso R. *Staphylococcus aureus* skin carriage and development of peritonitis in patients on continuous ambulatory peritoneal dialysis. Clin Nephrol. 1989;31(5):264–8.

153. Luzar MA, Coles GA, Faller B, Slingeneyer A, Dah GD, Briat C, Wone C, Knefati Y, Kessler M, Peluso F. *Staphylococcus aureus* nasal carriage and infection in patients on continuous ambulatory peritoneal dialysis. N Engl J Med. 1990;322(8):505–9.

154. Bode LGM, Kluytmans AJW, Wertheim HFL, Bogaers D, Vandenbroucke-Grauls CMJE, Roosendaal R, Troelstra A, Box ATA, Voss A, Van Der Tweel I, Belkum Van A, Verbrugh HA, Vos MC. Preventing surgical-site infections in nasal carriers of *Staphylococcus aureus*. N Engl J Med. 2010;362(1):9–17.

155. Schweizer ML, Chiang H-Y, Septimus E, Moody J, Braun B, Hafner J, Ward MA, Hickok J, Perencevich EN, Diekema DJ, Richards CL, Cavanaugh JE, Perlin JB, Herwaldt LA. Association of a bundled intervention with surgical site infections among patients undergoing cardiac, hip, or knee surgery. JAMA. 2015;313(21):2162.

156. Strippoli GFM. Catheter-related interventions to prevent peritonitis in peritoneal dialysis: a systematic review of randomized, controlled trials. J Am Soc Nephrol. 2004;15(10):2735–46.

157. Blowey DL, Warady BA, KS MF. The treatment of *Staphylococcus aureus* nasal carriage in pediatric peritoneal dialysis patients. Adv Perit Dial. 1994;10:297–9.

158. Crabtree JH, Hadnott LL, Burchette RJ, Siddiqi RA. Outcome and clinical implications of a surveil-lance and treatment program for *Staphylococcus aureus* nasal carriage in peritoneal dialysis patients. Adv Peritoneal Dial. 2000;16:271–5.

159. Webster J, Osborne S. Preoperative bathing or showering with skin antiseptics to prevent surgical site infection. Cochrane Database Syst Rev. 2015;20(2):CD004985.

160. Chlebicki MP, Safdar N, O'Horo JC, Maki DG. Preoperative chlorhexidine shower or bath for prevention of surgical site infection: a meta-analysis. Am J Infect Control. 2013;41:167–73.

161. Hall G. New directions in peritoneal dialysis patient training. Nephrol Nurs J. 2004;31:149.

162. Holloway M, Mujais S, Kandert M, Warady B. Pediatric peritoneal dialysis training: characteristics and impact on peritonitis rates. Perit Dial Int. 2001;21:401–4.

163. Bordin G, Casati M, Sicolo N, Zuccherato N, Eduati V. Patient education in peritoneal dialysis: an observational study in Italy. J Ren Care. 2007;33(4):165–71.

164. Bernadini J, Price J, Figueiredo A. Peritoneal dialysis training 2006. Perit Dial Int. 2006;26:625–32.

165. Crabtree JH, Fishman A. Laparoscopic epiplopexy of the greater omentum and epiploic appendices in the salvaging of dysfunctional peritoneal dialysis catheters. Surg Laparosc Endosc Percutan Tech. 1996;6(3):176–80.

166. Figueiredo AE, Goh BL, Johnson D, Mactier R, Ramalakshmmi S, Struijk DG. RA guidelines peritoneal access. Renal association – peritoneal access. 2009. http://www.renal.org/pages/pages/guidelines/current/peritoneal-ac. p. 1–10. Www.renal.org. The Renal Association, 2009. Web. 28 July 2016.

167. Kansal S, Rothers D. Modality consult following nursing led dialysis education improves peritoneal dialysis utilization. Am J Kidney Dis. 2015; 65:A46.

168. Kanute V, Patrick S. Improving outcomes in surgical placement of peritoneal dialysis catheters by educating nurses. Nephrol Nurs J. 2014;41(2):203.

169. Shetty A, Oreopoulos DG. Peritoneal dialysis: its indications and contraindications. Dialy Transplant. 2000;29:71–7.

170. Aksu N, Yavascan O, Anil M, Kara OD, Bal A, Anil AB. Chronic peritoneal dialysis in children with special needs or social disadvantage or both: contraindications are not always contraindications. Perit Dial Int. 2011;32:424–30.

171. Penner T, Crabtree JH. Peritoneal dialysis catheters with back exit sites. Perit Dial Int. 2013;33:93–6.

172. Berger JR, Jaikaransingh V, Hedayati Susan S. End-stage kidney disease in the elderly: approach to dialysis initiation, choosing modality, and predicting outcomes. Adv Chronic Kidney Dis. 2016;23(1):36–43.

173. Griva K, Yu Z, Chan S, Krisnasamy T, Yamin RBA, Zakaria FB, Wu SY, Oei E, Foo M. Age is not a contraindication to home-based dialysis – quality-of-life outcomes favour older patients on peritoneal dialysis

regimes relative to younger patients. J Adv Nurs. 2014;70(8):1902–14.

174. Paudel K, Namagondlu G, Samad N, Mckitty K, Fan SL. Lack of motivation: a new modifiable risk factor for peritonitis in patients undergoing peritoneal dialysis? J Ren Care. 2014;41:33–42.

175. Jones DR. Preoperative evaluation and perioperative management of the patient with renal failure. First Consult. Clinical Key Elsevier, 27 Jan 2014. Web.

176. Jalal D, Chonchol M, Targher G. Disorders of hemostasis associated with chronic kidney disease. Semin Thromb Hemost. 2010;36(01):034–40.

177. January CT, Wann LS, Alpert JS, Calkins H, Cigarroa JE, Cleveland JC, Conti JB, Ellinor PT, Ezekowitz MD, Field ME, Murray KT, Sacco RL, Stevenson WG, Tchou PJ, Tracy CM, Yancy CW. 2014 AHA/ACC/HRS guideline for the management of patients with atrial fibrillation: a report of the American College of Cardiology/American Heart Association Task Force on Practice Guidelines and the Heart Rhythm Society. Circulation. 2014;130(23):2071–104.

178. Chang M, Yu Z, Shenker A, Wang J, Pursley J, Byon W, Boyd RA, Lacreta F, Frost CE. Effect of renal impairment on the pharmacokinetics, pharmacodynamics, and safety of apixaban. J Clin Pharmacol. 2015;56:637–45.

179. Douketis JD, Spyropoulos AC, Kaatz S, et al. Perioperative bridging anticoagulation in patients with atrial fibrillation. N Engl J Med. 2015;373:823–33.

180. Garcia D, Alexander JH, Wallentin L, et al. Management and clinical outcomes in patients treated with apixaban vs warfarin undergoing procedures. Blood. 2014;124:3692–8.

181. Williams LA, Hunter JM, Marques MB, Vetter TR. Periprocedural management of patients on anticoagulants. Clin Lab Med. 2014;34:595–611.

182. Liew A, Douketis J. Perioperative management of patients who are receiving a novel oral anticoagulant. Intern Emerg Med. 2013;8:477–84.

183. Pernod G, Albaladejo P, Godier A, et al. Management of major bleeding complications and emergency surgery in patients on long-term treatment with direct oral anticoagulants, thrombin or factor-Xa inhibitors: proposals of the Working Group on Perioperative Haemostasis (GIHP) – March 2013. Arch Cardiovasc Dis. 2013;106:382–93.

184. Steinberg BA, Peterson ED, Kim S, Thomas L, Gersh BJ, Fonarow GC, Kowey PR, Mahaffey KW, Sherwood MW, Chang P, Piccini JP, Ansell J. Use and outcomes associated with bridging during anticoagulation interruptions in patients with atrial fibrillation: findings from the outcomes registry for better informed treatment of atrial fibrillation (ORBIT-AF). Circulation. 2015;131(5):488–94.

185. Chan KE, Giugliano RP, Patel MR, Abramson S, Jardine M, Zhao S, Perkovic V, Maddux FW, Piccini JP. Nonvitamin K anticoagulant agents in patients with advanced chronic kidney disease or on dialysis with AF. J Am Coll Cardiol. 2016;67:2888–99.

186. Kubitza D, Becka M, Mueck W, Halabi A, Maatouk H, Klause N, Lufft V, Dominic WD, Philipp T, Bruck H. Effects of renal impairment on the pharmacokinetics, pharmacodynamics and safety of rivaroxaban, an oral, direct factor Xa inhibitor. Br J Clin Pharmacol. 2010;70(5):703–12.

187. Connors JM. Antidote for factor Xa anticoagulants. N Engl J Med. 2015;373:2471–2.

188. American College of Surgeons. ACS NSQIP surgical risk calculator. ACS NSQIP Surgical Risk Calculator. American College of Surgeons National Surgical Quality Improvement Program, 2016. Web 12 July 2016.

189. Bilimoria KY, Liu Y, Paruch JL, Zhou L, Kmiecik TE, Ko CY, Cohen ME. Development and evaluation of the universal ACS NSQIP surgical risk calculator: a decision aid and informed consent tool for patients and surgeons. J Am Coll Surg. 2013;217(5):833–42. e1–3.

190. Birnie DH, Healey JS, Wells GA, Verma A, Anthony TS, Krahn AD, Simpson CS, Ayala-Paredes F, Coutu B, Leiria TLL, Essebag V. Pacemaker or defibrillator surgery without interruption of anticoagulation. N Engl J Med. 2013;368(22):2084–93.

191. Duggan EW, Klopman MA, Berry AJ, Umpierrez G. The Emory University perioperative algorithm for the management of hyperglycemia and diabetes in non-cardiac surgery patients. Curr Diab Rep. 2016;16(3):34.

Overview of Catheter Choices and Implantation Techniques

5

Pierpaolo Di Cocco, Edwina A. Brown, Vassilios E. Papalois, and Frank J.M.F. Dor

Decision-Making Algorithm for Peritoneal Dialysis (Patient-Centered)

The selection of dialysis modality is of great importance in planning a successful transition to renal replacement therapy in patients approaching end stage renal disease (ESRD). It is increasingly recognised that individuals, institutions, governments, and specialty societies may direct and subliminally influence the patient's selection/ choice of dialysis modality. The most visible and widespread effort in this regard is the CMS (Center for Medicare and Medicaid Services) FISTULA FIRST National Vascular Access Improvement Initiative [1, 2]. Similarly, the International Society for Peritoneal Dialysis is stressing the underutilization of the peritoneal dialysis modality, especially in the Western societies [3].

Rather than emphasizing the doctrine of one modality fitting all, it is ethically and morally a better model to consider a patient driven

P. Di Cocco, MD • E.A. Brown, MD
V.E. Papalois, MD • F.J.M.F. Dor, MD (✉)
West London Renal and Transplant Centre,
Imperial College Healthcare NHS Trust,
Hammersmith Hospital, 4th Floor Hammersmith
House, Du Cane Road, London W12 0HS, UK
e-mail: Pierpaolo.DiCocco@imperial.nhs.uk;
Edwina.Brown@imperial.nhs.uk;
Vassilios.Papalois@imperial.nhs.uk;
Frank.dor@imperial.nhs.uk

approach, keeping in mind quality of life, outcomes and costs. Consequently, the decision-making algorithm for two similar patients may vary, based on individual circumstances.

This chapter describes the types of peritoneal dialysis catheters and implantation techniques applied for peritoneal dialysis, technical considerations, and some of the related surgical complications.

Anatomy

A basic knowledge of the anatomy of the anterior abdominal wall and peritoneal cavity is necessary for a better understanding of the various techniques of catheter placement. The skin of the anterior abdominal wall is of moderate thickness and is relatively fixed on the underlying fascia and muscle layers (Fig. 5.1). The innervation of skin, fascia, muscles and parietal peritoneum of the anterior abdominal wall is segmental, mainly from the anterior primary rami of spinal nerves T6 to L1.

The main muscles of the abdominal wall are the rectus abdominis and pyramidalis muscles, which are anterior; the external and internal oblique muscles and the transversus abdominis muscle, which are lateral (Fig. 5.2). The fibers of the rectus run vertically; those of the external oblique muscle run inferior and anterior; those of the internal oblique muscle run superior and anterior, and those of the

© Springer International Publishing AG 2017
S. Haggerty (ed.), *Surgical Aspects of Peritoneal Dialysis*, DOI 10.1007/978-3-319-52821-2_5

Fig. 5.1 Section of the abdominal wall – coronal plane

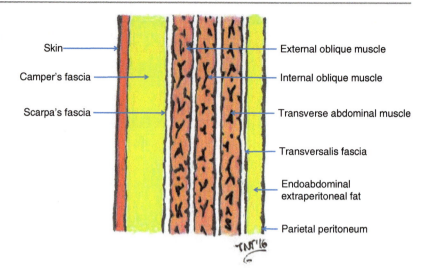

Skin
Camper's fascia
Scarpa's fascia

External oblique muscle
Internal oblique muscle
Transverse abdominal muscle
Transversalis fascia
Endoabdominal extraperitoneal fat
Parietal peritoneum

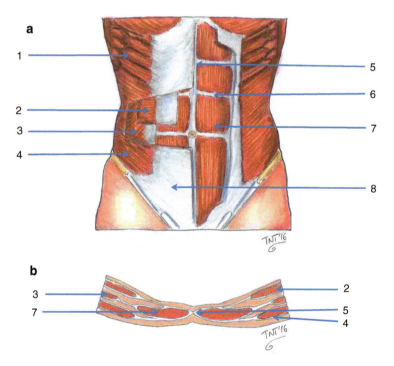

Fig. 5.2 Frontal (**a**) and transverse (**b**) planes of the abdominal wall muscles – *1* Serratus anterior; *2* Transversus abdominis; *3* Internal oblique; *4* External oblique; *5* Linea alba; *6* Tendinous intersection; *7* Rectus abdominis; *8* Aponeurosis of the external oblique

transversus run transversely. The major vessels and nerves pass downward and medially in the neurovascular plane, between the transversus abdominis and the internal oblique muscles (Fig. 5.3). Supplying the rectus muscle and firmly adherent to its posterior surface are the epigastric vessels. These could be potentially damaged, particularly during a lateral approach for surgical catheter insertion either with open or laparoscopic approaches. The rectus sheath appears as an elliptical tube with a strong anterior wall. The weaker posterior wall only extends to just below the level of the umbilicus.

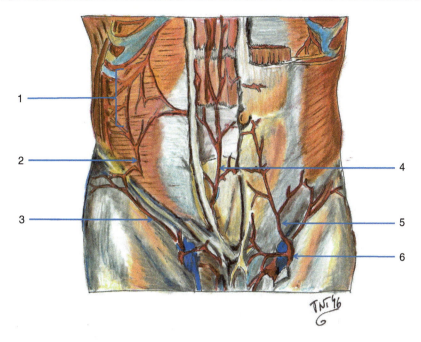

Fig. 5.3 Arterial anatomy of the abdominal wall – to be considered during PD catheter insertion – *1* Anastomoses with lower intercostal, subcostal and lumbar arteries; *2* Ascending branch of the deep circumflex artery; *3* Superficial circumflex iliac artery; *4* Inferior epigastric artery; *5* Superficial epigastric artery; *6* Femoral artery

Types of Peritoneal Catheters

(a) Acute peritoneal dialysis catheters

All catheters used for acute peritoneal dialysis are straight or slightly curved, relatively rigid tubing with numerous side holes at the distal end without any protective cuff. The implantation can be carried out with Seldinger percutaneous, open or laparoscopic insertion techniques. Acute peritoneal dialysis is still used in the management of acute and chronic renal failure in many developing countries [4, 5], where costs are a major limitation. In this setting, it is usually placed at the bedside under local anaesthesia, and catheters are used immediately after implantation. The absence of cuffs, a protection against bacterial migration, makes the incidence of peritonitis prohibitively high beyond 3 days of use; if extended dialysis is necessary the acute catheters are periodically replaced.

(b) Chronic peritoneal dialysis catheters

There are several types of catheters for chronic peritoneal dialysis; the basic structure is the same with an intraperitoneal portion, one or two cuffs, an inter-cuff segment and an external portion (Table 5.1). They are constructed from silicone rubber or polyurethane and are flexible, and atraumatic to the bowel. Catheters are available with barium impregnated either throughout or as a radiopaque stripe to assist in the radiologic localization of the intra-abdominal section. The silicone rubber or polyurethane surface promotes development of squamous epithelium in the subcutaneous tunnel around the catheter, at the exit site and within the abdominal wall. The presence of this epithelium increases resistance to bacterial penetration of the tissue near the skin exit and peritoneal entry sites. The Dacron cuffs provoke a local inflammatory response with fibrosis, which gives stability to the catheter and prevents bacterial migration from the skin surface into the subcutaneous tunnel and peritoneal cavity.

The intraperitoneal segment has multiple 0.5 mm perforations in the terminal part. Several modifications have been made to the intraperitoneal portion and to the tip of the catheters, with

Table 5.1 Characteristics of peritoneal dialysis catheters

Catheter type	Material	Cuffs	Shape of intra-abdominal segment	Inter-cuff shape	Characteristics
Tenkhoff catheters	Silicone	1–2	Straight/coiled	Straight/ Swan-Neck	
Toronto Western Hospital (TWH) or Oreopoulos-Zellerman catheter	Silicone	2	Straight	Straight	Dacron disc plus a silicone rubber bead (intraperitoneal segment)
Swan-Neck Missouri catheters	Silicone	1–2	Straight/ coiled[a]	Swan-Neck (bend 180° arc angle)	Bead and flange (intraperitoneal segment)
Pail-Handle (Cruz) catheter	Polyurethane	2	Coiled	Two bends (90° arc angle)	
Presternal Swan-Neck peritoneal catheter	Silicone	1–2	Straight/coiled	Arcuate inter-cuff shape	Titanium connector (between proximal and distal-end)
Moncrief-Papovich catheter	Silicone	2	Coiled	Arcuate inter-cuff shape	Larger external cuff (2.5 cm)
Ash (Advantage) catheter	Silicone	2	Straight		T-shaped

[a]Because in several patients infusion pain occurred due to a "jet effect" and/or tip pressure on the peritoneum, the intra-peritoneal segment of the catheters, was modified replacing a straight segment with a coiled one

the aim of obtaining an unrestricted flow of dialysate to and from the peritoneal cavity. This flow is most efficient if the catheter tip lies deep within the pelvis (also changes for dislocation/migration are less when placed deep in the pelvis). Catheter design and insertion techniques aim at the prevention of one- or two-way obstruction, tip displacement from the pelvis, common causes of catheter malfunction. Different catheter lengths are available for every patient size.

- Straight and coiled Tenkhoff catheters
- Toronto Western Hospital (TWH) or Oreopoulos-Zellerman catheter
- Straight and coiled Swan-Neck Missouri catheters
- Pail-Handle (Cruz) catheter
- Presternal Swan-Neck peritoneal catheter
- Moncrief-Papovich catheter
- Ash (Advantage) catheter
- Catheters designed for continuous flow peritoneal dialysis (CFPD)

Straight and Coiled Tenkhoff Catheters

The Tenckhoff catheter, first catheter with a widespread clinical use, is now available in different lengths, shapes and number of Dacron cuffs. It remains the most commonly used and the standard for comparison with other catheters. The catheter consists of a silicone rubber tube, bonded to one or two 1 cm cuffs. A barium-impregnated radiopaque strip assists in its radiological visualization. The intraperitoneal portion varies in length from 6.5 to 19.5 cm, with perforations (0.5 mm) in the terminal 2.5–9.5 cm [4, 6]. The intraperitoneal tip is in two shapes, coiled and straight [5].

Toronto Western Hospital (TWH) or Oreopoulos-Zellerman Catheter

The Toronto Western Hospital (TWH) or Oreopoulos-Zellerman catheter is a modified version of the Tenckhoff catheter [7]. The TWH1 and TWH2 are the two types available. Both catheter types have two flat silicone rubber discs attached to the catheter tip with the aim to be more stable in the pelvis. TWH2 has an additional modification consisting of a Dacron disc plus a silicone rubber bead in series with the pre-peritoneal cuff. The incorporation of a disc just superficial to the peritoneal closure is an attempt to prevent late dialysate increasing the area of peritoneal sealing. The catheter has two cuffs with a straight intra-abdominal and inter-cuff shape.

Straight and Coiled Swan-Neck Missouri Catheters

The Swan-Neck Missouri catheters are so called because of the permanent bend of the inter-cuff segment [8]. The inter-cuff shape, Swan-Neck, gives to the intraperitoneal and extraperitoneal segments an unforced downward direction. Several modifications have been described such as the number of cuffs (1 or 2), the distance between cuffs, the arc angle bend, increased from 80° to 180°, and the replacement of a straight intraperitoneal segment with a coiled one due to infusion pain ("jet effect" and/or tip pressure) on the peritoneum, occurred in several patients [9].

Pail-Handle (Cruz) Catheter

This catheter (polyurethane) has two right-angle bends of the inter-cuff segment: one to direct the intraperitoneal portion parallel to the parietal peritoneum and one to direct the subcutaneous portion towards the skin exit site. There are two cuffs and a coiled intra-abdominal segment. A single centre case series on 63 Pail-Handle catheters surgically implanted in 57 consecutive patients with a 5 year follow up, found a cumulative catheter survival rate of 80.8% at 12 months, 62.3% at 24 months and 48.1% at 51 months. An adverse outcome described in the study was related to the catheter adapter that caused large exit site wounds, predisposed to infection and catheter loss [10].

Presternal Swan-Neck Peritoneal Catheter

The swan neck pre-sternal catheter (silicon rubber) is composed of two flexible tubes joined by a titanium connector at the time of implantation. The exit site is located in the parasternal area. The catheter located on the chest was designed to reduce the incidence of exit site infections. The tube is bonded to two cuffs, and has a permanent bent (arc angle of 180°) of the inter-cuff segment (swan-neck). Both tubes have a radiopaque stripe that helps to achieve proper alignment of the tube during insertion and to facilitate radiological visualization of the intraperitoneal segment [11, 12].

Moncrief-Papovich Catheter

This catheter (silicone rubber) has several important structural changes compared to the Tenckhoff catheter. The structural changes are: a coiled internal segment, an arcuate bend in the subcutaneous segment similar to the swan-neck Missouri catheter and two Dacron cuffs. The external cuff is elongated from 1 to 2.5 cm. The catheter after implantation is locked with 1000 U of heparin, and the external segment is buried subcutaneously for a period of 4–8 weeks or longer to allow tissue ingrowth into the external cuff in a sterile environment. Subsequently, a small incision is made in the skin through which the external segment of the catheter is brought out [13, 14].

Ash (Advantage) Catheter

The Advantage catheter contains a straight portion that is held adjacent to the parietal peritoneum assuring a stable position, without extrusion of the deep cuff or exit site erosion. The intraperitoneal portion contains a short, perpendicular segment connected to two limbs with external grooves (flutes) to carry fluid into the catheter from the upper and lower abdomen. Due to the apposition of the grooved portion of this catheter against the parietal peritoneum, and the T shape of the catheter, the deep cuff of this catheter is fixed in position, and outward migration of the catheter is very unlikely. Based on the case series described by Ash, the placement of this type of catheter in 18 patients with 4 years of follow-up resulted in the absence of exit site erosion/infection, incisional hernia (peri-catheter) or leaks [15].

Catheters Designed for Continuous Flow Peritoneal Dialysis (CFPD)

Shinaberger and coll. [16], first described this technique in 1965, with the insertion of two peritoneal catheters at opposite sites of the peritoneal cavity. Other groups described this particular technique with mixed success [17–20]. A catheter for CFPD must provide separate conduits for infusing and draining the dialysate into and out of the peritoneal cavity at a high flow rate (100–250 mL/min) with good mixing of the peritoneal solution and minimal streaming and recirculation. The catheter should also be cosmetically acceptable (small diameter, minimal bulk), easy to implant and remove, biocompatible, reliable, and safe.

The simplest devices consist of two straight or curled barrels in a double-D or double-O configuration [21, 22]. The inflow barrel is shorter, and the drain barrel is longer and located in the most dependent pelvic area. Modifications to this basic design include the addition of discs placed in the distal intraperitoneal segment of the catheter to diffuse the inflow stream of dialysate and to improve mixing [23]. A recently introduced design describes a double-lumen catheter with maximum separation of the intraperitoneal limbs to minimize recirculation [24]. It consists of two tubes bonded together as they pass through the abdominal wall and into the peritoneum. The tubes once again separate intraperitoneally by 180° to form a double J, the cranial segment is shorter than the caudal, and both terminate with a fluted end.

Ash and coll. designed for this purpose a catheter with a T shaped configuration in order to maximally separates the tips of the double lumen [25].

Ronco and coll. designed a novel catheter for CFPD equipped with a thin walled silicone diffuser used to infuse the dialysate into the peritoneum. The holes on the round-tapered diffuser are positioned to allow dialysate to perpendicularly exit 360° from the diffuser, thereby reducing trauma to the peritoneal walls and allowing the dialysate to mix into the peritoneum. The fluid is then drained through the second lumen, whose tip is positioned in the lower pelvis [26].

Critical Comparison of Catheter Design

Despite all the different options, most programs limit their experience with one or two catheter types, making difficult a critical comparison. For simplicity and based on studies present in literature, the discussion on which catheter type offers better results focused mainly on the number of cuffs, single versus double, the configuration of the intraperitoneal portion, straight versus coiled, and of the inter-cuff shape, straight versus Swan-Neck. Lewis and coll. carried out a prospective randomized controlled study that favoured the double cuff over the single cuff Tenckhoff catheters, in terms of survival, time to the first peritonitis episode, and number of exit site infections [27]. Previous ISPD consensus opinion also supported the choice of double cuff Tenckhoff catheters [28]. However, Eklund and coll. in a prospective randomized controlled study found no differences in the number of peritonitis episodes, exit site infections, or in catheter survival between single and double cuff Tenckhoff catheters [29]. As mentioned earlier in the chapter, coiled catheters (intra-peritoneal segment) have been developed in order to achieve less infusion/pressure pain ("jet effect"), better flow, less catheter-related complications such as migration and omental wrapping. These theoretical advantages have been substantiated by some authors in randomised controlled trials [30–32], but not confirmed in two more recent meta-analyses [33, 34]. The meta-analysis conducted by Xie J and coll. suggested that coiled catheters might be more prone to migration and resultant dysfunction [33]. A more recent meta-analysis by Hagen and coll., including more studies and with the following outcomes of interest (catheter survival, drainage dysfunction, migration, leakage, exit-site infections, peritonitis, and catheter removal), found no differences when comparing straight versus swan neck and single versus double-cuffed catheters. Comparison of straight versus coiled-tip catheters demonstrated that survival was significantly different in favour of straight catheters (hazard ratio 2.05; confidence interval 1.10–3.79, $P = 0.02$). The conclusion of the authors was that for surgically inserted (open and laparoscopic) catheters, the removal rate and survival at 1 year were significantly in favour of straight catheters [34].

In our experience we primarily use double cuff Tenckhoff catheters, both straight and coiled (intraperitoneal portion) and with straight inter-cuff shape. **When critically comparing the different catheters we have to bear in mind that the most important aspect of preventing mechanical complications is probably attention to detail and the operative insertion technique used** [35].

Chronic Catheter Placement Procedures

Peritoneal dialysis catheters may be placed via a percutaneous, a laparoscopic, or an open surgical route. Open surgical and laparoscopic techniques are the most commonly performed worldwide. According to American data, the laparoscopic technique is now the most commonly used, compared to all other techniques [36].

(a) Percutaneous technique
(b) Peritoneoscopic technique
(c) Open surgical technique
(d) Laparoscopic technique

Seldinger Percutaneous Technique

First described in 1968 by Tenckhoff and Schechter, it is a percutaneous method of catheter placement. The authors reported a high incidence of catheter migration resulting in failure rates up to 65% at 2 years and risk of bowel or vessel injury [4]. Several other reports have shown adequate results, with dysfunction and leak rates below 7% [37–40] and a bowel perforation risk of 1–2% [38, 41]. Zappacosta et al. reserved the percutaneous catheter placement only in patients with no previous abdominal surgery, in view of the high risk of bowel perforation in presence of adhesions [37]. Aksu and coll. achieved excellent results in a pediatric population (108 peritoneal catheters percutaneously placed in 93 pediatric patients) with an overall incidence of catheter dysfunction of 14% over 10-year period and no cases of bowel perforation [42]. Varughese and coll. highlighted that the percutaneous insertion is now preferred in developing countries where costs play a major role [43]. Advantages and disadvantages of this technique are presented in the Table 5.2.

Technical Aspects

Percutaneous placement of peritoneal dialysis catheters, under local anaesthesia, uses a guidewire and a peel-away sheath applying the Seldinger technique.

Table 5.2 Pros and cons of percutaneous insertion

Pros	Cons
Procedure under local anaesthesia	Not all types of catheters can be inserted
Small incision (low risk of incisional hernia/fluid leakage)	Risk of intra-abdominal organ damage – risk of bleeding
Short operative times	Difficult precise positioning of the intra-peritoneal segment – risk of catheter malfunctioning
	No security at end of procedure that catheter is in correct position.
Low cost procedure	Does not allow to perform associated procedures (i.e. adhesiolysis, omentopexy, partial omentectomy)

- A small incision is made above the entrance site, most commonly in the midline.
- An 18-gauge needle is placed into the peritoneal cavity, which is then filled with air or 500 mL of saline. Absence of resistance or pain during this manoeuvre suggests proper positioning.
- A guide wire (usually 0.035-in.) is then advanced into the abdomen, this step can be done under XR guidance, and the needle is removed.
- A dilator and a peel-a-way sheath are advanced over the guidewire into the abdominal cavity. The dilator and wire are then removed, and the peritoneal dialysis catheter is placed in the peritoneal cavity and advanced through the sheath with a stylet until the proximal cuff is in the preperitoneal sheath.

The peel-a-way sheath and the stylet are then removed, and the correct position of the catheter is confirmed with fluoroscopy (Table 5.2).

Peritoneoscopic Technique

First described in 1981 by Ash [44], it is a technique of PD catheter insertion under local anaesthesia. The peritoneoscopic PD catheter insertion, commonly performed by nephrologists in an outpatient setting with all the associated potential benefits [45, 46], requires a specialized equipment (needlescope - Y-TEC, Medigroup, Inc. North Aurora, IL).

There are still limited data on outcomes for these catheters. Main concerns are relatively high dysfunction rates [47] and risk of bowel perforation [48, 49]. The vast majority of data on outcomes are coming from retrospective studies outside the United States [50, 51]; very recently Yorg and coll. reported in a retrospective series the Mount Sinai experience [52].

Technical Aspects

Peritoneoscopic placement of peritoneal dialysis catheters, under local anaesthesia, requires a needle trocar, a Quill guide, a needlescope (needlescope - Y-TEC, Medigroup, Inc. North Aurora, IL) and a Cuff Implanter Tool (Medigroup Inc., Oswego, IL).

A guidewire and a peel-away sheath applying the Seldinger technique.

- Needle trocar and surrounding Quill guide or sheath insertion through abdominal wall.
- Insufflation of the peritoneal cavity with room air [44] or NO [52].
- Needlescope insertion through the Quill guide, identification of the pelvis.
- The scope is removed; the guide is dilated to 6 mm to allow the PD catheter insertion.
- Deep cuff positioning below the anterior rectus sheath using a Cuff Implanter Tool (Medigroup Inc., Oswego, IL).
- Guide removal (Table 5.3).

Open Surgical Technique

First described in 1972 by Brewer, the open surgical peritoneal dialysis catheter placement has been until recent years the most commonly used in the adult and pediatric population [53, 54]. Advantages and disadvantages of this technique are presented in the Table 5.4. Since there is direct visualization of the peritoneum prior to insertion, the risk of bowel injury and bleeding is extremely low [53]. However, its main limitation is catheter malfunctioning; the reported incidence in some series is up to a 38% [55]. Two major factors that may be involved in catheter dysfunction are inadequate placement of the catheter tip into the pelvis, which

Table 5.3 Pros and cons of peritoneoscopic insertion

Pros	Cons
Procedure under local anaesthesia	Not all types of catheters can be inserted
Small incision (low risk of incisional hernia/ fluid leakage)	Risk of intra-abdominal organ damage – risk of bleeding
Short operative times	Does not allow to perform associated procedures (i.e. adhesiolysis, omentopexy, partial omentectomy)
Visualization of the abdominal cavity and more accurate placement of the tip of the catheter than with blind percutaneous or open surgical	Need for specialized equipment and expertise

Table 5.4 Pros and cons of open insertion

Pros	Cons
All types of catheters can be inserted	Larger incision compared to other techniques and consequent higher risk of incisional hernia/fluid leakage
Low risk of intra-abdominal organ damage	Risk of catheter malfunctioning – catheter migration, one-way or total obstruction
Low risk of bleeding	Limited space to perform associated procedures (i.e. adhesiolysis, omentopexy, partial omentectomy)
	Costs – surgeon and OR time No security at end of procedure that catheter is in correct position.

OR operating room

allows the catheter to migrate and become entrapped within the omentum, and the presence of intra-abdominal adhesions, which interfere with correct catheter placement [56–59]. Using the mini-laparotomy, it is difficult to visualize the entire peritoneal cavity, and to perform adhesiolysis should it be required; therefore, potentially poorer outcomes are to be expected in patients who have had prior abdominal surgery [60].

Technical Aspects

Open surgical placement of peritoneal dialysis catheters, under local or general anaesthesia, is performed via a mini-laparotomy.

- The skin incision, in a patient placed in supine position, is either sub-umbilical midline or ideally para-median [61]. Stegmayr and coll. introduced the paramedian approach and purse string sutures around the peritoneum and the catheter to reduce the incidence of leak rate [61].
- The subcutaneous layer is then dissected to the sheath of the rectus muscle. The anterior rectus sheath is opened, and the muscle fibers are split (muscle-splitting technique). The posterior sheath is incised, and the abdominal cavity is opened after dissecting the peritoneum.
- Placing the patient in Trendelemburg position allows a confortable peritoneal catheter placement deep in the peritoneal cavity; this manoeuvre can be done with or without a stylet.
- Omentectomy is commonly performed in the pediatric population [54, 62] (for more details

please refer to the section "Surgical Manoeuvres to Prevent Catheter Dysfunction")

- Some surgeons perform fixation of the intra-peritoneal catheter portion to the bladder, the parietal peritoneum, uterus or pelvic sidewall in order to minimize catheter dislocation (for more details please refer to the section "Surgical Manoeuvres to Prevent Catheter Dysfunction").
- The deep cuff is positioned within the rectus sheath; some surgeons place reinforcing sutures in order to prevent leakage of the dialysate [61].
- The posterior and anterior rectus sheaths are closed with absorbable sutures taking care to prevent catheter obstruction.
- A subcutaneous tunnel is then created and the distal cuff left at 2–4 cm from the exit site [28].
- Filling the abdomen with sterile saline - with no consensus about the amount of fluid that should be given – in order to check good in- and outflow at the end of the procedure and for eventual leakage (Table 5.4).

Laparoscopic Technique

Since its first description in the early 1990s, laparoscopic insertion of PD catheters has been increasingly used, an it is now in the United States the most commonly technique used [36]; its safety and feasibility in both adults and children have been documented in case series, retrospective reviews and comparative studies [50, 63–98]. Advantages and disadvantages of this technique are presented in the Table 5.5. The laparoscopic peritoneal catheter insertion without any associated intervention is referred in the literature as "basic laparoscopic technique". There is a growing body of evidence that the greatest benefit of laparoscopy is the minimization of catheter dysfunction securing optimal catheter position under direct vision, facilitating adhesiolysis, rectus sheath tunneling, omentopexy or omentectomy.

The use of these surgical manoeuvres is referred to as "advanced laparoscopic techniques" (for more details please refer to the section "Surgical Manoeuvres to Prevent Catheter Dysfunction") [50, 91, 99].

Technical Aspects

The laparoscopic peritoneal dialysis placement can be performed under general or local anaesthesia.

Standard laparoscopes of thirty degrees zero degrees, 3, 5, 8 and 10 mm ports have all been used in the studies present in the literature. One, two and three port techniques have all been described. Graspers and scissors should be available as well as ultrasonic dissecting instruments since adhesiolysis is sometimes necessary.

Minilaparoscopic instruments have also been used with equal success [72, 100–103]. Most authors recommend the use of the smallest available non-cutting ports to allow the quickest healing of the peritoneum, thus facilitating early start of PD and low leak rate; studies comparing leak rates and the size of trocars are lacking.

1. Procedure under general anaesthesia:
   - The patient is placed in a supine position.
   - For every technique, it is important to first place the PD catheter on the abdomen of the patient and determine optimal position, insertion site and exit site. There are even tools to assist with this.
   - The access to the peritoneal cavity is accomplished either by open Hassan trocar or by Veress needle insertion. In a review, Crabtree noted that 43% of authors used a peri-umbilical site (subcostal or supraumbilical) [60]. From the available literature, it is clear that the access to the peritoneal cavity is at discretion of the operating surgeon; most authors are now less in favour to the midline access [61].
   - After induction of pneumoperitoneum (max pressure 12–14 mmHg), a diagnostic laparoscopy is performed. An additional 5–8 mm trocar is placed under direct vision at the site of the planned exit-site position of the peritoneal dialysis catheter. For the description of the rectus sheath tunnelling technique, please refer to the section on Surgical Manoeuvres to Prevent Catheter Dysfunction.
   - If adhesions are present, adhesiolysis is usually performed.
   - A peritoneal dialysis catheter is then placed into the pouch of Douglas, with or without a stylet.
   - The distal cuff of the peritoneal dialysis catheter remains outside of the peritoneal cavity and is positioned either in the pre-peritoneal space or between the rectus sheaths.
   - The para-umbilical trocar is removed, and the catheter is then directed to its exit-site location.
   - A subcutaneous tunnel is created similarly to others implantation techniques.
   - The catheter is tested, and the abdomen is desufflated.
   - The trocar is removed, and the rectus fascia closed. Skin closure (Table 5.5).

Table 5.5 Pros and cons: Laparoscopic PD catheter insertion under general anaesthesia

Pros	Cons
Small incision(s) (low risk of incisional hernia/fluid leakage)	Need for general anaesthetic (can also be done under LA, but GA more common)
Allows to perform associated procedures (i.e. adhesiolysis, omentopexy, partial omentectomy)	Expertise in laparoscopic surgery
Low risk of intra-abdominal organ damage/low risk of bleeding	Not all types of catheters can be inserted
Immediate use possible	Need for special equipment (problem for 3rd World countries)
Precise positioning (under direct vision) of intraperitoneal segment.	
Cost-effective*	

*__Cost analysis__ When accounting for a year of postoperative management and treatment, laparoscopic insertion can be less costly than open insertion in the hands of an experienced and dedicated surgeon. Despite higher initial costs, PD catheter insertion under laparoscopic visualization can have lower total costs due to fewer postoperative complications [109]

Procedure Under Local Anaesthesia

It is reported the original technique described by Crabtree of laparoscopic dialysis catheter implantation using a two-port technique [104]. The infiltration with local anaesthetic of all abdominal wall layers until the peritoneum, for complete pain control, helium insufflation is used to create pneumoperitoneum; Keshvari and coll. described the technique using nitrous oxide (NO_2) [64]. Few characteristics make helium ideal in this setting: it is painless, thereby allowing the laparoscopic procedure to be performed under local anaesthesia [104]; non-flammable, thereby safe when using electrosurgical devices [105, 106]; inert, thereby increasingly utilized in high-risk patients [107, 108]. Contrary to paralyzed patients under general anaesthesia, patients under local anesthesia benefit from lower gas insufflation pressure (between 8 and 10 mmHg) and rates (0.5–2.0 L/min.). The peritoneal catheter is inserted through a para-median port site while continuously monitoring the implant procedure with a laparoscope from a second port location. The catheter–stylet assembly is then inserted and placed deep in the pelvis. The rectus sheath tunnelling technique is applied. The deep Dacron cuff is withdrawn until disappears above the peritoneum in the anterior rectus sheath. The stylet is removed from the catheter, the pneumoperitoneum is allowed to deflate, and the laparoscope is removed. The catheter is tested with the patient in reverse Trendelemburg position; a standard 1-L bag of normal saline is observed for unimpeded inflow and drainage by gravity. A residual of 250–300 mL is left in the abdomen to reduce the likelihood of intraperitoneal structures sucking up against the catheter toward the end of the drainage process. At the conclusion of a successful irrigation, the entire system is flushed with 20 mL of heparin (100 U/mL) (Table 5.6).

Surgical Manoeuvres to Prevent Catheter Dysfunction

Adhesiolysis

Previous abdominal surgery and consequent peritoneal adhesion formation represent a unique challenge and a major factor in PD catheter dysfunction [110]. Although no studies specifically compared PD catheter placement and adhesiolysis to PD catheter placement alone, adhesiolysis is considered essential in optimising primary PD catheter function. In this context, the laparoscopic approach is particularly beneficial, allowing identification and lysis of the adhesions [65, 111]. Adhesiolysis can be performed using ultrasonic shears or regular laparoscopic scissors [60] and it has been employed in several large case series [63, 78, 80–82, 85, 111] and some authors described similar catheter function rates in patients with adhesions as those with a virgin abdomen [60, 112, 113].

Suture Fixation

Catheter tip migration away from the pelvis is a common cause for catheter failure as the intraperitoneal portion of the catheter functions best

Table 5.6 Pros and cons: Laparoscopic PD catheter insertion under local anaesthesia

Pros	Cons
No need for general anaesthesia	Not all types of catheters can be inserted
Small incision (low risk of incisional hernia/fluid leakage)	Need for special equipment
Allows to perform associated procedures (i.e. adhesiolysis, partial omentectomy)	Expertise in laparoscopic technique
Low risk of intra-abdominal organ damage/low risk of bleeding	Need for special equipment (problem for 3rd World countries)
Immediate use possible	
Precise positioning (under direct vision) of the intraperitoneal segment.	
Cost-effective[a]	

[a]*Cost analysis* When accounting for a year of postoperative management and treatment, laparoscopic insertion can be less costly than open insertion in the hands of an experienced and dedicated surgeon. Despite higher initial costs, PD catheter insertion under laparoscopic visualization can have lower total costs due to fewer postoperative complications [109]

when in the pelvis [48, 49, 68]. Several authors reported suture fixation of the catheter tip to the bladder, uterus or pelvic sidewall in an attempt to prevent catheter tip migration in either open or laparoscopic approach [14, 59, 61, 62, 64]. Potential harms of suture fixation are not easy catheter removal and internal hernias or adhesions [93]. Other authors showed a relatively high dysfunction rate after suture fixation (12–14%), possibly due to the inability of the catheter to "float" into the largest area of PD fluid [14, 77, 93]. However, the lack of comparative studies on peritoneal catheter insertion with and without suture fixation leaves the decision on suture fixation to the operating surgeon, based on his personal experience.

Rectus Sheath Tunneling

Many authors have used rectus sheath tunneling, also described as extraperitoneal or preperitoneal tunneling, as a way to prevent catheter migration and decrease the incidence of fluid leak [78, 79, 82, 91, 94]. The technique, applied during laparoscopic insertion, involves visualizing the insertion device (sheath, blunt trocar or grasper) as it comes through the rectus muscle but before it enters the peritoneal cavity. Once the device is seen just above the posterior rectus sheath and peritoneum, it is tunnelled 4–6 cm toward the midline pelvis before actually penetrating and entering the peritoneal cavity. In addition, this technique has the advantage over suture fixation of not requiring extra trocars for suturing. Several studies using laparoscopic insertion and rectus sheath tunnel showed dysfunction rates between 4% and 8.6% and leak rates from 0% to 12.5% [78, 79, 82, 91, 94]. In a recent review article, Frost and Bagul recommend that rectus sheath tunneling and placement of the deep cuff in the rectus sheath are far more important than suture fixation in reducing catheter tip migration [99]. However, randomized trials comparing suture fixation to rectus sheath tunneling have not been performed.

Omentopexy and Omentectomy

The omentum is a well-known source of catheter dysfunction; omentectomy has been described in adults and children as a way to reduce this complication. With the open technique the omentum is pulled up through the incision and excised [54, 114–122]. McIntosh described an alternative technique, omentopexy, which consists in suturing the omentum to the abdominal wall [119]. Although omentectomy is feasible during laparoscopic PD catheter insertion [69, 111, 118, 120–122], it is more time consuming and has an increased risk of bleeding [65]; therefore, laparoscopic omentopexy seems to be favoured [67, 82, 94, 112, 113]. Omentopexy techniques can be accomplished with trans-abdominal suture passer or with intracorporeal suturing. An alternative technique described by Goh consists of omental folding in order to shorten it [122].

Critical Comparison of Different Implantation Techniques

Percutaneous – Peritoneoscopic Versus Surgical (Open or Laparoscopic)

Several single centre experiences compared percutaneous and open surgical peritoneal dialysis catheter insertion. Besides the general agreement that percutaneous insertion is particularly well suited for high-risk patients, who cannot tolerate general anaesthesia [42, 117, 118, 123, 124], comparative results yield to a different results. While older studies including a retrospective single center study by Nicholson and coll. found that catheter survival was significantly better after open surgical insertion compared to percutaneous insertion [115]. Gadallah and coll. in a prospective randomized study on percutaneous versus open placement of peritoneal dialysis catheters showed that the placement modality did not affect catheter survival; however, early mechanical complications, including technical failures, occurred more frequently in the percutaneous group [116]. More recent studies show that percutaneous placement of PD catheter offers an effective and safe alternative surgical technique in selected patients (such as no previous abdominal operation, BMI < 28 kg/m²) [123–126]; a meta-analysis comparing open surgery/laparoscopic and percutaneous PD catheter insertion reports no difference in the 1-year catheter survival rate [127].

Open Versus Laparoscopic

A number of randomized prospective studies [88, 92, 95, 96, 128, 129] comparing open surgical versus laparoscopic peritoneal catheter insertion justified systematic reviews [130] and meta-analyses [131, 132].

The systematic review of randomized controlled trials conducted by Strippoli and coll. included any randomized controlled trial of different catheter types and catheter-related interventions used to prevent peritonitis or exit-site and tunnel infection in PD. The subgroup analysis on surgical approaches included three trials (248 patients in total) comparing laparoscopic versus open surgical catheter insertion, could not demonstrate any advantage of one technique over the other, with respect to the risk of peritonitis, catheter removal or replacement, technical failure and all-cause mortality [130].

Xie and coll. performed a meta-analysis of four randomized controlled trials and a systematic review of ten observational studies to compare laparoscopy with open placement of peritoneal dialysis catheter. The authors extracted data on the following reported outcomes: operation time, duration of hospital stay, incidence-rate of catheter-related complications (such as infection, dialysate leak, catheter migration, outflow obstruction, bleeding, blockage and hernia). According to this analysis open surgery needs a shorter operative time and simpler equipment requirement but has a similar effect to the laparoscopic technique. Therefore, the authors conclude that laparoscopic catheter placement has no

superiority to open surgery; on the other hand, they state that further trials that focus on long-term outcomes are needed, taking into account the rapid development of the advanced laparoscopic technique, which may reduce further the complication rates [131].

Hagen and coll. performed a meta-analysis of three randomized controlled trials [85, 87, 88] and eight cohort studies [88, 90, 91, 93, 96, 101, 133, 134], comparing laparoscopic versus open surgical peritoneal catheter insertion. Contrarily to the study conducted by Xie and coll. [131], the authors did not include studies assessing different techniques (peritoneoscopic and percutaneous insertion) and studies including pediatric patients. The following outcome measures were included: incidence of peritonitis, exit-site/tunnel infection, leakage, catheter migration, catheter removal for complications, need for revision and catheter survival. The results of this meta-analysis reveal the potential benefits of laparoscopic PD-catheter insertion with better one-year catheter survival and less migration rates compared to the open surgical insertion [132].

The conclusion of both meta-analyses [131, 132] is the need of studies with larger numbers of patients and long-term follow up in order to be able to evaluate the true value of laparoscopy in PD-catheter insertion; a large randomized controlled trial is currently under way [129].

Limitations of Comparative Studies

Small numbers, single centre experiences and other confounding factors bias the studies comparing insertion techniques. The expertise of the operators, which may vary significantly, the exclusion of high-risk patients, such as those with history of prior abdominal surgery, in some insertion techniques, the different definitions of complications (for example some papers split up catheter migration and outflow obstruction as causes of catheter dysfunction), make comparative studies less accurate and difficult to interpret. Finally, the follow-up periods vary greatly, but generally tended to be short making it difficult to compare data on one technique versus another. For peritoneal access, the only strong recommendation that can be made is that all the techniques, percutaneous, open surgical, and laparoscopic insertion procedures, when performed by experienced/dedicated operators, are feasible and safe with acceptable outcomes.

Timing? When to Start PD After Catheter Insertion

The timing of commencement of dialysis after catheter insertion has not been studied in randomized controlled trials, although one is currently underway in Australia [135]. There is general consensus worldwide to observe a break in period of at least 2 weeks for both adult and children. [28, 135–140] (see table). Over the last decade, urgent-start PD has gained considerable interest in the United States. Urgent-start PD refers to an approach that involves initiation of PD therapy earlier than 2 weeks after PD catheter insertion. Treatment is performed with low fill volumes in the supine position using a cycler to avoid peri-catheter leak. Numerous clinical experiences with urgent-start PD have been published or discussed at scientific meetings [141–150].

With all the limitations of a single center including a small number of patients, Ghaffari recently described the feasibility and efficacy of an urgent-start peritoneal dialysis program [141].

| British Renal Association (2009) | Whenever possible, that catheter insertion should be performed at least 2 weeks before starting peritoneal dialysis. Small dialysate volumes in the supine position can be used if dialysis is required earlier (2B). |
| European Dialysis and Transplant Association – European Renal Association (2005) | Whenever possible, the implantation should be at least 2 weeks before starting peritoneal dialysis. Small dialysate volumes in the supine position can be used if dialysis is required earlier (Evidence C) |

Australian: Caring for Australasians with Renal Impairment (CARI) (2004)	When possible, peritoneal dialysis should not be commenced until at least 2 weeks after the insertion of the dialysis catheter (Suggestions are based on level III and IV studies)
International Society for Peritoneal Dialysis (ISPD)	When possible, peritoneal dialysis should not be commenced until at least 2 weeks after the insertion of the dialysis catheter
Kidney Disease Outcomes Quality Initiative (KDOQI)	No recommendations.
Canadian Society of Nephrology	No recommendations.

Surgical Complications and Management

(a) Hernia
(b) Hemorrhage
(c) Perforation
(d) Catheter-related (fluid leak, one-way or total obstruction, migration)
(e) Others (chyloperitoneum, genital edema, peritoneal-vaginal leak)

Hernia

Hernias represent one of the most frequent non-infectious complications of PD and will be extensively treated in a separate chapter [15].

Hemorrhage

Hemorrhage secondary to peritoneal catheter insertion can be classified as intraperitoneal and extraperitoneal.

Intraperitoneal bleeding (intraabdominal bleeding) may be secondary to trauma of omental or mesenteric vessels during the manipulation of the catheter tip into the pelvis, adhesiolysis or omentectomy. During a percutaneous insertion this is usually recognised as bloodstaining of the draining fluid. This complication may occur or be recognised only postoperatively and usually presents with bloody staining of the dialysate effluent. If the bleeding is minimal and the patient is hemodynamically stable, conservative management is indicated. Obviously, in case of severe bleeding and/or hemodynamic instability, patient should be taken back to theatres as emergency. During open and/or laparoscopic insertion it is easier to recognise and treat this complication.

Extraperitoneal bleeding may occur from the inferior epigastric vessels, subcutaneous vessels or skin edges. If the bleeding is difficult to control, the epigastric vessels can be tied off with ligature above and below the site of trauma. Bleeding from subcutaneous vessels and skin edges is in the vast majority of cases self-limiting or stops with conservative management; large hematomas may require surgical intervention in case of patient discomfort and potential source of infection [151].

Perforation

Intra-abdominal perforation is a described complication during peritoneal catheter insertion; it is more common during percutaneous insertion. The most commonly injured organs are bowel and bladder. Perforation of viscera by erosion of the peritoneal catheter is extremely rare. This complication is facilitated by episodes of peritonitis, an empty peritoneal cavity, the use of steroids, or the presence of vasculitis.

Lesions to the bladder occur more frequently in patients with chronic urinary outflow obstruction; some authors advocate the use of a urinary catheter to limit its occurrence. Urine in the peritoneal cavity may give rise to signs of peritonitis. A small laceration may close spontaneously draining the bladder with a urethral catheter. A large laceration may require a surgical repair followed by urethral catheterization.

The risk of bowel perforation is higher in patients with intra-abdominal adhesions from previous surgery or peritonitis. The most common mechanism of injury is advancement of the catheter against resistance into a bowel loop, fixed in the peritoneal cavity by adhesions; the pathogenetic mechanism previously described is characteristic of the percutaneous placement. During laparoscopic or open insertion, the insertion under direct vision makes this complication extremely rare.

After catheter insertion, perforation may present in a variety of ways. The patient without experiencing abdominal signs may pass large volumes of dialysate per rectum if the catheter is placed into the lumen of the bowel. Alternatively the run-out may be cloudy and contain mixed bacterial organisms with signs of peritonitis. Several courses of action are possible. In the absence of clinical signs and symptoms, the catheter may be left in free drainage for few days to allow an intra-peritoneal track to form, then it may be removed; few weeks are usually required before attempting a new catheter insertion.

In case of peritonitis or when conservative management fails, a diagnostic laparoscopy or laparotomy is mandatory.

Catheter-Related (Fluid Leak, One-Way or Total Obstruction)

Fluid Leak

Fluid leak is defined as the appearance of dialysate fluid through the wound(s) or he catheter exit site. It can be divided in early and late, depending upon its appearance soon after the insertion or at later stage. The wide variety of its incidence (from 0% to 27%) present in the literature mostly depends on the technique of implantation (percutaneous vs peritoneoscopic vs open vs laparoscopic) and the definition of leak (early vs late) [85, 86, 89, 100, 152–154]. The vast majority are represented by early leaks. The pathogenesis is due to a defect in the peritoneal closure around the catheter or other peritoneal defects created during insertion [154]. Preventive measures reported in the literature are the observation of a break-in period of about 2 weeks [89, 91]; in this period the wound can heal properly and ingrowth of fibrous tissue can anchor the catheter. If the start cannot be delayed, it would be reasonable reducing the dialysate volume (500–1000 mL in adults) for the initial period. There is also evidence that the laparoscopic insertion and the application of advanced techniques such as rectus sheath tunneling could further reduce the incidence of this complication [50].

One-Way or Total Obstruction

Catheter obstruction is one of the most common complications of peritoneal catheters; it usually occurs in the early postoperative phase and presents in the form of one-way (outflow) or total (inflow/outflow) obstruction. Its incidence varies widely depending on the catheter type and the technique applied. One-way obstruction presents when peritoneal fluid runs into the peritoneal cavity but only drains slowly or does not drain at all; total obstruction presents with inability to flush the catheter. The most common cause of obstruction and consequently catheter malfunctioning is catheter tip migration away from the pelvis [57, 58]. As described before, preventive surgical techniques have been applied in order to reduce its incidence, such as suture fixation of the catheter tip [58, 88, 118] and rectus sheath tunneling. The latter seems to yield the most promising results [99]. Other potential causes of obstruction are omental wrapping, presence of adhesions, full rectum or bladder, obstruction of the lumen with clots or fibrin [62].

The management of catheter obstruction depends on the cause. History and physical examination are important to identify the nature of the problem (sudden vs gradual) and to rule out constipation. A plain abdominal X-ray will give further information regarding constipation and will show the position of the catheter tip. If negative, further studies such as catheterography [155] or CT peritoneography [156, 157] followed by diagnostic laparoscopy [158] are indicated.

Non-operative treatments of malfunctioning PD catheters include laxatives or enemas, catheter flushing, intraluminal heparin or fibrinolytic agents [159–161]. Several procedures under fluoroscopic guidance have been described to reposition displaced catheters [162–165]. The manipulation of catheters with intraluminal instruments may predispose to visceral damage,

bacterial contamination [166] and it is ineffective in case of adhesions or omental wrapping. Patients with malfunctioning peritoneal dialysis catheters not responding to non-operative treatments require operative management. The laparoscopic approach is particularly beneficial in this context, allowing catheter repositioning [167], adhesiolysis [67], omentectomy or omentopexy [89, 120] or catheter replacement when the obstruction can not be resolved [168].

Others (Chyloperitoneum, Genital Edema, Peritoneal-Vaginal Leak)

Chyloperitoneum

Chyloperitoneum is a rare but well-described complication in patients on peritoneal dialysis [169]. One case series reported an incidence of 0.5% [170]. It has been described after laparoscopic [169–171] and percutaneous [172] PD catheter placement. Its pathogenesis is unclear but has been hypothesized that could be secondary to injury of fine lymphatic vessels. The complication is usually recognised postoperatively when the dialysate has a milky white, turbid appearance and contains triglyceride levels that exceed those in the plasma [173]. Most cases resolve spontaneously within weeks but may require temporary cessation of PD. In persistent chyloperitoneum, conservative management consists of low fat diet to reduce the turbidity of the triglyceride-rich lymphatic flow; supplements with medium-chain triglycerides, absorbed directly into the portal system instead of intestinal lymphatics. Some authors achieved good results with Orlistat, a reversible inhibitor of pancreatic and gastric lipases, and octreotide, a somatostatin analogue, but the overall clinical experience with these agents is limited for this indication [174, 175]. Surgery may be indicated and some authors have advocated a laparoscopic approach [176].

Genital Edema

Genital, scrotal or labial, edema is typically secondary to two main causes: a patent processus vaginalis or a subcutaneous tissue leak of dialysate.

The most common pathogenetic cause is a patent processus vaginalis, which usually allows the flow of dialysate in the genital area and it is too small for the formation of a true hernia.

Patients with subcutaneous leaks will often have signs of leak in the subcutaneous tissue of the lower abdomen with evidence of these changes continuing into the genital area, such as palpable thickness of the tissue or visible peau d'orange appearance of the surrounding skin.

To differentiate between these presentations and to confirm the diagnosis, a CT peritoneogram or nuclear medicine scan can be useful. In CT peritoneography, 150 mL of contrast can be added to the 2 L dialysate bag and infused into the patient. The patient is asked to remain active for 30–60 min and then undergo a CT scan of the abdomen and processus vaginalis. Similarly, Tc-99m can be infused with the dialysate and after a similar period the patient undergoes to peritoneal scintigraphy.

In patients diagnosed with a patent processus vaginalis, surgical correction is usually required to resolve the genital edema, if a trial of night exchanges with dry days fails. [177]

Peritoneal-Vaginal Leak

This complication develops when the fallopian tubes act as conduits for antegrade passage of dialysate in the uterine cavity. The leak can be stopped by bilateral tubal ligation [178]. If the women wish to maintain fertility and transplantation is planned, temporary conversion to hemodialysis may be considered.

Bibliography

1. AV Fistula First Breakthrough Coalition. National Vascular Access Improvement Initiative (NVAII). Available at: http://www.fistulafirst.org/ Accessed 18 Jan 2009.
2. National Vascular Access Improvement Project. CMS launches "Fistula First" initiative to improve care and quality of life for hemodialysis patients. Press release April 14, 2004. http://www.cms.hhs.gov/aaps/media/press/release.asp?counter=1007.
3. van Biesen W, Veys N. Norbert Lameire and Raymond Vanholder Why less success of the peritoneal dialysis programmes in Europe? Nephrol Dial Transplant. 2008;23(5):1478–81.
4. Tenckhoff J, Schechter H. A bacteriologically safe peritoneal access device. Trans Am Soc Artif Intern Organs. 1968;14:181–7.
5. Ash SR, Nichols WK. Placement, repair and removal of chronic peritoneal catheters. In: Gokal R, Nolph KD, editors. Textbook of peritoneal dialysis. Boston: Kluwer Academic; 1994.
6. Diaz-Buxo JA, Geissinger WT. Single versus double cuff Tenckhoff catheters. Perit Dial Bull. 1984;4:100.
7. Oreopoulos DG, Izatt S, Zellerman G, et al. A prospective study of the effectiveness of three permanent peritoneal catheters. Proc Clin Dial Transplant Forum. 1976;6:96–100.
8. Twardowski ZJ, Nichols WK, Khanna R, Nolph KD. Swan-neck Missouri peritoneal dialysis catheters: design, insertion and break-in (video). Columbia: University of Missouri, Academic Support Center; 1993.
9. Twardowski ZJ, Prowant BF, Nichols WK, et al. Six-year experience with swan-neck catheter. Peril Dial Int. 1992;12:384–9.
10. Crabtree JH, Siddiqi RA, Chung JJ, Greenwald LT. Long-term experience with polyurethane, pail handle, coiled tip peritoneal dialysis catheters. ASAIO J. 1998;44(4):309–13.
11. Twardowski ZJ, Prowant BF, Pickett B, et al. Four-year experience with swan-neck pre-sternal peritoneal dialysis catheter. Am J Kidney Dis. 1996;27:99–105.
12. Twardowski ZJ. Presternal peritoneal catheter. Adv Ren Replace Ther. 2002;9(2):125–32.
13. Moncrief JW, Popovich RP, Broadrick LJ. New peritoneal access technique for CAPD (Abstract). Perit Dial Int. 1991;11(Suppl 1):A180.
14. Moncrief JW, Popovich RP, Broadrick LJ, He ZZ, Simmons EE, Tate RA. The Moncrief-Popovich catheter: a new peritoneal access technique for patients on peritoneal dialysis. ASAIO J. 1993;39(1):62–5.
15. Ash SR. Experience with a new catheter design. Twenty-first conference on dialysis proceedings. New Orleans. LA, 19–21 Feb 2001, p. 303–5.
16. Shinaberger JH, Shear L, Barry KG. Peritoneal extracorporeal recirculation dialysis: a technique for improving efficiency of peritoneal dialysis. Invest Urol. 1965;2:555–65.
17. Lange K, Treser G, Mangalat J. Automatic continuous high flow rate peritoneal dialysis. Arch Klin Med. 1968;214:201–6.
18. Raja RM, Kramer MS, Rosenbaum JL. Recirculating peritoneal dialysis with Sorbent Redy cartridge. Nephron. 1976;16:134–42.
19. Kabitz C, Stephen RL, Jacobsen SC, et al. Reciprocating peritoneal dialysis. Dial Transplant. 1978;7:211–4.
20. Kraus MA, Shasha SM, Nemas M, et al. Ultrafiltration peritoneal dialysis and recirculating peritoneal dialysis with a portable kidney. Dial Transplant. 1983;12:385–8.
21. Mineshima M, Watanuki M, Yamagata K, et al. Development of continuous recirculating peritoneal dialysis using a double lumen catheter. ASAIO J. 1992;38:M377–81.

22. Diaz–Buxo JA, Folden TI. Optimization of peritoneal dialysis: a bioengineering approach. Semin Dial. 1999;12:S97–100.

23. Passlick–Deetjen J, Quellhorst E. Continuous flow peritoneal dialysis (CFPD): a glimpse into the future. Nephrol Dial Transplant. 2001;16:2296–9.

24. Diaz–Buxo JA. Streaming, mixing, and recirculation: role of the peritoneal access in continuous flow peritoneal dialysis (clinical considerations). Adv Perit Dial. 2002;18:87–90.

25. Ash SR, Janle EM. Continuous flow-through peritoneal dialysis: comparison of efficiency to IPD, TPD and CAPD in an animal model. Perit Dial Int. 1997;17:365–72.

26. Ronco C, Gloukhoff A, Dell'Aquila R, Levin NW. Catheter design for continuous flow peritoneal dialysis. Blood Purif. 2002;20:40–4.

27. Lewis MA, Smith T, Postlethwaite RJ, Webb NJ. A comparison of double-cuffed with single-cuffed Tenckhoff catheters in the prevention of infection in pediatric patients. Adv Perit Dial. 1997;13:274–6.

28. Gokal R, Alexander S, Ash S, Chen TW, Danielson A, Holmes C, Joffe P, Moncrief J, Nichols K, Piraino B, Prowant B, Slingeneyer A, Stegmayr B, Twardowski Z, Vas S. Peritoneal catheters and exit-site practices toward optimum peritoneal access: 1998 update. (Official report from the International Society for Peritoneal Dialysis). Perit Dial Int. 1998;18:11–33.

29. Eklund B, Honkanen E, Kyllönen L, Salmela K, Kala AR. Peritoneal dialysis access: prospective randomized comparison of single-cuff and double-cuff straight Tenckhoff catheters. Nephrol Dial Transplant. 1997;12(12):2664–6.

30. Swartz R, Messana J, Rocher L, Reynolds J, Starmann B, et al. The curled catheter: dependable device for percutaneous peritoneal access. Perit Dial Int. 1990;10:231–5.

31. Nielsen PK, Hemmingsen C, Friis SU, Ladefoged J, Olgaard K. Comparison of straight and curled Tenckhoff peritoneal dialysis catheters implanted by percutaneous technique: a prospective randomized study. Perit Dial Int. 1995;15:18–21.

32. Johnson DW, Wong J, Wiggins KJ, Kirwan R, Griffin A, et al. A randomized controlled trial of coiled versus straight swan-neck Tenckhoff catheters in peritoneal dialysis patients. Am J Kidney Dis. 2006;48:812–21.

33. Xie J, Kiryluk K, Ren H, et al. Coiled versus straight peritoneal dialysis catheters: a randomized controlled trial and meta-analysis. Am J Kidney Dis. 2011;58(6):946–55.

34. Hagen SM, Lafranca JA, IJzermans JN, Dor FJ. A systematic review and meta-analysis of the influence of peritoneal dialysis catheter type on complication rate and catheter survival. Kidney Int. 2014;85(4):920–32.

35. Hagen SM, Lafranca JA, Steyerberg EW, IJzermans JN, Dor FJ. Laparoscopic versus open peritoneal dialysis catheter insertion: a meta-analysis. PLoS ONE. 2013;8(2):e56351.

36. Distribution of 2007–2014 CMS Part B Claims for CPT 49324 (Laparoscopy) and all other methods (Open and percutaneous needle-guidewire) – physician/supplier procedure summary master file 2007–2014 Medicare, Baltimore, MD – Centers for Medicare and Medicaid Services, Department of Health and Human Services.

37. Zappacosta AR, Perras ST, Closkey GM. Seldinger technique for Tenckhoff catheter placement. ASAIO Trans. 1991;37:13–5.

38. Napoli M, Russo F, Mastrangelo F. Placement of peritoneal dialysis catheter by percutaneous method with the Veress needle. Adv Perit Dial. 2000;16:165–9.

39. Banli O, Altun H, Oztemel A. Early start of CAPD with the Seldinger technique. Perit Dial Int. 2005;25:556–9.

40. Allon M, Soucie JM, Macon EJ. Complications with permanent peritoneal dialysis catheters: experience with 154 percutaneously placed catheters. Nephron. 1998;48:8–11.

41. Mellotte GJ, Ho CA, Morgan SH, Bending MR, Eisinger AJ. Peritoneal dialysis catheters: a comparison between percutaneous and conventional surgical placement techniques. Nephrol Dial Transplant. 1993;8:626–30.

42. Aksu N, Yavascan O, Anil M, Kara OD, Erdogan H, Bal A. A ten-year single centre experience in children on chronic peritoneal dialysis – significance of percutaneous placement of peritoneal dialysis catheters. Nephrol Dial Transplant. 2007;22:2045–51.

43. Varughese S, Sundaram M, Basu G, Tamilarasi V, John GT. Percutaneous continuous ambulatory peritoneal dialysis (CAPD) catheter insertion – a preferred option for developing countries. Trop Doct. 2010;40:104–5.

44. Ash S, Wolf GC, Bloch R. Placement of the Tenckhoff peritoneal dialysis catheter under peritoneoscopic visualization. Dial Transplant. 1981;10:383–5.

45. Goh BL, Ganeshadeva YM, Chew SE, Dalimi MS. Does peritoneal dialysis catheter insertion by interventional nephrologists enhance peritoneal dialysis penetration? Semin Dial. 2008;21:561–6.

46. Li PK, Chow KM. Importance of peritoneal dialysis catheter insertion by nephrologists: practice makes perfect. Nephrol Dial Transplant. 2009;24:3274–6.

47. Maffei S, Bonello F, Stramignoni E, Forneris G, Iadarola GM, Borca M, Quarello F. Two years of experience and 119 peritoneal dialysis catheters placed with peritoneoscopy control and Y-TEC system. Minerva Urol Nefrol. 1992;44:63–7.

48. Nahman Jr NS, Middendorf DF, Bay WH, McElligott R, Powell S, Anderson J. Modification of the percutaneous approach to peritoneal dialysis catheter placement under peritoneoscopic visualization: clinical results in 78 patients. J Am Soc Nephrol. 1992;3:103–7.

49. Asif A, Byers P, Vieira CF, Merrill D, Gadalean F, Bourgoignie JJ, Leclercq B, Roth D, Gadallah MF. Peritoneoscopic placement of peritoneal dialysis catheter and bowel perforation: experience of an interventional nephrology program. Am J Kidney Dis. 2003;42:1270–4.

50. Haggerty S, Roth S, Walsh D, Stefanidis D, Price R, Fanelli RD, Penner T, Richardson W, SAGES Guidelines Committee. Guidelines for laparoscopic peritoneal dialysis access surgery. Surg Endosc. 2014;28(11):3016–45.

51. Kelly J, McNamara K, May S. Peritoneoscopic peritoneal dialysis catheter insertion. Nephrology (Carlton). 2003;8:315–7.

52. Al Azzi Y, Zeldis E, Nadkarni GN, Schanzer H, Uribarri J. Outcomes of dialysis catheters placed by the Y-TEC peritoneoscopic technique: a single-center surgical experience. Clin Kidney J. 2016;9(1):158–61.

53. Brewer TE, Caldwell FT, Patterson RM, Flanigan WJ. Indwelling peritoneal (Tenckhoff) dialysis catheter. Experience with 24 patients. JAMA. 1972;219:1011–5.

54. Washburn KK, Currier H, Salter KJ, Brandt ML. Surgical technique for peritoneal dialysis catheter placement in the pediatric patient: a North American survey. Adv Perit Dial. 2004;20:218–21.

55. Brandt ML, Brewer ED. Peritoneal catheter placement in children. In: Nissenson A, Fine RN, editors. Handbook of dialysis therapy. Philadelphia: Saunders (Elsevier Inc.); 2008. p. 1295–301.

56. Rubin J, Adair CM, Raju S, Bower JD. The Tenckhoff catheter for peritoneal dialysis – an appraisal. Nephron. 1982;32:370–4.

57. Cronen PW, Moss JP, Simpson T, Rao M, Cowles L. Tenckhoff catheter placement: surgical aspects. Am Surg. 1985;51:627–9.

58. Bullmaster JR, Miller SF, Finley Jr RK, Jones LM. Surgical aspects of the Tenckhoff peritoneal dialysis catheter. A 7 year experience. Am J Surg. 1985;149:339–42.

59. Olcott C, Feldman CA, Coplon NS, Oppenheimer ML, Mehigan JT. Continuous ambulatory peritoneal dialysis. Technique of catheter insertion and management of associated surgical complications. Am J Surg. 1983;146:98–102.

60. Crabtree JH. The use of the laparoscope for dialysis catheter implantation: valuable carry-on or excess baggage? Perit Dial Int. 2009;29:394–406.

61. Stegmayr BG. Lateral catheter insertion together with three purse-string sutures reduces the risk for leakage during peritoneal dialysis. Artif Organs. 1994;18:309–13.

62. Swartz RD. Chronic peritoneal dialysis: mechanical and infectious complications. Nephron. 1985;40:29–37.

63. Maio R, Figueiredo N, Costa P. Laparoscopic placement of Tenckhoff catheters for peritoneal dialysis: a safe, effective, and reproducible procedure. Perit Dial Int. 2008;28:170–3.

64. Keshvari A, Najafi I, Jafari-Javid M, Yunesian M, Chaman R, Taromlou MN. Laparoscopic peritoneal

dialysis catheter implantation using a Tenckhoff trocar under local anesthesia with nitrous oxide gas insufflation. Am J Surg. 2009;197:8–13.

65. Mattioli G, Castagnetti M, Verrina E, Trivelli A, Torre M, Jasonni V, Perfumo F. Laparoscopic-assisted peritoneal dialysis catheter implantation in pediatric patients. Urology. 2007;69:1185–9.

66. Milliken I, Fitzpatrick M, Subramaniam R. Single-port laparoscopic insertion of peritoneal dialysis catheters in children. J Pediatr Urol. 2006;2:308–11.

67. Kurihara S, Akiba T, Takeuchi M, Nakajima K, Inoue H, Yoneshima H. Laparoscopic mesenterioadhesiotomy and Tenckhoff catheter placement in patients with predisposing abdominal surgery. Artif Organs. 1995;19:1248–50.

68. Harissis HV, Katsios CS, Koliousi EL, Ikonomou MG, Siamopoulos KC, Fatouros M, Kappas AM. A new simplified one port laparoscopic technique of peritoneal dialysis catheter placement with intra-abdominal fixation. Am J Surg. 2006;192:125–9.

69. Wang JY, Hsieh JS, Chen FM, Chuan CH, Chan HM, Huang TJ. Secure placement of continuous ambulatory peritoneal dialysis catheters under laparoscopic assistance. Am Surg. 1999;65:247–9.

70. Watson DI, Paterson D, Bannister K. Secure placement of peritoneal dialysis catheters using a laparoscopic technique. Surg Laparosc Endosc. 1996;6:35–7.

71. Ogunc G. Videolaparoscopy with omentopexy: a new technique to allow placement of a catheter for continuous ambulatory peritoneal dialysis. Surg Today. 2001;31:942–4.

72. Haggerty SP, Zeni TM, Carder M, Frantzides CT. Laparoscopic peritoneal dialysis catheter insertion using a Quinton percutaneous insertion kit. JSLS. 2007;11:208–14.

73. Comert M, Borazan A, Kulah E, Ucan BH. A new laparoscopic technique for the placement of a permanent peritoneal dialysis catheter: the preperitoneal tunneling method. Surg Endosc. 2005;19:245–8.

74. Barone GW, Lightfoot ML, Ketel BL. Technique for laparoscopy-assisted complicated peritoneal dialysis catheter placement. J Laparoendosc Adv Surg Tech A. 2002;12:53–5.

75. Al-Dohayan A. Laparoscopic placement of peritoneal dialysis catheter (same day dialysis). JSLS. 1999;3:327–9.

76. Al-Hashemy AM, Seleem MI, Al-Ahmary AM, Bin-Mahfooz AA. A two-port laparoscopic placement of peritoneal dialysis catheter: a preliminary report. Saudi J Kidney Dis Transpl. 2004;15:144–8.

77. Brownlee J, Elkhairi S. Laparoscopic assisted placement of peritoneal dialysis catheter: a preliminary experience. Clin Nephrol. 1997;47:122–4.

78. Caliskan K, Nursal TZ, Tarim AM, Noyan T, Moray G, Haberal M. The adequacy of laparoscopy for continuous ambulatory peritoneal dialysis procedures. Transplant Proc. 2007;39:1359–61.

79. Leung LC, Yiu MK, Man CW, Chan WH, Lee KW, Lau KW. Laparoscopic management of Tenckhoff

catheters in continuous ambulatory peritoneal dialysis. A one port technique. Surg Endosc. 1998;12:891–3.

80. Manouras AJ, Kekis PB, Stamou KM, Konstadoulakis MM, Apostolidis NS. Laparoscopic placement of Oreopoulos-Zellerman catheters in CAPD patients. Perit Dial Int. 2004;24:252–5.

81. Nijhuis PH, Smulders JF, Jakimowicz JJ. Laparoscopic introduction of a continuous ambulatory peritoneal dialysis (capd) catheter by a two-puncture technique. Surg Endosc. 1996;10:676–9.

82. Yan X, Zhu W, Jiang CM, Huang HF, Zhang M, Guo HQ. Clinical application of one-port laparoscopic placement of peritoneal dialysis catheters. Scand J Urol Nephrol. 2010;44:341–4.

83. Ko J, Ra W, Bae T, Lee T, Kim HH, Han HS. Two-port laparoscopic placement of a peritoneal dialysis catheter with abdominal wall fixation. Surg Today. 2009;39:356–8.

84. Bar-Zohar D, Sagie B, Lubezky N, Blum M, Klausner J, Abu-Abeid S. Laparoscopic implantation of the Tenckhoff catheter for the treatment of end-stage renal failure and congestive heart failure: experience with the pelvic fixation technique. Isr Med Assoc J. 2006;8:174–8.

85. Schmidt SC, Pohle C, Langrehr JM, Schumacher G, Jacob D, Neuhaus P. Laparoscopic-assisted placement of peritoneal dialysis catheters: implantation technique and results. J Laparoendosc Adv Surg Tech A. 2007;17:596–9.

86. Crabtree JH, Burchette RJ. Effective use of laparoscopy for long-term peritoneal dialysis access. Am J Surg. 2009;198:135–41.

87. Poole GH, Tervit P. Laparoscopic Tenckhoff catheter insertion: a prospective study of a new technique. Aust N Z J Surg. 2000;70:371–3.

88. Soontrapornchai P, Simapatanapong T. Comparison of open and laparoscopic secure placement of peritoneal dialysis catheters. Surg Endosc. 2005;19:137–9.

89. Attaluri V, Lebeis C, Brethauer S, Rosenblatt S. Advanced laparoscopic techniques significantly improve function of peritoneal dialysis catheters. J Am Coll Surg. 2010;211(6):699–704.

90. Ogunc G, Tuncer M, Ogunc D, Yardimsever M, Ersoy F. Laparoscopic omental fixation technique versus open surgical placement of peritoneal dialysis catheters. Surg Endosc. 2003;17:1749–55.

91. Crabtree JH, Fishman A. A laparoscopic method for optimal peritoneal dialysis access. Am Surg. 2005;71(2):135–43.

92. Wright MJ, Bel'eed K, Johnson BF, Eadington DW, Sellars L, Farr MJ. Randomized prospective comparison of laparoscopic and open peritoneal dialysis catheter insertion. Perit Dial Int. 1999;19:372–5.

93. Draganic B, James A, Booth M, Gani JS. Comparative experience of a simple technique for laparoscopic chronic ambulatory peritoneal dialysis catheter placement. Aust N Z J Surg. 1998;68:735–9.

94. Blessing Jr WD, Ross JM, Kennedy CI, Richardson WS. Laparoscopic-assisted peritoneal dialysis catheter placement, an improvement on the single trocar technique. Am Surg. 2005;71:1042–6.

95. Jwo SC, Chen KS, Lee CC, Chen HY. Prospective randomized study for comparison of open surgery with laparoscopic-assisted placement of Tenckhoff peritoneal dialysis catheter – a single center experience and literature review. J Surg Res. 2010;159:489–96.

96. Gajjar AH, Rhoden DH, Kathuria P, Kaul R, Udupa AD, Jennings WC. Peritoneal dialysis catheters: laparoscopic versus traditional placement techniques and outcomes. Am J Surg. 2007;194:872–5; discussion 875–876.

97. Daschner M, Gfrorer S, Zachariou Z, Mehls O, Schaefer F. Laparoscopic Tenckhoff catheter implantation in children. Perit Dial Int. 2002;22:22–6.

98. Jwo SC, Chen KS, Lin YY. Video-assisted laparoscopic procedures in peritoneal dialysis. Surg Endosc. 2003;17:1666–70.

99. Frost JH, Bagul A. A brief recap of tips and surgical manoeuvres to enhance optimal outcome of surgically placed peritoneal dialysis catheters. Int J Nephrol. 2012;251584

100. Ogunc G. Minilaparoscopic extraperitoneal tunneling with omentopexy: a new technique for CAPD catheter placement. Perit Dial Int. 2005;25:551–5.

101. Batey CA, Crane JJ, Jenkins MA, Johnston TD, Munch LC. Minilaparoscopy-assisted placement of Tenckhoff catheters: an improved technique to facilitate peritoneal dialysis. J Endourol. 2002;16:681–4.

102. Varela JE, Elli EF, Vanuno D, Horgan S. Minilaparoscopic placement of a peritoneal dialysis catheter. Surg Endosc. 2003;7:2025–7.

103. Yun EJ, Meng MV, Brennan TV, McAninch JW, Santucci RA, Rogers SJ. Novel microlaparoscopic technique for peritoneal dialysis catheter placement. Urology. 2003;61:1026–8.

104. Crabtree JH, Fishman A. A laparoscopic approach under local anesthesia for peritoneal dialysis access. Perit Dial Int. 2000;20:757–65.

105. Bhoyrul S, Mori T, Way LW. Radially expanding dilatation. A superior method of laparoscopic trocar access. Surg Endosc. 1996;10:775–8.

106. Fleming RYD, Dougherty TB, Feig BW. The safety of helium for abdominal insufflation. Surg Endosc. 1997;11:230–4.

107. McMahon AJ, Baxter JN, Murray W, Imrie CW, Kenny G, O'Dwyer PJ. Helium pneumoperitoneum for laparoscopic cholecystectomy: ventilatory and blood gas changes. Br J Surg. 1994;81:1033–6.

108. Neuberger TJ, Andrus CH, Wittgen CM, Wade TP, Kaminski DL. Prospective comparison of helium versus carbon dioxide pneumoperitoneum. Gastrointest Endosc. 1996;43:38–41.

109. Davis WT, Dageforde LA, Moore DE. Laparoscopic versus open peritoneal dialysis catheter insertion cost analysis. J Surg Res. 2014;187(1):182–8.

110. Chen S-Y, Chen T-W, Lin S-H, Chen C-J, Yu J-C, Lin C-H. Does previous abdominal surgery increase postoperative complication rates in continuous

ambulatory peritoneal dialysis? Perit Dial Int. 2007;27:557–9.

111. Wang JY, Chen FM, Huang TJ, Hou MF, Huang CJ, Chan HM, Cheng KI, Cheng HC, Hsieh JS. Laparoscopic assisted placement of peritoneal dialysis catheters for selected patients with previous abdominal operation. J Invest Surg. 2005;18:59–62.

112. Lu CT, Watson DI, Elias TJ, Faull RJ, Clarkson AR, Bannister KM. Laparoscopic placement of peritoneal dialysis catheters: 7 years experience. ANZ J Surg. 2003;73:109–11.

113. Crabtree JH, Burchette RJ. Effect of prior abdominal surgery, peritonitis, and adhesions on catheter function and long-term outcome on peritoneal dialysis. Am Surg. 2009;75:140–7.

114. Henderson S, Brown E, Levy J. Safety and efficacy of percutaneous insertion of peritoneal dialysis catheters under sedation and local anaesthetic. Nephrol Dial Transplant. 2009 Nov;24(11):3499–504.

115. Nicholson ML, Donnelly PK, Burton PR, Veitch PS, Walls J. Factors influencing peritoneal catheter survival in continuous ambulatory peritoneal dialysis. Ann R Coll Surg Engl. 1990;72:368–72.

116. Gadallah MF, Pervez A, el-Shahawy MA, Sorrells D, Zibari G, McDonald J, Work J. Peritoneoscopic versus surgical placement of peritoneal dialysis catheters: a prospective randomized study on outcome. Am J Kidney Dis. 1999;33(1):118–22.

117. Keshvari A, Fazeli MS, Meysamie A, Seifi S, Taromloo MK. The effects of previous abdominal operations and intraperitoneal adhesions on the outcome of peritoneal dialysis catheters. Perit Dial Int. 2008;30:41–5.

118. Numanoglu A, Rasche L, Roth MA, McCulloch MI, Rode H. Laparoscopic insertion with tip suturing, omentectomy, and ovariopexy improves lifespan of peritoneal dialysis catheters in children. J Laparoendosc Adv Surg Tech A. 2008;18:302–5.

119. McIntosh G, Hurst PA, Young AE. The 'omental hitch' for the prevention of obstruction to peritoneal dialysis catheters. Br J Surg. 1985;72:880.

120. Crabtree JH, Fishman A. Laparoscopic omentectomy for peritoneal dialysis catheter flow obstruction: a case report and review of the literature. Surg Laparosc Endosc Percutan Tech. 1999;9:228–33.

121. Crabtree JH, Fishman A. Selective performance of prophylactic omentopexy during laparoscopic implantation of peritoneal dialysis catheters. Surg Laparosc Endosc Percutan Tech. 2003;13:180–4.

122. Goh YH. Omental folding: a novel laparoscopic technique for salvaging peritoneal dialysis catheters. Perit Dial Int. 2008;28:626–31.

123. Medani S, Shantier M, Hussein W, Wall C, Mellotte G. A comparative analysis of percutaneous and open surgical techniques for peritoneal catheter placement. Perit Dial Int. 2012;32(6):628–35.

124. Ozener C, Bihorac A, Akoglu E. Technical survival of CAPD catheters: comparison between percutaneous and conventional surgical placement techniques. Nephrol Dial Transplant. 2001;16:1893–9.

125. Nicholas J, Thomas M, Adkins R, Sandhu K, Smith S, Odum J, Dasgupta I. Percutaneous and surgical peritoneal dialysis catheter placements have comparable outcomes in the modern era. Perit Dial Int. 2014;34:552–6.

126. Medani S, Hussein W, Shantier M, Flynn R, Wall C, Mellotte G. Comparison of percutaneous and open surgical techniques for first-time peritoneal dialysis catheter placement in the unbreached peritoneum. Perit Dial Int. 2015;35(5):576–85.

127. Tullavardhana T, Akranurakkul P, Ungkitphaiboon W, Songtish D. Surgical versus percutaneous techniques for peritoneal dialysis catheter placement: a meta-analysis of the outcomes. Ann Med Surg (Lond). 2016;10:11–8.

128. Lo WK, Lui SL, Li FK, Choy BY, Lam MF, et al. A prospective randomized study on three different peritoneal dialysis catheters. Perit Dial Int. 2003;23(Suppl 2):S127–31.

129. Hagen SM, van Alphen AM, Ijzermans JN, Dor FJ. Laparoscopic versus open peritoneal dialysis catheter insertion, the LOCI-trial: a study protocol. BMC Surg. 2011;(11):35.

130. Strippoli GFM, Tong A, Johnson D, et al. Catheter-related interventions to prevent peritonitis in peritoneal dialysis: a systematic review of randomized, controlled trials. J Am Soc Nephrol. 2004;15:2735–46.

131. Xie H, Zhang W, Cheng J, He Q. Laparoscopic versus open catheter placement in peritoneal dialysis patients: a systematic review and meta-analysis. BMC Nephrol. 2012;13(1):69.

132. Hagen SM, Lafranca JA, Steyerberg EW, IJzermans JN, Dor FJ. Laparoscopic versus open peritoneal dialysis catheter insertion: a meta-analysis. PLoS One. 2013;8(2):e56351.

133. Lund L, Jonler M. Peritoneal dialysis catheter placement: is laparoscopy an option? Int Urol Nephrol. 2007;39:625–8.

134. Li JR, Chen WM, Yang CK, Shu KH, Ou YC, et al. A novel method of laparoscopy-assisted peritoneal dialysis catheter placement. Surg Laparosc Endosc Percutan Tech. 2011;21:106–10.

135. The CARI Guidelines. Evidence for peritonitis treatment and prophylaxis: timing of commencement of dialysis after peritoneal dialysis catheter insertion. Nephrology (Carlton). 2004;9(Suppl 3):S76–7.

136. Dombros N, Dratwa M, Feriani M, Gokal R, Heimburger O, Krediet R, Plum J, Rodrigues A, Selgas R, Struijk D, Verger C. European best practice guidelines for peritoneal dialysis. 3 peritoneal access. Nephrol Dial Transplant. 2005;20(Suppl 9):ix8–ix12.

137. Figueiredo A, Goh BL, Jenkins S, Johnson DW, Mactier R, et al. Clinical practice guidelines for peritoneal access. Perit Dial Int. 2010;30:424–9.

138. Ranganathan D, Baer R, Fassett RG, et al. Randomised controlled trial to determine the appropriate time to initiate peritoneal dialysis after

insertion of catheter to minimise complications (Timely PD study). BMC Nephrol. 2010;11:11.

139. Cheng YL, Chau KF, Choi KS, et al. Peritoneal catheter related complications: a comparison between hemodialysis and intermittent peritoneal dialysis in the break-in period. Adv Perit Dial. 1996;12:231–5.

140. Patel UD, Mottes TA, Flynn JT. Delayed compared with immediate use of peritoneal catheter in pediatric peritoneal dialysis. Adv Perit Dial. 2001;17: 253–9.

141. Ghaffari A. Urgent-start peritoneal dialysis: a quality improvement report. Am J Kidney Dis. 2012;59(3):400–8.

142. Casaretto A, Rosario R, Kotzker WR, Pagan-Rosario Y, Groenhoff C, Guest S. Urgent-start peritoneal dialysis: report from a U.S. private nephrology practice. Adv Perit Dial. 2012;28:102–5.

143. Lobbedez T, Lecouf A, Ficheux M, Henri P, Hurault de Ligny B, Ryckelynck JP. Is rapid initiation of peritoneal dialysis feasible in unplanned dialysis patients? A single-centre experience. Nephrol Dial Transplant. 2008;23(10):3290–4.

144. Moran J, Shapiro M, Ghafferi A, Milligan T, Swanzy K. Urgent-start peritoneal dialysis: a clinical process improvement report. Presented at: 33rd Annual Dialysis Conference; Seattle, WA. 9–12 Mar 2013.

145. McClernon M. Rapid PD start: single-center experience in 30 patients—nursing perspective. Presented at: 33rd Annual Dialysis Conference; Seattle, WA, 2013.

146. Balsera C, Majirsky J, Malone L. Urgent start program: an alternative protocol. Presented at: 33rd Annual Dialysis Conference; Seattle, WA. 2013. – Hartley J. Rapid PD start: single-center experiences in 30 patients—administrator perspective. Presented at: 33rd Annual Dialysis Conference; Seattle, WA, 2013.

147. Jayavelu B, Cohen R, Kumar V. Rapid-start PD: single center experience in 30 patients—clinical perspective. Presented at: 33rd Annual Dialysis Conference; Seattle, WA, 2013.

148. Ludden R. Rapid PD start: single-center experience in thirty patients—renal dietician's perspective. Presented at: 33rd Annual Dialysis Conference; Seattle, WA, 2013.

149. Flanigan S. Rapid PD start: single-center experience in 30 patients—social worker perspective. Presented at: 33rd Annual Dialysis Conference; Seattle, WA, 2013.

150. Povlsen JV, Ivarsen P. How to start the late referred ESRD patient urgently on chronic APD. Nephrol Dial Transplant. 2006;21(Suppl 2):ii56–9.

151. Twardowski ZJ, Nichols WK. Peritoneal dialysis access and exit site including surgical aspects. In: Gokal R, Khanna R, Krediet R, Nolph K, editors. Textbook of peritoneal dialysis. 2nd ed. Dordrecht: Kluwer Academic; 2000. p. 307–61.

152. Ponce SP, Pierratos A, Izatt S, et al. Comparison of the survival and complications of three permanent peritoneal dialysis catheters. Perit Dial Bull. 1982;2:82–6.

153. Francis DMA, Donnelly PK, Veitch PS, et al. Surgical aspects of continuous ambulatory peritoneal dialysis: 3 years experience. Br J Surg. 1984;71:225–9.

154. Ash SR, Daugirdas JT. Peritoneal access devices. In: Daugirdas JT, Blake PG, Ing TS, editors. Handbook of dialysis. Dordrecht: Kluver Academic; 2001. p. 309–43.

155. Scabardi M, Ronco C, Chiaramonte S, Feriani M, Agostini F, La Greca G. Dynamic catheterography in the early diagnosis of peritoneal catheter malfunction. Int J Artif Organs. 1992;15:358–64.

156. Hollett MD, Marn CS, Ellis JH, Francis IR, Swartz RD. Complications of continuous ambulatory peritoneal dialysis: evaluation with CT peritoneography. AJR Am J Roentgenol. 1992;159: 983–9.

157. Cakir B, Kirbas I, Cevik B, Ulu EM, Bayrak A, Coskun M. Complications of continuous ambulatory peritoneal dialysis: evaluation with CT. Diagn Interv Radiol. 2008;14:212–20.

158. Ovnat A, Dukhno O, Pinsk I, Peiser J, Levy I. The laparoscopic option in the management of peritoneal dialysis catheter revision. Surg Endosc. 2002;16: 698–9.

159. Stadermann MB, Rusthoven E, van de Kar NC, Hendriksen A, Monnens LA, Schroder CH. Local fibrinolytic therapy with urokinase for peritoneal dialysis catheter obstruction in children. Perit Dial Int. 2002;22:84–6.

160. Shea M, Hmiel SP, Beck AM. Use of tissue plasminogen activator for thrombolysis in occluded peritoneal dialysis catheters in children. Adv Perit Dial. 2001;17:249–52.

161. Zorzanello MM, Fleming WJ, Prowant BE. Use of tissue plasminogen activator in peritoneal dialysis catheters: a literature review and one center's experience. Nephrol Nurs J. 2004;31:534–7.

162. Dobrashian RD, Conway B, Hutchison A, Gokal R, Taylor PM. The repositioning of migrated Tenckhoff continuous ambulatory peritoneal dialysis catheters under fluoroscopic control. Br J Radiol. 1999; 72:452–6.

163. Savader SJ, Lund G, Scheel PJ, Prescott C, Feeley N, Singh H, Osterman Jr FA. Guide wire directed manipulation of malfunctioning peritoneal dialysis catheters: a critical analysis. J Vasc Interv Radiol. 1997;8:957–63.

164. Jones B, McLaughlin K, Mactier RA, Porteous C. Tenckhoff catheter salvage by closed stiff-wire manipulation without fluoroscopic control. Perit Dial Int. 1998;18:415–8.

165. Gadallah MF, Arora N, Arumugam R, Moles K. Role of Fogarty catheter manipulation in management of migrated, nonfunctional peritoneal dialysis catheters. Am J Kidney Dis. 2000;35:301–5.

166. Korten G, Arendt R, Brugmann E, Klein B. Relocation of a peritoneal catheter without surgical intervention. Perit Dial Bull. 1983;3:46.

167. Hughes CR, Angotti DM, Jubelirer RA. Laparoscopic repositioning of a continuous ambulatory peritoneal dialysis (CAPD) catheter. Surg Endosc. 1994;8(9): 1108–9.

168. Zakaria HM. Laparoscopic management of malfunctioning peritoneal dialysis catheters. Oman Med J. 26:171–4. Surg Endosc 2011;8:1108-1109.

169. Cheung CK, Khwaja A. Chylous ascites: an unusual complication of peritoneal dialysis. A case report and literature review. Perit Dial Int. 2008;28: 229–31.

170. García Falcón T, Rodríguez-Carmona A, Pérez Fontán M, Fernández Rivera C, Bouza P, Rodríguez Lozano I, et al. Complications of permanent catheter implantation for peritoneal dialysis: incidence and risk factors. Adv Perit Dial. 1994;10:206–9.

171. Levy RI, Wenk RE. Chyloperitoneum in a peritoneal dialysis patient. Am J Kidney Dis. 2001;38:E12.

172. Ramos R, Gonzalez MT, Moreso F, et al. Chylous ascites: an unusual complication of percutaneous peritoneal catheter implantation. Perit Dial Int. 2006;26:722–3.

173. Aalami O, Allen D, Organ C. Chylous ascites: a collective review. Surgery. 2000;128:761–78.

174. Chen J, Lin RK, Hassanein T. Use of Orlistat (Xenical) to treat chylous ascites. J Clin Gastroenterol. 2005;39:831–3.

175. Lee PH, Lin CL, Lai PC, Yang CW. Octreotide therapy for chylous ascites in a chronic dialysis patient. Nephrology. 2005;10:344–7.

176. Geary B, Wade B, Wollman W, El-Galley R. Laparoscopic repair of chylous ascites. J Urol. 2004; 171:1231–2.

177. Khanna R, Oreopoulos DG, Dombros N, et al. Continuous ambulatory dialysis after 3 years: still a promising treatment. Perit Dial Bull. 1981;1:24–34.

178. Whiting M, Smith N, Agar JWN. Vaginal peritoneal dialysate leakage per fallopian tubes. Perit Dial Int. 1995;15(1):85.

Surgical Considerations for Open Placement of Peritoneal Dialysis Catheters

Monika A. Krezalek

The Early History of Peritoneal Dialysis

Georg Ganter first suggested the use of peritoneal membrane for the purpose of dialysis in 1923 after demonstrating its efficacy in an animal model of uremia following ureter ligation [1]. At the same time, Tracy Putnam published his research on the solute exchange potential of the peritoneal membrane [2]. In 1946, Frank, Seligman and Fine reported first instance of successful use of peritoneal irrigation as the treatment for acute renal failure [3]. Following these discoveries, intermittent peritoneal dialysis was used for the treatment of acute renal failure for short-term replacement of kidney function. Peritoneal dialysis for management of chronic kidney failure did not become popular until much later, due to the fears of underdialysis, malnutrition, and frequent complications of peritonitis. In 1959, Maxwell et al. described a technique of peritoneal dialysis similar to what is used today, utilizing commercial solutions and disposable tubing [4]. In 1968 Tenckhoff and Schechter revolutionized the field when they published a novel indwelling catheter implantation method using Dacron cuffed silicone catheters that allowed for long-term peritoneal dialysis in six

patients with end-stage renal failure [5]. Finally, in 1976 Popovich, Moncrief and colleagues introduced the concept of continuous ambulatory peritoneal dialysis (CAPD). The authors demonstrated that patients could free themselves of the constraints of a hemodialysis machine and perform dialysis independently, avoiding dietary restrictions and improving their daily life. By 1980, CAPD was established as a proven method of renal replacement therapy [6].

Recent Trends in Peritoneal Dialysis and Catheter Implantation Techniques

Continuous ambulatory peritoneal dialysis has clear and undeniable benefits over hemodialysis, including improved patient autonomy, quality of life, preservation of residual renal function, slight survival advantage during the first 2 years of peritoneal dialysis, preservation of vascular access, as well as economic benefit of lower costs [7–14]. Despite these benefits and continued improvement in outcomes, peritoneal dialysis utilization in the United States has declined. Peritoneal dialysis use waned from 15% in mid-1980 to 8% in 2010, with slight increase to 9% over the recent years [15, 16]. These rates remain low when compared to other countries [17]. Peritoneal catheters are placed using variety of modalities by surgeons, nephrologists and interventional radiologists. The technique used

M.A. Krezalek, MD
Department of General Surgery,
The University of Chicago, 5841 S Maryland,
MC6030, Chicago, IL 60637, USA
e-mail: monika.krezalek@uchospitals.edu

© Springer International Publishing AG 2017
S. Haggerty (ed.), *Surgical Aspects of Peritoneal Dialysis*, DOI 10.1007/978-3-319-52821-2_6

for catheter placement plays an important role in the success of peritoneal dialysis, as mechanical complications related to implantation are among the leading causes of failure of peritoneal dialysis and need to switch to hemodialysis [18, 19]. Open surgical catheter insertion was first described in 1972 by Brewer and colleagues and maintained the status of the most commonly used modality for over 30 years. However, with introduction of less invasive techniques, its use has fallen to 27% in the United States [20]. Nevertheless, it still remains the main technique used at certain hospitals worldwide and for certain patient populations. In the remainder of the chapter we focus on the open peritoneal dialysis catheter insertion technique and how it compares to the other currently used modalities in terms of their technique and outcomes.

Patient Selection and Pre-operative Preparation for Open Technique

Contraindications to adult peritoneal dialysis include significant defects of the anterior abdominal wall, abdominal wall or intraperitoneal infections, loss of peritoneal function, inflammatory bowel disease, and patient's inability to perform daily dialysis care [21, 22]. Severe intra-abdominal adhesions and obesity have been frequently cited as relative contraindication to CAPD, and remain as such for open peritoneal dialysis catheter placement. However, with the increased use of laparoscopy, safe peritoneal dialysis catheter implantation is now possible for both of these patient populations.

Regardless of the technique used, it is imperative to mark the patient in the pre-operative waiting area while they are standing and laying supine. The belt line should be marked and the exit site should be planned above or below the beltline in direct line of patient's vision to ensure comfort and ease of peritoneal dialysis in the future (Fig. 6.1). An extended catheter with pre-sternal exit site should be considered for obese patients and patients with ostomies, to further assist with visualization and ease of CAPD. Patients should be examined for presence of abdominal wall and inguinal hernias, and if noted,

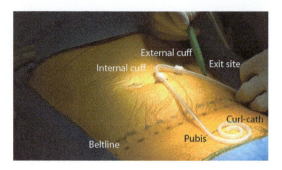

Fig. 6.1 Optimal peritoneal dialysis catheter positioning. Patient's beltline is marked preoperatively, while supine and standing to ensure ease of future dialysis. Following sterile preparation, the distal end of the catheter (in this case curl-cath) is aligned with the pubis. The insertion site is marked to the left of midline at the site of the distal cuff. Exit site is planned at least 2–3 cm caudal to the proximal cuff

laparoscopy should be considered. Bladder decompression with a Foley catheter should be utilized to prevent inadvertent placement of the catheter within the bladder. Cathartics should be given pre- and post-operatively to prevent constipation.

Catheter Types and Their Advantages

Tenckhoff peritoneal dialysis catheter, made of flexible silicone tubing, is the most commonly used catheter presently. A wide variety of peritoneal dialysis catheters are available and they vary based on the configuration of the extraperitoneal and intraperitoneal catheter segments.

The most commonly used designs of the extraperitoneal catheter segment differ based on the number of cuffs and on the angle of the subcutaneous portion. Peritoneal dialysis catheters are equipped with one or two Dacron cuffs that are located at the proximal catheter end. Majority of surgeons prefer to use double cuffed catheters due to the reported lower risk of infectious complications [23, 24]. The cuff allows for tissue ingrowth, effectively fixing the catheter in place, guarding against leaks and infections. The superficial cuff rests in the subcutaneous tissue, at least 2–3 cm from the exit site; while the distal cuff lays within the rectus muscle (Fig. 6.2). The orientation of the subcutaneous segment can be

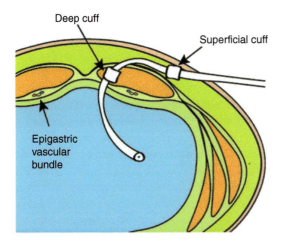

Deep cuff

Superficial cuff

Epigastric vascular bundle

Fig. 6.2 Peritoneal dialysis catheter trajectory as it passes through the anterior abdominal wall during open insertion technique. The catheter is inserted to the left of midline with a curved subcutaneous tunnel. The location of the distal cuff should be at least 2–3 cm from the exit site to prevent cuff extrusion. The distal cuff is located within the rectus muscle above the peritoneum and medial to the epigastric vascular bundle

straight or permanently bent in a swan neck configuration. Some studies show that swan neck catheters have lower rates of mechanical catheter dysfunction from decreased torque on the intraabdominal portion of the catheter, resulting in lower rates of catheter migration [25, 26]. Furthermore, swan neck catheters may lead to lower rates of exit site infections when compared to upward directed straight catheters [24]. In general, catheter exit site should always be directed downward or laterally to minimize infection.

The design of the intraperitoneal segment of the catheter optimizes dialysate exchange, while minimizing the risk of migration and obstruction by peritoneal surfaces, bowel, or omentum. The intraperitoneal design is either straight or coiled, with a number of side openings facilitating easy dialysate exchange [27]. Some studies show that coiled catheters result in less discomfort to the patient during dialysate infusion, which is thought to be due to dispersion of the inflow force. However, current evidence is conflicting in terms of dysfunction rates and catheter survival in regards to intraperitoneal catheter design [24, 26, 28, 29].

Technique of Open Peritoneal Dialysis Catheter Insertion

Open surgical peritoneal dialysis catheter placement is performed using a mini-laparotomy incision. Historically, patients were placed under general anesthesia for catheter insertion, however in the mid-1980, the trend shifted to the predominant use of local anesthesia and conscious sedation reducing the length of surgical recovery and anesthetic complications [30]. Initially, catheters were placed using a midline infraumbilical vertical or transverse incision, or supraumbilical incision in those patients with prior celiotomy scars and obese abdomen. Although the catheter trajectory was slightly off-midline as it passed through the rectus muscle, the midline insertion technique resulted in high rates of peritoneal fluid leakage, cuff extrusion and herniation [31, 32]. In order to reduce these complications, paramedian incision was adopted as the new standard in adult patient population [32–34]. Currently, midline skin incision with a paramedian trajectory through the rectus muscle is still utilized in the pediatric population due to their smaller size and thinner abdominal wall [35].

Following sterile preparation, the catheter is positioned over the abdomen, preferentially to the left of the midline. Positioning of the peritoneal dialysis catheter on the left side is thought to result in lower incidence of catheter migration due to downward directed peristaltic waves of the left colon [36]. The distal portion of the catheter is positioned over the pubis (Fig. 6.1). The insertion site is planned at the level of the distal Dacron cuff. The exit site is planned 2–3 cm away from the proximal cuff to prevent cuff extrusion and directed downward to minimize the risk of tunnel infection. Once marking is complete, the insertion site is infiltrated with local anesthetic and a 4–5 cm incision is made and carried down to the anterior rectus sheath which is sharply opened. Muscle fibers are split bluntly to expose the posterior rectus sheath and the peritoneum, which are also entered sharply. Patient should be placed in a Trendelenburg position, effectively shifting the bowel cephalad and freeing up the pelvis. The catheter is then inserted with the help of a stylet

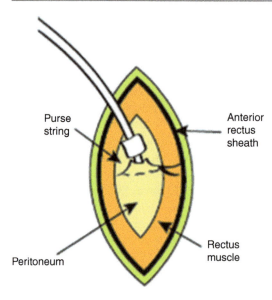

Fig. 6.3 Peritoneal dialysis catheter deep cuff is secured within the rectus muscle. Purse string suture is used to secure the catheter at the level of the peritoneum and the anterior rectus sheath

and blindly directed towards the pelvis. Catheter is secured to the peritoneum using a purse string suture to prevent peritoneal fluid leaks and minimize the risk of peritonitis and tunnel infection. Peritoneal purse string is generally placed just below the distal Dacron cuff when double cuffed catheter is used (Fig. 6.3). The anterior rectus sheath is also tightly closed around the catheter with purse string suture, trapping the distal cuff within the rectus muscle [34]. The extraperitoneal catheter segment is tunneled in the subcutaneous space following the previously marked trajectory towards the exit site. Care is taken to position the proximal Dacron cuff at least 2–3 cm from the exit site to prevent cuff extrusion (Fig. 6.1). Finally, catheter is tested with saline infusion, skin is closed and sterile dressing applied.

In patients who are found to have a large omentum, a partial omental resection (omentectomy) can be performed through the mini-laparotomy incision. Alternatively and to avoid the risk of bleeding complications with omentectomy, "omental hitch" (omentopexy) has been described with open peritoneal dialysis catheter placement. During omentopexy, the bulky omentum is displaced from the pelvis and anchored to the

anterior abdominal wall in the epigastric region [37], which may necessitate a larger incision.

According to the International Society for Peritoneal Dialysis Clinical Practice Guidelines, catheter insertion should be planned at least 2 weeks before peritoneal dialysis start, to allow for tissue healing, catheter incorporation, as well as patient training [38]. In cases when earlier start is necessary, peritoneal dialysis can be initiated with small dialysate volumes in the supine position [39]. However, catheter-related mechanical complications may be higher with earlier peritoneal dialysis start following open insertion technique [40].

Complications of Open Peritoneal Dialysis Catheter Placement

The most common complications of open peritoneal dialysis catheter placement technique include infections, peri-catheter dialysate leakage, and mechanical catheter dysfunction. Infectious complications related to the catheter placement are defined as occurring within 2 weeks of surgery and include peritonitis and tunnel infections. Technique-related mechanical catheter problems include (1) catheter inflow and outflow obstruction due to omental entrapment, adhesions and fibrin plugs, (2) catheter migration into the upper abdomen, often resulting in pain with dialysate infusion and possible obstruction, (3) peritoneal fluid leakage around the catheter, which may predispose to infectious complications. Rare intraoperative complications include bowel or bladder perforation and bleeding from inadvertent vascular injury, requiring extension of the laparotomy incision for management and abandonment of the peritoneal dialysis catheter placement due to excessive risk of peritonitis.

Comparison with Other Insertion Techniques

One benefit of open peritoneal dialysis catheter insertion is the ability to perform the operation under local anesthesia and conscious sedation with faster recovery and lesser risk to the patient.

Compared to blind percutaneous insertion, placement of the catheter under direct surgical vision permits limited intra-operative peritoneal assessment, lowering rates of undiagnosed bowel injury.

Traditional open peritoneal dialysis catheter insertion techniques as described above, have been historically associated with high catheter dysfunction rates up to 38% due to the blind placement of the catheter towards the pelvis and the inability to perform complete lysis of adhesions. These catheter problems include mechanical issues, such as obstruction to dialysate flow due to catheter entrapment in the omentum or adhesions, pain and flow obstruction related to catheter migration, and peri-catheter fluid leakage.

When compared to blind percutaneous bedside peritoneal dialysis catheter insertion using Seldinger technique, open technique results in similar or improved catheter outcomes, depending on the series being reviewed. Nicholson et al. published the results of their large cohort comparing percutaneous to open midline peritoneal dialysis catheter insertion, showing a significant improvement in catheter survival with the use of open technique [41]. Blind percutaneous technique has been historically associated with highest rates of catheter malposition and failure rates up to 65%, as well as increased risks of hemorrhage and injury to the bowel [5]. However, others show acceptable rates of dysfunction and low rates of bowel injury, comparable to open technique [42–46]. Percutaneous technique benefits include faster recovery and ambulation, less delays associated with scheduling of an operation, as well as cost saving benefits. It has been recommended for low risk patients in developing countries with poor resources [47].

Fluoroscopic-guided peritoneal dialysis catheter placement method also utilizes Seldinger technique, with the peritoneal entry of the access needle confirmed by instillation of contrast under fluoroscopy, as well as confirmation of guide wire location in the pelvis. Ultrasound guidance is often used as an adjunct to avoid injury to the inferior epigastric vessels. Catheter-related outcomes appear to be similar to those with open peritoneal dialysis catheter insertion method,

depending on the series being reviewed [48–51]. Additionally, hollow viscous perforation rates range from 0% to 4.4% [48, 52].

The use of basic laparoscopy was incorporated to visualize the peritoneum, perform lysis of adhesions when necessary, and direct the catheter tip towards the pelvis under direct vision. Basic laparoscopy, as will be seen in later chapters, is associated with slightly lower catheter dysfunction rates, up to 14% [53, 54]. In order to further lower catheter dysfunction rates and thus improve peritoneal dialysis failure rates, additional laparoscopic maneuvers such as catheter fixation, rectus sheath tunnel and omentopexy have been used, either alone or in combination, collectively called the advanced laparoscopic technique. Utilization of the advanced laparoscopic technique has been shown to result in even lower rates of catheter dysfunction. This is especially true when combination of these techniques is used, with dysfunction rates of 4.7% [55, 56]. Nonetheless, the available data comparing these modalities in terms of catheter dysfunction is sparse, conflicting and difficult to compare between studies because of lack of standardization and large heterogeneity of the insertion techniques used.

Current Recommendations for Open Peritoneal Dialysis Catheter Insertion

Open peritoneal dialysis catheter placement technique is ideal for patients who are not good candidates for general anesthesia due to their co-morbidities. Patients suspected of having peritoneal adhesive disease due to history of prior operations may not be good candidates for open peritoneal dialysis catheter insertion method due to the difficulty with ensuring proper catheter placement in the pelvis and risk of intra-operative complications, such as bowel injury and bleeding. Therefore, patients with history of prior intra-abdominal operations should be considered for laparoscopic approach to peritoneal dialysis catheter placement, when possible. Patients with obese abdomen or evidence of anterior abdominal wall or inguinal hernias should also be considered for laparoscopy, as hernia repair can be performed simultaneously with catheter placement. Ultimately, the choice of the technique rests with the surgeon, depending on their experience. Open peritoneal dialysis catheter insertion technique remains a safe and viable option for certain patient populations.

References

1. Teschner M, Heidland A, Klassen A, et al. Georg Ganter – a pioneer of peritoneal dialysis and his tragic academic demise at the hand of the Nazi regime. J Nephrol. 2004;17(3):457–60.
2. Putnam TJ. The living peritoneum as a dialyzing membrane. Am J Physiol. 1923;63:548–65.
3. Frank HA, Seligman AM, Fine J. Treatment of uremia after acute renal failure by peritoneal irrigation. JAMA. 1946;130:703–5.
4. Maxwell MH, Rockney RE, Kleeman CR, et al. Peritoneal dialysis. 1. Technique and applications. JAMA. 1959;170(8):917–24.
5. Tenckhoff H, Schechter H. A bacteriologically safe peritoneal access device. Trans Am Soc Artif Intern Organs. 1968;14:181–7.
6. Nolph KD, Sorkin M, Rubin J, et al. Continuous ambulatory peritoneal dialysis: three-year experience at one center. Ann Intern Med. 1980;92(5):609–13.
7. Rubin HR, Fink NE, Plantinga LC, et al. Patient ratings of dialysis care with peritoneal dialysis vs hemodialysis. JAMA. 2004;291(6):697–703.
8. Juergensen E, Wuerth D, Finkelstein SH, et al. Hemodialysis and peritoneal dialysis: patients' assessment of their satisfaction with therapy and the impact of the therapy on their lives. Clin J Am Soc Nephrol CJASN. 2006;1(6):1191–6.
9. Moist LM, Port FK, Orzol SM, et al. Predictors of loss of residual renal function among new dialysis patients. J Am Soc Nephrol JASN. 2000;11(3):556–64.
10. Tam P. Peritoneal dialysis and preservation of residual renal function. Perit Dial Int J Int Soc Perit Dial. 2009;29(Suppl 2):S108–10.
11. Fenton SS, Schaubel DE, Desmeules M, et al. Hemodialysis versus peritoneal dialysis: a comparison of adjusted mortality rates. Am J Kidney Dis Off J Natl Kidney. 1997;30(3):334–42.
12. Heaf JG, Løkkegaard H, Madsen M. Initial survival advantage of peritoneal dialysis relative to haemodialysis. Nephrol Dial Transplant Off Publ Eur Dial Transpl Assoc Eur Ren Assoc. 2002;17(1):112–7.
13. Klarenbach SW, Tonelli M, Chui B, et al. Economic evaluation of dialysis therapies. Nat Rev Nephrol. 2014;10(11):644–52.
14. Shih Y-CT, Guo A, Just PM, et al. Impact of initial dialysis modality and modality switches on Medicare expenditures of end-stage renal disease patients. Kidney Int. 2005;68(1):319–29.
15. Mehrotra R, Kermah D, Fried L, et al. Chronic peritoneal dialysis in the United States: declining utilization despite improving outcomes. J Am Soc Nephrol JASN. 2007;18(10):2781–8.
16. Dalal P, Sangha H, Chaudhary K. In peritoneal dialysis, is there sufficient evidence to make "PD first" therapy? Int J Nephrol. 2011;2011:239515.
17. United States Renal Data System. 2015 USRDS annual data report: epidemiology of kidney disease in the United States. Bethesda: National Institutes of Health, National Institute of Diabetes and Digestive and Kidney Diseases; 2015.
18. Mujais S, Story K. Peritoneal dialysis in the US: evaluation of outcomes in contemporary cohorts. Kidney Int Suppl. 2006;103:S21–6.
19. Shahbazi N, McCormick BB. Peritoneal dialysis catheter insertion strategies and maintenance of catheter function. Semin Nephrol. 2011;31(2):138–51.
20. Brewer TE, Caldwell FT, Patterson RM, et al. Indwelling peritoneal (Tenckhoff) dialysis catheter. Experience with 24 patients. JAMA. 1972;219(8):1011–5.
21. Shetty A, Oreopoulos DG. Peritoneal dialysis: its indications and contraindications. Dial Transplant. 2000;29(2):71–7.
22. NKF KDOQI Guidelines [Internet]. Cited 12 June 2016. Available from: http://www2.kidney.org/professionals/KDOQI/guideline_upHD_PD_VA/.
23. Dell'Aquila R, Chiaramonte S, Rodighiero MP, et al. Rational choice of peritoneal dialysis catheter. Perit Dial Int J Int Soc Perit Dial. 2007;27(Suppl 2):S119–25.
24. Flanigan M, Gokal R. Peritoneal catheters and exit-site practices toward optimum peritoneal access: a review of current developments. Perit Dial Int J Int Soc Perit Dial. 2005;25(2):132–9.
25. Gadallah MF, Mignone J, Torres C, et al. The role of peritoneal dialysis catheter configuration in preventing catheter tip migration. Adv Perit Dial Conf Perit Dial. 2000;16:47–50.
26. Lye WC, Kour NW, van der Straaten JC, et al. A prospective randomized comparison of the Swan neck, coiled, and straight Tenckhoff catheters in patients on CAPD. Perit Dial Int J Int Soc Perit Dial. 1996;16(Suppl 1):S333–5.
27. Peppelenbosch A, van Kuijk WHM, Bouvy ND, et al. Peritoneal dialysis catheter placement technique and complications. NDT Plus. 2008;1(Suppl 4):iv23–8.
28. Nielsen PK, Hemmingsen C, Friis SU, et al. Comparison of straight and curled Tenckhoff peritoneal dialysis catheters implanted by percutaneous technique: a prospective randomized study. Perit Dial Int J Int Soc Perit Dial. 1995;15(1):18–21.
29. Johnson DW, Wong J, Wiggins KJ, et al. A randomized controlled trial of coiled versus straight swanneck Tenckhoff catheters in peritoneal dialysis patients. Am J Kidney Dis Off J Natl Kidney. 2006;48(5):812–21.

30. Robison RJ, Leapman SB, Wetherington GM, et al. Surgical considerations of continuous ambulatory peritoneal dialysis. Surgery. 1984;96(4):723–30.

31. Cronen PW, Moss JP, Simpson T, et al. Tenckhoff catheter placement: surgical aspects. Am Surg. 1985;51(11):627–9.

32. Helfrich GB, Pechan BW, Alijani MR, Barnard WF, Rakowski TA, Winchester JF. Reduction of catheter complications with lateral placement. Perit Dial Bull. 1983;3(4):S2–4.

33. Spence PA, Mathews RE, Khanna R, et al. Improved results with a paramedian technique for the insertion of peritoneal dialysis catheters. Surg Gynecol Obstet. 1985;161(6):585–7.

34. Stegmayr BG. Paramedian insertion of Tenckhoff catheters with three purse-string sutures reduces the risk of leakage. Perit Dial Int J Int Soc Perit Dial. 1993;13(Suppl 2):S124–6.

35. Brandt ML, Brewer ED. Chapter 91 – Peritoneal catheter placement in children A2 – Nissenson, Allen R. In: Fine RN, editor. Handbook of dialysis therapy. 4th ed [Internet]. Philadelphia: W.B. Saunders; 2008. Cited 7 June 2016. p. 1295–301. Available from: http://www.sciencedirect.com/science/article/pii/B978141604197950096X.

36. Twardowski ZJ, Nolph KD, Khanna R, et al. The need for a "Swan Neck" permanently bent, arcuate peritoneal dialysis catheter. Perit Dial Int. 1985;5(4):219–23.

37. McIntosh G, Hurst PA, Young AE. The "omental hitch" for the prevention of obstruction to peritoneal dialysis catheters. Br J Surg. 1985;72(11):880.

38. Figueiredo A, Goh B-L, Jenkins S, et al. Clinical practice guidelines for peritoneal access. Perit Dial Int. 2010;30(4):424–9.

39. Dombros N, Dratwa M, Feriani M, et al. European best practice guidelines for peritoneal dialysis. 3 peritoneal access. Nephrol Dial Transplant Off Publ Eur Dial Transpl Assoc Eur Ren Assoc. 2005;20(Suppl 9):ix8–ix12.

40. Povlsen JV, Ivarsen P. How to start the late referred ESRD patient urgently on chronic APD. Nephrol Dial Transplant Off Publ Eur Dial Transpl Assoc Eur Ren Assoc. 2006;21(Suppl 2):ii56–9.

41. Nicholson ML, Donnelly PK, Burton PR, et al. Factors influencing peritoneal catheter survival in continuous ambulatory peritoneal dialysis. Ann R Coll Surg Engl. 1990;72(6):368–72.

42. Zappacosta AR, Perras ST, Closkey GM. Seldinger technique for Tenckhoff catheter placement. ASAIO Trans Am Soc Artif Intern Organs. 1991;37(1):13–5.

43. Napoli M, Russo F, Mastrangelo F. Placement of peritoneal dialysis catheter by percutaneous method with the Veress needle. Adv Perit Dial Conf Perit Dial. 2000;16:165–9.

44. Allon M, Soucie JM, Macon EJ. Complications with permanent peritoneal dialysis catheters: experience with 154 percutaneously placed catheters. Nephron. 1988;48(1):8–11.

45. Mellotte GJ, Ho CA, Morgan SH, et al. Peritoneal dialysis catheters: a comparison between percutaneous and conventional surgical placement techniques. Nephrol Dial Transplant Off Publ Eur Dial Transpl Assoc Eur Ren Assoc. 1993;8(7):626–30.

46. Medani S, Shantier M, Hussein W, et al. A comparative analysis of percutaneous and open surgical techniques for peritoneal catheter placement. Perit Dial Int J Int Soc Perit Dial. 2012;32(6):628–35.

47. Varughese S, Sundaram M, Basu G, et al. Percutaneous continuous ambulatory peritoneal dialysis (CAPD) catheter insertion – a preferred option for developing countries. Trop Doct. 2010;40(2):104–5.

48. Buffington M. Peritoneal dialysis catheter placement techniques. Open Urol Nephrol J. 2012;5(1):4–11.

49. Moon J-Y, Song S, Jung K-H, et al. Fluoroscopically guided peritoneal dialysis catheter placement: long-term results from a single center. Perit Dial Int J Int Soc Perit Dial. 2008;28(2):163–9.

50. Vaux EC, Torrie PH, Barker LC, et al. Percutaneous fluoroscopically guided placement of peritoneal dialysis catheters – a 10-year experience. Semin Dial. 2008;21(5):459–65.

51. Reddy C, Dybbro PE, Guest S. Fluoroscopically guided percutaneous peritoneal dialysis catheter placement: single center experience and review of the literature. Ren Fail. 2010;32(3):294–9.

52. Abdel-Aal AK, Gaddikeri S, Saddekni S, et al. Technique of peritoneal catheter placement under fl> uroscopic guidance. Radiol Res Pract. 2011;2011:e141707.

53. Draganic B, James A, Booth M, et al. Comparative experience of a simple technique for laparoscopic chronic ambulatory peritoneal dialysis catheter placement. Aust N Z J Surg. 1998;68(10):735–9.

54. Gajjar AH, Rhoden DH, Kathuria P, et al. Peritoneal dialysis catheters: laparoscopic versus traditional placement techniques and outcomes. Am J Surg. 2007;194(6):872. -875-876

55. Crabtree JH, Burchette RJ. Effective use of laparoscopy for long-term peritoneal dialysis access. Am J Surg. 2009;198(1):135–41.

56. Attaluri V, Lebeis C, Brethauer S, et al. Advanced laparoscopic techniques significantly improve function of peritoneal dialysis catheters. J Am Coll Surg. 2010;211(6):699–704.

Fluoroscopic Guided Percutaneous Insertion of PD Catheters

Ahmed Kamel Abdel Aal, Nael Saad,
Wael Darwish, Nael Saad,
and Amr Soliman Moustafa

Introduction

Patients suffering from chronic kidney disease (CKD) progressing to end-stage renal disease (ESRD) undergoing renal replacement therapy may elect to use peritoneal dialysis (PD) or hemodialysis (HD) or pursue pre-emptive renal transplantation. The overall costs for patients receiving PD have been shown to be an average of $20,000 (US) per year lower than for patients receiving in-center HD, the savings to dialysis providers incentivized the use of PD. Despite this

A.K.A. Aal, MD, MSc, PhD (✉)
Department of Radiology, University of Alabama at Birmingham, 619 19th Street South,
Birmingham, AL 35249, USA
e-mail: akamel@uabmc.edu

N. Saad, MD
Department of Radiology, Mallinckrodt Institute of Radiology, Washington University in Saint Louis,
510 S. Kingshighway Blvd, Campus Box 8131,
St. Louis, MO 63110, USA

W. Darwish, MD
Department of Radiology, National Cancer Institute,
Cairo, Egypt
e-mail: doctorwaeldarwish@gmail.com

N. Saad, MD
Department of Radiology, Washington University,
Saint Louis, MO, USA
e-mail: nsaad@wustl.edu

A.S. Moustafa, MD, MSc
Department of Radiology, University of Arkansas for Medical Science, Little Rock, AR, USA
e-mail: dr.asoliman.md@gmail.com

fact, data still shows that more than 90% of ESRD patients receive in-center HD treatments, while patients on PD and home HD combined account for only 10% of these patients [1]. In addition to the favorable economic landscape for PD, the patient-centric factors that may make PD a favorable dialysis option are the ability to perform dialysis at home, largely during the night time allowing for more flexibility during the daytime, less interference with employment schedule, ability to travel, and less dietary restrictions, compared to in-center HD [2]. Recent comparisons of early and late survival between PD and HD suggest an early survival advantage to starting dialysis with PD and a similar longer term survival at 5 years [3, 4].

Therefore, PD offers patients a home dialysis modality which may afford unique life style benefits, allow for greater ease of travel and work accommodation, and is a less costly dialysis modality. These factors have led for some clinicians to adopt a "PD First" position and to consider PD not just for the elective start to dialysis but for more urgent initiation of dialysis in patients presenting late in the course of their disease [2, 5, 6]. The recent interest in "urgent-start PD" raised awareness of the need to more expeditious placement of PD catheters to avoid unnecessary use of temporary vascular access catheters for HD in patients whom would otherwise be considered good candidates for PD.

Therefore, one of the most crucial infrastructure requirements for an urgent-start peritoneal

S. Haggerty (ed.), *Surgical Aspects of Peritoneal Dialysis*, DOI 10.1007/978-3-319-52821-2_7

dialysis program is PD catheter placement within 24–48 h of patient presentation [7]. This requirement faces obstacles in some busy academic institutions and private practices that use laparoscopic PD catheter insertion where there is suboptimal accessibility to surgical services for PD catheter placement due to backlog and waiting lists resulting in difficulties in surgical clinics and operating room scheduling.

These operational inefficiencies drew attention to a different technique for PD catheter placement by interventional radiologists and nephrologists using fluoroscopy and ultrasound guidance [8–13]. This technique is increasingly described and provides a minimally invasive, cost-effective approach to catheter placement which avoids general anesthesia or operating room logistical barriers. Therefore, placement of PD catheters by interventional radiologists and interventional nephrologists may be increasingly requested by nephrology practices, as recent publications have demonstrated the favorable impact of Radiologic placement of PD catheter on PD practices.

In this chapter, the authors will describe in details the technique for placement of PD catheters using ultrasound and fluoroscopic guidance. The technical aspects described in this chapter are believed to represent key steps used in the establishment of high-volume IR-based PD catheter placement programs. The authors will describe the roles of ultrasound and fluoroscopy, provide additional technical comments, and describe pre- and post-procedure care.

Techniques of PD Catheter Placement

Peritoneal dialysis catheter placement can be performed in the operating room by surgeons or by minimally-invasive techniques in radiology suites and outpatient procedure centers. Surgical placement has evolved from simple open laparotomy to basic laparoscopic and advanced laparoscopic techniques that include tunneling of catheter segments within the rectus muscle sheath, adhesiolysis and omentopexy [14, 15].

Percutaneous techniques have included blind placement with rigid trochar or a modified Seldinger technique, and the use of a peritoneoscope [14, 16]. The Seldinger technique has evolved to include initial ultrasound guidance of the introducer needle and subsequent fluoroscopic guidance for guide wire placement and catheter positioning [10, 12]. Successful catheter placement has been described with all of the above techniques and ultimate outcomes may be largely due to the experience and skill of the operator.

Placement by laparotomy and basic laparoscopic techniques has resulted in 82–87% 2-year patency rate [14, 17]. Recently, surgical advances in laparoscopic techniques improved the PD catheter placement technique to involve rectus sheath tunneling of the catheter prior to entering of the abdominal cavity combined with adhesiolysis and/or omentopexy, if required. These advanced laparoscopic techniques have been reported to provide 96–99% 5-year patency rate [14, 15].

Despite the improved results with newer surgical approaches, many institutions have increased placement of PD catheter using Interventional Radiology (IR) techniques. Use of ultrasound (US) and fluoroscopic guidance has made this procedure safe and cost effective and a reasonable alternative to traditional surgical catheter placement. Technical success and patency rates from IR placed catheters appear to be equivalent to basic laparoscopic results [12].

Patient Selection and Pre-procedure Preparation

A history and physical examination is performed directed at known conditions that may generally contraindicate PD catheter placement such as hernias, presence of abdominal mesh, organomegaly, prior transplanted kidney, abdominal infection, or past abdominal or pelvic surgeries. In patients with prior pelvic surgery, PD catheter is better placed with laparoscopic technique since adhesiolysis and omentopexy procedures can be performed in the same setting. If the patient is on anticoagulants they are held they should be held before the procedure according to the type of the anticoagulant and the institution/hospital protocol.

In non-urgent placements a bowel preparation is recommended to reduce colonic distension and reduce post-operative constipation that may affect catheter function. On the night prior to the procedure an enema may be administered. Avoiding phosphate or magnesium containing enemas in patients with advanced kidney disease is mandatory. Bisacodyl suppositories may substitute for enemas. If patients have chronic constipation, oral laxatives may also be administered several days before the procedure. Post-procedure instructions to avoid constipation are also discussed with the patient.

The patient is kept fasting for at least 6 h before the procedure since conscious sedation will be administered. Pre-procedure antibiotics are administered intravenously with either cefazolin 1000 mg. Vancomycin 1000 mg is used if the patient is allergic to cephalosporin or penicillin [14, 18]. The antibiotics are administered 1 h prior to the procedure. The patient is asked to fully empty the bladder and if the patient has bladder dysfunction, a Foley catheter can be used to ensure full bladder drainage.

Pre-procedure Abdominal Site Marking

Marking of the entry and exit sites of the catheter is performed in the pre-procedure area. The site marking can be performed with a non-sterile PD catheter or using commercially available stencils. The belt line is noted in sitting and standing position while patients are fully dressed. With the patient in the recumbent position, the upper border of the PD catheter curl is aligned to upper border of the symphysis pubis. After aligning the catheter curl with the symphysis pubis as outlined above, the catheter length from the curled end to the deep rectus Dacron cuff determines the entry site location on the skin, which should be 2–4 cm lateral to the midline. The exit site is then marked on the skin such that the superficial cuff within the subcutaneous tunnel is at least 2–4 cm away from the exit site (Fig. 7.1). The location of the catheter curl

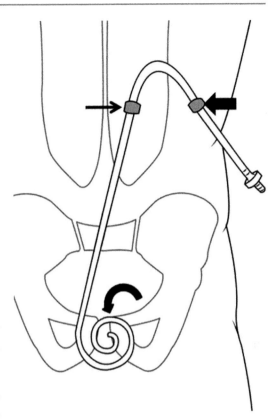

Fig. 7.1 Diagram showing abdominal site marking done before the procedure. The location of the catheter curl in relation to the symphysis pubis is an important determination as catheters that extend too deep in the pelvis may result in infusion or drain pain during PD exchanges. When marking the entry site (*small arrow*) and exit site (*large arrow*), it is essential to align the upper border of the PD catheter curl with the upper border of the symphysis pubis (*curved arrow*)

in relation to the symphysis pubis is an important determination, since catheters that extend too deep into the pelvis may result in infusion or drain pain during the PD exchanges. In the obese patient there may be substantial movement of the abdominal pannus so marking in the upright position to allow for the pannus being dependent, may assist in catheter localization. There is no consensus on left versus right side catheter placement.

Catheter Selection

A variety of body configurations of patients has resulted in modification of the standard Tenckhoff

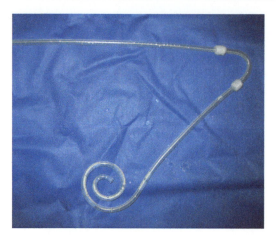

Fig. 7.2 Photograph showing a swan neck (*pre-curved*), double-cuff, curled catheter

catheter in terms of the length and presence of a pre-formed bend (swan neck) in the subcutaneous section of the catheter to assist in creation of a downward facing exit site and avoidance of the beltline. The chosen catheter design would allow for pelvic location of the distal catheter (keeping it out of reach of omentum) and appropriate exit location that is easily accessible for the patients and away from belt line or skin crease/folds. Three standard variations of the Tenckhoff catheters are: straight intercuff segment, pre-formed bend between cuffs (Swan neck design) and a modular (two-piece) extended system to produce upper abdominal or chest exit-site locations. The literature is not consistent regarding superiority of either configuration (straight versus Swan neck configuration).

The authors' preferred catheter is the Swan neck (pre-curved), double-cuff, curled catheter (Fig. 7.2). The authors feel that the swan neck design aids in orienting the catheter caudally into the pelvis. The curled distal portion of the catheter adds additional mass to encourage the distal catheter to remain low in the pelvis and therefore helps prevent cephalad migration of the distal end of the catheter. The curled tubing and numerous inflow/outflow holes diffuse the dialysate gently into and out of the patient. The two catheter cuffs are anchored preperitoneal and subcutaneously. The pre-peritoneal cuff (deep cuff) is anchored within the anterior rectus sheath to

reduce the possibility of dialysate leakage from the peritoneal cavity. The subcutaneous cuff (superficial cuff) is placed deep subcutaneously about 2–4 cm from the catheter exit site, to avoid cuff infection or extrusion. Both cuffs anchor the catheter via tissue in-growth and serve as a barrier to infection. The catheter is prepared by placing the catheter in a surgical bowl filled with saline and manually compressing the Dacron cuffs to extrude any air within the cuffs that may inhibit tissue in-growth.

Catheter Placement Procedure

Intra-procedure Preparation and Monitoring

The patient is placed supine on the angiographic table in the procedure room. Preliminary ultrasound of the abdomen is performed to help determine the safest puncture site (entry site) and plan for the subcutaneous tunnel and the catheter exit site. The *puncture site* is defined as the site of the initial needle stick but, due to caudal angling of the needle, the entry site into the peritoneum is 2–3 cm inferior. The *subcutaneous tunnel* is defined as the tunnel through which the catheter will be passed under the skin. The *exit site* is defined as the site on the skin where the catheter will exit from the subcutaneous tunnel. The safest puncture site should be determined by gray-scale ultrasound, color-Doppler ultrasound and fluoroscopy. Gray-scale ultrasound will determine the site on the anterior abdominal wall that does not have bowel loops underneath, or has the maximum separation between the anterior abdominal wall and the bowel loops, to minimize the risk of inadvertent bowel puncture. On gray-scale ultrasound, the subcutaneous tissue is visualized as a superficial hypoechoic band and the rectus abdominis muscle is visualized as a deeper hypoechoic band with linear high specular echoes. The parietal peritoneum is visualized as a thin echogenic linear streak just posterior to the rectus abdominis muscle. The air-filled bowel loops demonstrate ring-down artifact caused by air (Fig. 7.3), while the fluid-filled bowel loops will appear hypoechoic. Both air and fluid-filled bowel

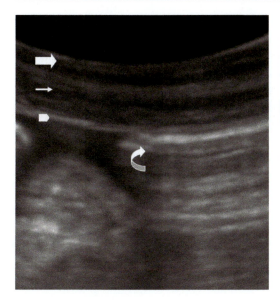

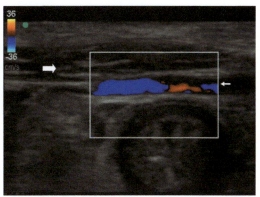

Fig. 7.4 Color Doppler ultrasound image shows the inferior epigastric artery (*small arrow*) coursing through the rectus abdominis muscle (*large arrow*)

Fig. 7.3 Gray scale ultrasound image showing the different layers of the anterior abdominal wall. The subcutaneous fat appears as a superficial hypoechoic band (*large arrow*). The rectus abdominis muscle appears as a deeper hypoechoic structure with linear high specular echoes (*small arrow*). The peritoneum appears as a thin linear hyperechoic streak deep to the rectus abdominis muscle (*arrowhead*). The air-filled bowel loops demonstrate ringdown artifact caused by air (*curved arrow*)

loops might demonstrate motion on real time ultrasound confirming their nature. Color Doppler or Power Doppler ultrasound can then be used to confirm the absence of any large arteries, mainly the inferior epigastric artery and its branches, coursing through or deep to the anterior abdominal wall (Fig. 7.4). If these are present, then a search for a different puncture site should be attempted to avoid transecting these arteries which can result in abdominal wall or intra-abdominal hematoma. A site in the mid-rectus abdominis muscle is preferred for placement of the catheter compared to the thinner lateral or medial aspects of the rectus abdominis muscle since one of the cuffs of the catheter will be implanted in the muscle. In the authors' experience, scanning for a safe puncture site that is 2–4 cm lateral and superior to the umbilicus is usually optimal. The subcutaneous tunnel usually makes a gentle lateral and inferior course towards the exit site which is located lateral and inferior to the initial puncture site. All planned sites should be marked with a pen.

The hair on the anterior abdominal wall in the involved area is then shaved. The abdomen is then prepped with an antiseptic scrub and then sterilely draped to provide exposure to the initial puncture site and the expected exit site. Mild or moderate sedation is performed using intravenous midazolam hydrochloride and fentanyl citrate. Vital sign parameters (pulse, blood pressure, oxygen saturation) and bedside electrocardiogram are continuously monitored during the procedure by the operating physician and a dedicated nurse. Anesthesiology assistance is not routinely required but may be considered in the case of patients requiring CPAP ventilation or on chronic narcotics. If on CPAP, those patients should bring their own home devices to the procedure.

Ultrasound Guidance

As mentioned, ultrasound guidance should be used in all cases for the initial puncture to ensure safe entry into the peritoneal cavity. The use of gray-scale and Doppler ultrasound allows for visualization and avoidance of bowel and vascular structures such as the inferior epigastric artery. The safest initial puncture site is again confirmed using ultrasound. Local anesthesia using 1% lidocaine is infiltrated within the skin, subcutaneous, and deep tissues of the anterior abdominal wall at the anticipated puncture site.

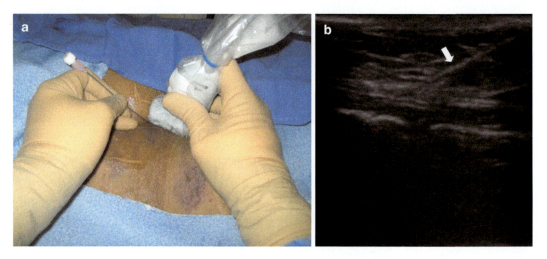

Fig. 7.5 (**a**) Photograph showing a 21 gauge micropuncture needle advanced in a caudal direction towards the pelvis at a 45° angle from the skin surface using ultrasound guidance. (**b**) Ultrasound image showing needle puncture of the peritoneum using ultrasound guidance

A 21 gauge micropuncture needle is usually used. Alternatively, a blunt tip needle such as an 18 gauge Hawkins-Adkins needle or a Veress needle can be used. Using ultrasound guidance, the needle is advanced in a caudal direction towards the pelvis at a 45° angle from the skin surface and slightly laterally (Fig. 7.5). Taking a caudal and lateral tract through the rectus sheath, helps direct the catheter in the caudal direction which has been associated with less cephalic catheter migration in the surgical literature [14, 15]. The parietal peritoneal layer is well-innervated and the patient usually experiences transient discomfort as the needle traverses the parietal peritoneum. A 22 gauge, 15 cm Chiba needle can be used in the obese patient and the curved low frequency probe can be used to assess for the needle passing into the peritoneal cavity, if the linear probe cannot provide visualization.

Fluoroscopic Guidance

Following the ultrasound-guided entry into the peritoneal cavity, approximately 3–5 mL of nonionic contrast material can be injected and visualized under fluoroscopy. The free spread of contrast material around the bowel loops confirms successful entry into the peritoneal cavity (Fig. 7.6). Contrast outlining the mucosal folds of

the small bowel or the colonic haustra indicates inadvertent puncture of bowel. If bowel perforation occurs, the procedure is terminated in order to avoid catheter infection and peritonitis. The patient can be managed conservatively or treated with oral Ciprofloxacin 500 mg twice daily for 2 weeks after which the patient can return for a second attempt.

After visual confirmation of successful entry into the peritoneal cavity, a 0.018 in. nitinol wire that accompanies the original micro-introducer kit is threaded into the peritoneal cavity (Fig. 7.7). The nitinol wire is left in place and the 21 gauge needle is then exchanged over the nitinol wire for the 4 or 5 French microsheath included in the microintroducer kit (Fig. 7.8). The wire and inner stiffener of the sheath are then removed and contrast may again be injected through the sheath to confirm that the sheath is in the peritoneal cavity. A 0.035 in. guide wire, preferably a stiff glide wire, is advanced through the sheath and directed toward the pelvis under fluoroscopic guidance. During advancement, the wire is negotiated through the path of least resistance around bowel and omentum to reach the pelvis. Alternately, when a larger bore needle (Veress-type) is used for entry, a 0.035 in. guide wire can be directly introduced through the needle. The 0.035 in. wire is ideal as it allows for manipulation around the bowel and is stiff enough to allow catheter traction during the final catheter placement.

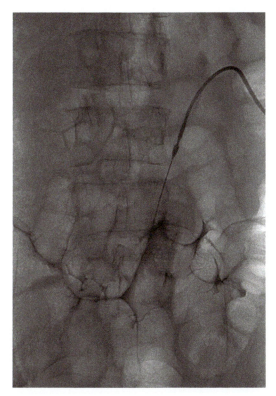

Fig. 7.6 Fluoroscopic image after injection of 5 ml of non-ionic contrast material into the peritoneal cavity showing free spread of contrast material outlining the outer surface of the bowel loops and confirming successful entry into the peritoneal cavity

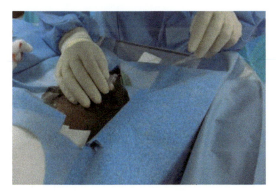

Fig. 7.7 Photograph showing a 0.018 in. nitinol wire threaded through the introducer needle into the peritoneal cavity

If advancement of the wire down to the pelvic cavity is difficult or problematic due to adhesions from prior surgery, a 4 or 5 French angled-tip catheter together with the guide wire can be used to negotiate down into the pelvic cavity. The 4-French

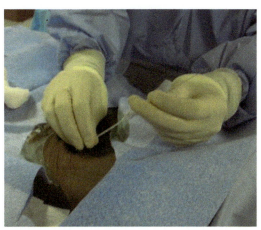

Fig. 7.8 Photograph showing a 4-French microsheath introduced over the 0.018 nitinol wire

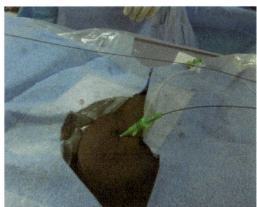

Fig. 7.9 Photograph showing the placement of a 6-French introducer sheath over the stiff glide wire

microsheath is then exchanged over the wire for a 6-French introducer sheath with a sidearm (Fig. 7.9). Contrast may again be injected through the sidearm of the introducer sheath to confirm location of the sheath in the peritoneal cavity. A 2–4 cm incision is made at the site of entry of the introducer sheath followed by blunt dissection down to the rectus abdominis muscle using a finger or curved hemostat (Fig. 7.10). Three hundred to 1000 mL of normal saline may be infused through the sidearm of the introducer sheath to separate the bowel loops and facilitate the passage of the catheter into the peritoneum.

The sheath is then removed and the tract is serially dilated over the wire with an 8-French, then

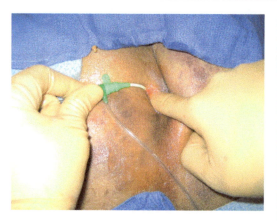

Fig. 7.10 Photograph showing a 2 cm incision made at the site of entry of the introducer sheath followed by blunt dissection with a finger down to the rectus abdominis muscle

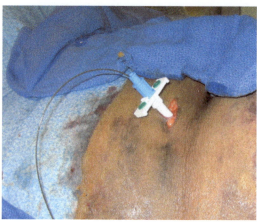

Fig. 7.12 Photograph shows placement of 16-French pull-apart sheath over the stiff glide wire

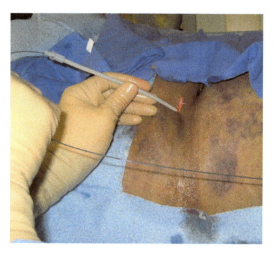

Fig. 7.11 Photograph showing dilatation of the tract using a 14-French hydrophilic dilator over the stiff glide wire

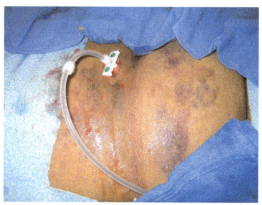

Fig. 7.13 Photograph showing the peritoneal dialysis catheter advanced over the stiff glide wire within the pull-apart sheath after removing the inner dilator of the sheath

12-French, then 14-French dilator (Fig. 7.11). Dilatation should be done under fluoroscopic visualization and the dilators should be directed caudally towards the pelvic cavity in the same direction as the original needle stick in order to avoid the wire and the dilator being pushed in the subcutaneous tissue superficial to the rectus abdominis muscle, rather than through the muscle into the peritoneal cavity. A 16-French, 15 cm peel-apart sheath, that is typically included in the peritoneal catheter kit, is advanced into the peritoneal cavity over the wire in the deep pelvic direction (Fig. 7.12).

The dialysis catheter is then removed from the saline bowl and the curled end of the catheter is advanced over the guide wire within the peel-apart sheath after removing the inner dilator of the sheath (Fig. 7.13). The catheters contain a radio-opaque strip that helps to visually orient the catheter to maintain a straight alignment as it is being advanced over the wire, to avoid twisting of the catheter during advancement. The radio-opaque strip also helps the Interventional Radiologist orient the catheter curl towards the same side of the needle stick. The catheter is advanced until the deep Dacron cuff reaches the rectus abdominis muscle surface. At this point,

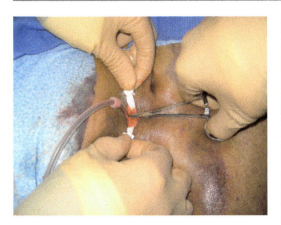

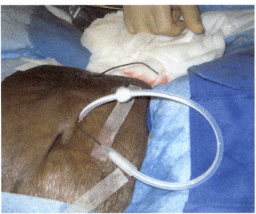

Fig. 7.14 Photograph showing the pull-apart sheath being split and pulled in an upward fashion by the assistant, while the primary Interventional Radiologist applies a downward pressure on the peritoneal catheter using a blunt curved hemostat to keep the deep Dacron cuff inside the substance of the rectus abdominis muscle

Fig. 7.15 Photograph showing tunneling of the peritoneal dialysis catheter towards the exit site in a gentle lateral-inferior arc

both the catheter and the sheath are advanced together for 1 cm over the guide wire to ensure that the deep Dacron cuff is located within the substance of the rectus abdominis muscle. The next step may require coordination between the primary operating Interventional Radiologist and an assistant. The pull-apart sheath is split and pulled in an upward fashion by the assistant, while the primary Interventional Radiologist applies a downward pressure on the peritoneal catheter using a blunt curved hemostat or large DeBakey forceps without teeth held only on the cuff and not the catheter, to keep the deep Dacron cuff inside the substance of the rectus abdominis muscle (Fig. 7.14).

The catheter exit site is then anesthetized with 1% lidocaine. This exit site is typically 4 cm lateral and inferior to the original peritoneal entry site. It is important that the catheter exiting the skin should be directed in a downward and lateral position to prevent water, perspiration, bacteria and skin debris from pooling in the exit site at the skin-catheter interface [18]. The exit site is also chosen to allow for the superficial Dacron cuff to be at least 2–4 cm away from the skin exit site and not closer, to reduce the chance of subsequent cuff extrusion. A small 5 mm incision is made at the planned exit site, easily performed as a stab incision with a 12 F scalpel. The subcuta-

neous tissue between the planned exit site and the initial peritoneal entry site, where the catheter will be tunneled, is then also anesthetized with 1% lidocaine. It is important not to make an incision that is significantly larger than the size of the catheter since suturing at the exit site is strictly prohibit due to the high risk of infection.

The proximal end of the catheter is then attached to a tunneling stylet that is included in the catheter kit. The catheter is tunneled toward the exit site in a gentle lateral-then-inferior arc. The catheter is brought out of the exit site allowing the superficial Dacron cuff to be 2–4 cm away from the skin exit site. Caution should be exercised during the tunneling process to avoid displacement of the deep Dacron cuff from the rectus abdominis muscle (Fig. 7.15).

The catheter adapter, included in the catheter kit, is attached to the outer end of the catheter and 20 mL of non-ionic contrast material may be injected through the catheter under fluoroscopic visualization to exclude any catheter kink in the subcutaneous tunnel or at the peritoneal entry site, and to confirm the proper location of the curled distal tip within the pelvic portion of the peritoneal cavity (Fig. 7.16).

The catheter should then be tested for functional patency, by injecting up to 1 l of normal saline through the catheter to demonstrate free infusion and draining of fluid. A portion of the infused normal saline may be retained in the peritoneal cavity

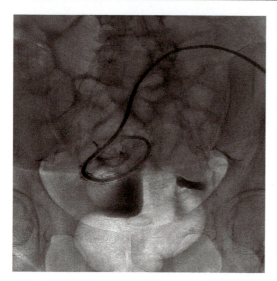

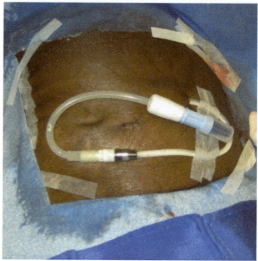

Fig. 7.16 Fluoroscopic image shows non-ionic contrast injected through the catheter under fluoroscopic visualization to exclude any catheter kinking in the subcutaneous tunnel or peritoneal entry site, and to confirm the proper location of the curled distal tip within the pelvic portion of the peritoneal cavity

Fig. 7.17 Photograph showing transfer set connected to a titanium adapter

due to the patient's recumbent position with pooling of fluid in the deep pelvic gutter. Alternately, and less time consuming, is the infusion of a single 20 mL infusion of fluid followed by inspection of the column of fluid within the catheter observing for respiratory variation. If drained fluid is blood tinged additional flushing can be done until clear.

Incision Closure and Dressing

The entrance incision is closed in two layers. The subcutaneous tissue of the incision is closed and sutured with 2-0 Vicryl absorbable suture followed by skin closure with 4-0 Monocryl absorbable suture. Topical skin adhesive may be applied to the sutured skin. Sutures are explicitly avoided at the exit site to avoid infection.

An extension catheter, which serves as the transfer set for the dialysis solution provider, is attached to the adapter to close the catheter system and maintain a sterile distal capping of the catheter (Fig. 7.17). The catheter and transfer set are entirely covered with gauze and then covered with a transparent, semi-occlusive dressing. The

gauze underneath the transparent dressing is important to absorb any moisture and to prevent contact between the catheter and the dressing, which might lead to catheter dislodgement while removing the dressing before the dialysis session.

The initial dressing placed during the procedure should be exchanged by a health care provider using sterile technique at 7 days and then sterilely redressed with similar bandage for an additional 7 days [14, 19]. Ideally the initial bandage change should be performed by an experienced peritoneal dialysis nurse while observing sterile procedure and wearing a mask and sterile gloves. The catheter exit site and incision are cleaned with only normal saline. Betadine and hydrogen peroxide solutions should be avoided due to cytotoxicity. Sterile gauze and semi-occlusive Tegaderm dressings should be re-applied using the same technique described above. After the 2 week interval, the exit-site care can be initiated by the patient with exit site prophylaxis with mupirocin cream or gentamicin [14, 20, 21]. If the PD catheter is to be used acutely, the transfer set can be excluded from the dressing to allow easy access to the transfer set cap and facilitate connection to the dialysate bag or cycler. Immersion bathing is prohibited for 21 days except for sponge baths and the exit site should be kept dry until complete healing which typically occurs after 21 days. Heavy lifting of more than 5 kg should be avoided for 4 weeks after the procedure to prevent dislodgment of the deep cuff from the rectus abdominis muscle.

Outcomes

PD catheter placement by interventional radiologists has been advocated as a cost-effective, efficient, and safe procedure [22]. The procedure still carries the risk of tunnel infection and peritonitis, bowel perforation, major and minor leaks, and primary catheter dysfunction [23]. However, several publications reporting on catheter outcomes have documented similar outcomes between catheters placed by traditional surgical techniques and catheters placed by IR using fluoroscopic imaging techniques.

A prospective randomized non-inferiority study reported 113 PD catheter insertions randomly assigned to laparoscopic placement under general anesthesia by a surgeon or fluoroscopic guided placement under local anesthesia by interventional radiologists [24]. Individuals were eligible if they were ≥18 years and suitable for both laparoscopic and radiological PD catheter insertions. Exclusion criteria included severe obesity [body mass index (BMI) >35], previous abdominal surgery or a history consistent with adhesions, severe medical comorbidity precluding general anaesthesia, bleeding diatheses, anticoagulation, HIV infection, ongoing corticosteroid or immunosuppressant use, severe psychiatric disease and definite plans for live donor kidney transplantation. The composite endpoint of complication-free survival by day 365 was reported and included all mechanical and infectious complications. The authors also assessed occurrence of catheter removal, death from any cause, pain during the procedure, time required for the procedure, time required in the procedure room, length of admission and direct hospital costs. They reported superior complication-free catheter survival in the interventional radiology group compared to the surgical group. The

interventional radiology group had significantly reduced hospital costs. The authors concluded that PD catheter placement by IR was clinically non-inferior and was a cost-effective alternative to traditional surgical catheter placement.

Another study compared 1-year outcomes in 52 fluoroscopically placed catheters versus 49 surgically placed catheters [25]. Although the differences in complication rates between the two techniques did not reach statistical significance there was a trend towards greater leakage, malfunction, malposition and bleeding in the surgical group. Additional reports suggest equivalency of outcomes by the traditional surgical and percutaneous techniques [26, 27]. A retrospective study reported 286 PD catheter insertions of which 153 catheters were placed using laparoscopic technique under general anesthesia by a surgeon and 133 were placed using fluoroscopic guided technique under local anesthesia by interventional radiologists [28]. All patients who received catheters radiologically or laparoscopically, either as first or repeat procedures, were included. Exclusion criteria were age younger than 18 years, catheter placement for reasons other than the treatment of ESKD, and open surgical procedures. There was no significant difference in the unadjusted 365-day complication-free catheter survival or overall catheter survival between the two groups. Patient survival was better in the laparoscopic group which was interpreted by the authors to be due to the preferential selection of the radiologic insertion for frail patients.

Only the newer and less utilized advanced laparoscopic placement techniques appear to have superior outcomes to fluoroscopically placed catheters [17].

In conclusion, PD catheter placement by interventional radiologists is a cost effective, minimally invasive alternative to traditional surgical and laparoscopic placement in the operating room under general anesthesia. In many centers, this alternative may offer a more expeditious way to schedule and place peritoneal dialysis access. IR placement with ultrasound and fluoroscopic guidance offers enhanced safety and confirmation of catheter placement into the pelvis. IR catheter placement in the late-referred ESRD patient may allow for urgent initiation of PD and avoidance of temporary vascular access catheters.

References

1. United States Renal System. USRDS 2012. Annual data report, vol. 2. Bethesda: National Institutes of Health. p. 157.
2. Chaudhary K, Sangha H, Khanna R. Peritoneal dialysis first: rationale. Clin J Am Soc Nephrol. 2011;6:447–56.
3. Mehrotra R, Chiu Y, Kalantar-Zadeh K, et al. Similar outcomes with hemodialysis and peritoneal dialysis in patients with end-stage renal disease. Arch Intern Med. 2011;171:110–8.
4. Kumar VA, Sidell MA, Jones JP, Vonesh EF. Survival of propensity matched incident peritoneal and hemodialysis patients in a United States health care system. Kidney Int. 2014;86:1016–22.
5. Ghaffari A. Urgent-start peritoneal dialysis: a quality improvement report. Am J Kidney Dis. 2012;59:400–8.
6. Arramreddy R, Zheng S, Saxena AB, Liebman SE, Wong L. Urgent-start peritoneal dialysis: a chance for a new beginning. Am J Kidney Dis. 2014;63:390–5.
7. Ghaffari A, Kumar V, Guest S. Infrastructure requirements for an urgent-start peritoneal dialysis program. Perit Dial Int. 2013;33:611–7.
8. Abdel-aal AK, Gaddikeri S, Saddekni S. Technique of peritoneal catheter placement under fluoroscopic guidance. Radiol Res Pract. 2011;2011:141707.
9. Reddy C, Dybbro PE, Guest S. Fluoroscopically guided percutaneous peritoneal dialysis catheter placement: single center experience and review of the literature. Ren Fail. 2010;32:294–9.
10. Abdel-aal AK, Joshi AK, Saddekni S, Maya ID. Fluoroscopic and sonographic guidance to place peritoneal catheters: how we do it. Am J Roentgenol. 2009;192:1085–9.
11. Savader SJ. Percutaneous radiologic placement of peritoneal dialysis catheters. J Vasc Interv Radiol. 1999;10:249–56.
12. Savader SJ, Geschwind J, Lund GB, Scheel PJ. Percutaneous radiological placement of peritoneal dialysis catheters: long-term results. J Vasc Interv Radiol. 2000;11:965–70.
13. Abdel-aal AK, Dybbro P, Hathaway P, et al. Best practices consensus protocol for peritoneal dialysis catheter placement by interventional radiologists. Perit Dial Int. 2014;34:481–93.
14. Abdel Aal AK, Dybbro P, Hathaway P, Guest S, Neuwirth M, Krishnamurthy V. Best practice consensus protocol for peritoneal dialysis catheter placement by interventional radiologists. Perit Dial Int. 2014;34(5):481–93.
15. Crabtree JH, Burchette RJ. Effective use of laparoscopy for long-term peritoneal dialysis access. Am J Surg. 2009;198:135–41.
16. Ash SR. Chronic peritoneal dialysis catheters: overview of design, placement, and removal procedures. Semin Dial. 2003;16:323–34.
17. Crabtree JH, Fishman A. A laparoscopic method for optimal peritoneal dialysis access. Am J Surg. 2005;71:135–43.
18. Crabtree JH, Burchette RJ. Prospective comparison of downward and lateral peritoneal dialysis catheter tunnel-tract and exit-site directions. Perit Dial Int. 2006;26(6):677–83.
19. Dombros N, Dratwa M, Feriani M, Gokal R, Heimburger O, Krediet R, et al. European best practice guidelines for peritoneal dialysis. 3 peritoneal access. Nephrol Dial Transplant. 2005;20(Suppl 9):ix8–ix12.
20. Bernardini J, Bender F, Florio T, Sloand J, Palmmontalbano L, Fried L, et al. Randomized, double-blind trial of antibiotic exit site cream for prevention of exit site infection in peritoneal dialysis patients. J Am Soc Nephrol. 2005;16:539–45.
21. Piraino B, Bernardini J, Brown E, Figueiredo A, Johnson DW, Lye WC, et al. ISPD position statement on reducing the risks of peritoneal dialysis-related infections. Perit Dial Int. 2011;31:614–30.
22. Brunier G, Hiller JA, Drayton S, Pugash RA, Tobe SW. A change to radiological peritoneal dialysis catheter insertion: three-month outcomes. Perit Dial Int. 2010;30:528–33.
23. Ghaffari A. Urgent-start peritoneal dialysis: a quality improvement report. Am J Kidney Dis. 2012;59:400–8.
24. Voss D, Hawkins S, Poole G, Marshall M. Radiological versus surgical implantation of first catheter for peritoneal dialysis: a randomized non-inferiority trial. Nephrol Dial Transplant. 2012;27:4196–204.
25. Rosenthal MA, Yang PS, Liu IA, Sim JJ, Kujubu DA, Rasgon SA, et al. Comparison of outcomes of peritoneal dialysis catheters placed by the fluoroscopically guided percutaneous method versus directly visualized surgical method. J Vasc Interv Radiol. 2008;19:1202–7.
26. Medani S, Shantier M, Hussein W, Wall C, Mellotte G. A comparative analysis of percutaneous and open surgical techniques for peritoneal catheter placement. Perit Dial Int. 2012;32(6):628–35.
27. Georgiades CS, Geschwind JF. Percutaneous peritoneal dialysis catheter placement for the management of end-stage renal disease: technique and comparison with the surgical approach. Tech Vasc Interv Radiol. 2002;5:103–7.
28. Maher E, Wholley MJ, Abbas SA, Hawkins SP, Marshall MR. Fluoroscopic versus laparoscopic implantation of peritoneal dialysis catheters: a retrospective cohort study. J Vasc Interv Radiol. 2014;25:895–903.

Advanced Laparoscopic Insertion of Peritoneal Dialysis Catheters

8

Ivy N. Haskins and Steven Rosenblatt

Introduction

One in ten adult Americans, or an estimated 20 million people, have some form of chronic kidney disease [1]. From the years 1980 through 2009, the incidence of end-stage renal disease (ESRD) requiring renal replacement therapy (RRT) increased by 600% [1]. More interesting than these statistics is the fact that the use of peritoneal dialysis (PD) has been steadily declining in the United States [2, 3]. In 1980, the incidence of PD in patients with ESRD was 15% while current reports estimate that only 7% of patients with ESRD are utilizing this form of dialysis [2, 3].

A variety of hypotheses have been proposed to help understand the decline in the use of PD nationally. Most of these explanations center around the perceived, or even real, differences in morbidity and mortality rates between those patients who undergo hemodialysis (HD) and those patients who are started on PD [2–4]. However, it has been our experience that finding surgeons who are willing to place peritoneal dialysis (PD) catheters is even more of a contributing factor.

Prior to the publication of best-demonstrated practices of PD catheter placement, this was a

procedure that was fraught with high rates of non-function. These poor results subsequently led to a decline in surgeon and patient enthusiasm for this form of dialysis. Indeed, the long-term success of PD is predicated on the proper placement of a PD catheter. In this chapter, we will discuss the indications for laparoscopic PD catheter placement, our surgical technique, and outcomes with this type of renal replacement therapy.

Indications and Patient Selection for Laparoscopic PD Catheter Placement

The transition of the patient with chronic kidney disease (CKD) to dialysis therapy is an often overwhelming and life changing event for patients and their families alike. Our role as surgeons is to make this transition as seamless as possible. The best way to ensure successful initiation of PD is early assessment of the patient with CKD [4]. In order for this evaluation to occur, surgeons must work in coordination with the PD team, including the nephrologists and the PD nurses, so that patient referral and evaluation is not delayed.

In general, patients should be evaluated by a general surgeon well in advance of the estimated time of dialysis initiation. PD catheter placement and the initiation of PD are rarely performed on an emergent basis. Without proper foresight, patients who originally planned to start with PD may unexpectedly experience a precipitous

I.N. Haskins, MD • S. Rosenblatt, MD, FACS (✉)
Digestive Disease and Surgical Institute,
The Cleveland Clinic Foundation,
9500 Euclid Avenue, A100, Cleveland,
OH 44195, USA
e-mail: ihaskins@gwu.edu; rosenbs@ccf.org

© Springer International Publishing AG 2017
S. Haggerty (ed.), *Surgical Aspects of Peritoneal Dialysis*, DOI 10.1007/978-3-319-52821-2_8

decline in their renal function. In such situations, emergent HD is initiated and the transition thereafter from HD to PD is logistically challenging [4]. Therefore, it cannot be overemphasized that careful planning and communication with all members of the team are crucial.

The advantages of the laparoscopic approach to PD placement are multifold and include techniques to prevent catheter tip migration and catheter occlusion, management of intra-abdominal adhesions, and identification and possible preemptive repair of abdominal wall hernias not previously diagnosed [4]. Integrating laparoscopy into the surgical placement of PD catheters helps to minimize the risk of long-term complications which in turn provides for durable, and uninterrupted, access to the peritoneal cavity. Because of these advantages, we firmly believe that laparoscopic PD placement should be the standard of care for all ESRD patients able to tolerate general anesthesia and pneumoperitoneum.

Laparoscopic PD Catheter Placement Technique

This section will detail the operative technique for PD catheter placement at our institution. Like all surgical procedures, there is more than one safe and effective technique for PD catheter placement and our method should be adapted for surgeon comfort with the described techniques and institutional restrictions. In summary, the steps to successful PD catheter placement include:

1. Use of a double-cuff Tenkhoff type catheter
2. Careful determination of insertion incision, subcutaneous tunnel configuration, and exit site location
3. Paramedian insertion site
4. Rectus sheath tunneling of the catheter
5. Prophylactic omentopexy (as needed)
6. Prophylactic adhesiolysis (as needed)
7. Location of the deep catheter cuff within the rectus sheath
8. Location of the superficial subcutaneous catheter cuff at least two centimeters from the exit site

Patient Positioning and Induction of Anesthesia

Patients are brought to the operating room and placed supine on the operating room table. General anesthesia is induced at the discretion of the anesthesia team with the usual considerations for those patients with ESRD. Unless contraindicated by the presence of a graft or fistula, we prefer to tuck both arms. Tucking the arms is particularly helpful when laparoscopic adhesiolysis is necessary as this facilitates the ability of both the surgeon and the camera operator to be on the same side of the table. A footboard is mandatory, as the patient will eventually be placed into the steep reverse Trendelenburg position. The abdomen is then widely shaved, prepped, and draped.

Although there are many different catheters available, we strictly utilize the basic Tenckhoff type double-cuffed catheters with a straight segment or swan neck arc bend between the cuffs. The decision as to which type of catheter we use is patient dependent. The straight catheter is used far more often in our practice, mainly due to patient body habitus. An important consideration for catheter type is the location of the patient's belt line. Ideally, the catheter should exit the abdominal wall either above or below the belt line for patient comfort. Similarly, the presence of incisions, ostomies, and more commonly skin folds in obese patients must be taken into consideration when determining the exit site in order to minimize the risk of catheter malfunction or infection.

Catheter Mapping

Catheter mapping, just like venous mapping for arteriovenous fistula formation, is crucial to the success of PD catheter placement [5]. Some institutions prefer to use catheter stencils for this portion of the procedure. However, we prefer to use the catheter itself as a guide. There may be an inherent variability of the catheter lengths and dimensions based on the manufacturer of the

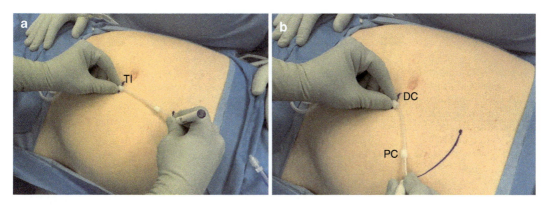

Fig. 8.1 Catheter mapping. The transverse incision (*TI*) is marked overlying the left rectus muscle (**a**). The distal cuff (*DC*) is held in place while an arc is made on the abdominal wall using the proximal cuff (*PC*) (**b**)

catheter. Therefore, only the stencil that corresponds with the particular catheter to be placed during surgery should be used to produce accurate preoperative mapping [5].

Regardless of which type of catheter is being placed, determining the location of the insertion incision for the intramuscular tunnel is the first step in PD catheter placement. Under sterile conditions, the tip of the curled portion of the catheter is placed overlying the pubis. Using gentle upwards traction, and taking care not to place undue tension on the catheter, the location of the distal cuff (that which is closest to the curled portion) is marked with a sterile marker overlying the rectus muscle. Traditionally, this incision has been placed over the left rectus muscle but this location is dependent on prior surgical wounds, the presence of a stoma, and any existing skin breakdown. Should any of these conditions be present on the left side of the abdomen, then the PD catheter may be placed on the right side to minimize the risk of catheter malfunction and infection.

Next, and while still using the catheter as our guide, the planned exit site is marked out. When a Swan neck catheter is placed, the exit site is determined by the natural curve of the catheter into the lower abdomen, again keeping in mind the location of the belt line, incisions or skin folds. Determining the exit site with a straight catheter is a bit more complex. First, the catheter is grasped two centimeters above the proximal cuff while the distal cuff is held in place at the previously marked rectus muscle incision site. Moving the proximal cuff as if it were a compass, a gentle arc is created

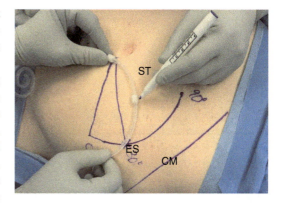

Fig. 8.2 Exit site marking. The exit site (*ES*) is at a 30° angle to the distal cuff /transverse incision. In order to determine the trajectory of the subcutaneous tract (*ST*), the catheter is grasped four centimeters from the proximal cuff and aligned with the previously identified ES. Care is taken to ensure that the ES is far enough away from the costal margin (*CM*)

in the upper abdomen using a sterile marker from 90° to 0° with respect to the distal cuff. A point 30° from the distal cuff is then marked on the arc, which serves as the planned exit site (Fig. 8.1).

In order to minimize the potential for cuff extrusion, it is imperative to keep the subcutaneous cuff at least two centimeters from the exit site. To this end, the catheter is grasped four centimeters from the proximal cuff, a gentle bend is created with the catheter, and this point is aligned with the previously determined exit site (Fig. 8.2). This line defines the planned path for subcutaneous tunneling of the portion of the PD catheter between the proximal and distal cuffs, while

Fig. 8.3 Preoperative mapping. The landmark for preoperative mapping is the transverse incision (*TI*). Distal to the TI is the site of the preperitoneal tract (*PPT*) while proximal to the TI is the catheter exit site (*ES*) and subcutaneous tract (*ST*) for the proximal portion of the catheter

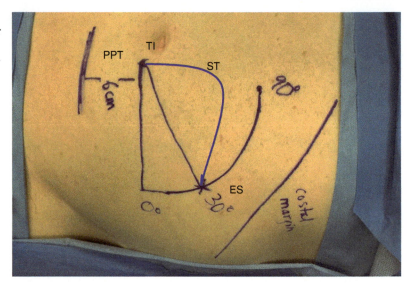

keeping the proximal cuff well away from the skin. In planning the location of the catheter exit site, it is imperative to always be cognizant as to the location of the costal margin so that this position is not too close to the rib.

Finally, the length of the rectus sheath tunnel must be marked. A six-centimeter rectus sheath tunnel is normally developed, although a shorter four-centimeter tunnel may be required for obese patients. The proximal extent of the intramuscular tunnel is the planned location of the deep PD catheter cuff. A ruler is used to mark 4–6 cm distal to this site (towards the pubis) based on the patient's body habitus (Fig. 8.3).

Entrance into the Abdominal Cavity

Unless otherwise contraindicated due to previous surgery or skin issues, we prefer to place a five-millimeter trocar in the right upper quadrant. It is important to avoid periumbilical incisions, as this location does not provide for adequate visualization of the tunnel, and may lead to future hernia. Entrance into the abdomen is performed using a 5 mm, 0-degree scope as well as an optical viewing trocar. Once the abdomen has been accessed, CO_2 insufflation is begun and the 0-degree scope is switched out for a 30-degree scope. A careful diagnostic laparoscopy is performed.

Before the placement of additional trocars, the location of adhesions and/or previously undiagnosed hernias is appreciated. Additional 5 mm trocars are placed as necessary for adhesiolysis or herniorrhaphy. If no adhesions are present, then a second 5 mm port is routinely placed in the right lower quadrant. Further details regarding lysis of adhesions and concurrent hernia repair are described in further detail below.

Lysis of Adhesions

Adhesions lead to abdominal and pelvic compartmentalization that can cause incomplete dialysate drainage during PD. Similarly, such scarring can prevent visualization of the posterior abdominal wall where the intramuscular tunnel is to be created. For these reasons, adhesions in the pelvis and lower abdominal wall should be addressed at the time of PD catheter placement. Please keep in mind that excessive adhesiolysis is oftentimes not beneficial for PD catheter function and therefore more superior adhesions can be left alone [4]. Indeed, upper abdominal adhesions between the omentum and the abdominal wall may sometimes serve as a natural omentopexy, keeping the omentum out of the retrovesical space.

If indicated, our practice is to perform adhesiolysis using sharp dissection without the use of an energy device, if possible. Although this method is a bit more tedious, we feel that it minimizes the risk of thermal injury to other intra-abdominal structures. Previous abdominal or pelvic surgery should not be a deterrent to attempting laparoscopic PD catheter placement. However, it is important to realize that intra-peritoneal adhesions are sometimes so severe that the PD catheter cannot be safely placed. Therefore, the possibility that catheter placement may not be feasible should be discussed in detail prior to surgical intervention with any patient who has a history of previous major abdominal and/or pelvic surgery. Nevertheless, we do not feel that prior abdominal surgery is a contraindication to catheter placement as it is impossible to predict the extent of adhesive disease preoperatively [6, 7].

Omentopexy and Resection of Epiploic Appendages

Catheter obstruction or dislodgement is most often caused by the omentum falling into the retrovesicular space and less frequently by the epiploic appendages occluding the PD catheter. Because catheter obstruction is the most common reason for abandonment of PD for HD, it is imperative to preemptively address these causes at the time of PD catheter placement.

In order to determine if the patient requires an omentopexy, the patient is placed into the steep reverse Trendelenburg position. If the omentum falls into the retrovesicular space, then the omentum will have to be retracted out of the deep pelvis. It should be noted that omentopexy is at least equivalent to omentectomy for the management of the omentum in these cases. As omentopexy has decreased associated morbidity, it is the preferred option for the management of the omentum [4].

In order to perform an omentopexy, the patient is placed back into the supine position and a small stab incision is made in the left upper quadrant with an 11-blade scalpel. This incision is usually above the planned PD catheter exit site. The omentum is then retracted into the upper abdomen using a laparoscopic soft bowel grasper. A suture passer with a nonabsorbable suture is used to take several bites of the omentum. The

suture is then grasped with a Maryland forceps and the suture passer is withdrawn. Through the same skin incision, but with a different trajectory through the fascia, the suture is handed back to the suture passer and brought out through the skin. The stitch is then used to secure the omentum to the abdominal wall and out of the pelvis (Fig. 8.4). Great care must be maintained in order to remain well away from the transverse colon during this portion of the procedure. The efficacy of the omentopexy is confirmed by placing the patient back into the steep reverse Trendelenburg position to ensure that the omentum no longer falls into the retrovesicular space. If the omentum still falls into the pelvis, then the omentopexy should be redone, either at a point superior to the original incision or with a larger bite of omentum secured to the abdominal wall.

Epiploic appendages are fat-filled projections most commonly found in the region of the sigmoid colon [4]. When small, these appendages do not interfere with PD catheter function. However, these attachments can be up to 15 centimeters in length. The longer the epiploic appendage, the more mobile it is, and the more likely it is to lead to PD catheter occlusion. When these structures are noted to interfere with PD catheter function, there are two options for their management. Firstly, the epiploics can be removed with the use of an energy device. A bowel grasper holds the appendage in place while the energy device is used to amputate it from the colon. Care must be taken to ensure that the site of resection is far enough away from the colon so that the colon does not sustain inadvertent thermal injury. These appendages should be removed either through a 10-mm port or with the assistance of a specimen collection bag if more than one appendage is removed. Far easier in our opinion is to simply secure one or two of the epiploics to the lateral abdominal wall in a manner, which is very similar to an omentopexy (Fig. 8.5). Again, through a two-millimeter stab incision, the suture passer and a permanent suture can be used to 'lasso' the distal epiploics and secure them to the upper and lateral abdominal wall. Again, great care has to be maintained when performing this procedure in order to prevent injury to the colon.

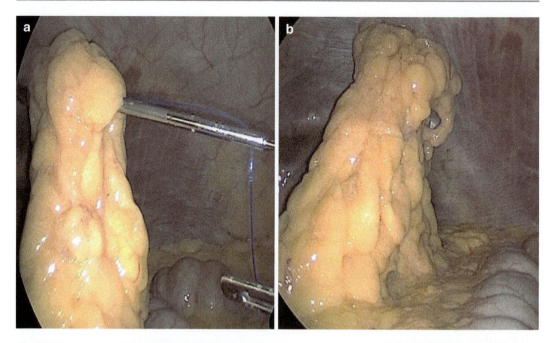

Fig. 8.4 Omentopexy. Omentum is grasped with a small bowel grasper into the left upper quadrant. A suture passer is passed through the omentum (**a**) which is then secured to the abdominal wall (**b**)

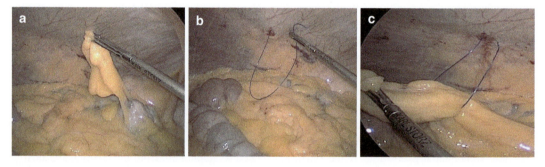

Fig. 8.5 Management of epiploic appendages. Large epiploics (**a**) are pulled up to the abdominal wall using a small bowel grasper. The suture passer is not passed through the epiploic itself. Rather, the epiploic is passed through a loop of suture (**b**) and secured to the abdominal wall (**c**). Care should be taken to ensure that the colon is identified and excluded from any epiploic lasso

Hernia Repair

Careful consideration must be given to repairing previously undiagnosed abdominal wall or inguinal hernias that are detected at the time of laparoscopy, due to the risk of hernia enlargement or symptom progression with the initiation of PD. The decision to proceed with hernia repair must be considered in the context of the specific risks and benefits of hernia repair in this patient population. Specifically, hernia repair with mesh increases the potential for catheter non-function from omental and bowel adhesions as well as mesh infection should the patient experience PD catheter-associated peritonitis [8, 9]. On the other hand, hernia repair utilizing primary suture repair has led to an unacceptably high rate of recurrence in our experience, except when the hernia defects are quite small. Surgeons must be mindful of these very real risks when deciding how best to manage previously undiagnosed abdominal wall and inguinal hernias at the time of laparoscopy.

After taking all risks and benefits of concomitant hernia repair at the time of PD catheter placement into account, the laparoscopic approach has been the preferred approach when an unexpected defect is identified. Traditionally, abdominal wall hernias are sutured closed and reinforced with synthetic mesh placed into the peritoneal cavity, if indicated by the size of the hernia. Inguinal hernias are repaired using a standard transabdominal preperitoneal (TAPP) approach with synthetic mesh reinforcement. TAPP is preferred to total extra-peritoneal repair (TEP) as the preperitoneal dissection required with TEP repair often interferes with the intramuscular catheter tunnel.

Over time however, it has become our practice to simply avoid repairing hernias when they are discovered at the time of PD catheter placement. Rather, the presence of a ventral or inguinal hernia is documented in the operative report at the time of PD catheter placement. Should the hernia enlarge or become symptomatic, it may be repaired at a later date. This approach allows for mesh to be placed in the preperitoneal space during ventral hernia repair, which absolves the risk of catheter malfunction from adhesive disease to the mesh previously discussed. Furthermore, symptomatic inguinal hernias can be repaired using an open technique, which prevents the risk of pelvic adhesion formation that may occur following a TAPP repair.

Tunneling and PD Catheter Placement

As previously stated, we prefer to place PD catheters to the left of the umbilicus, although there is no literature to support one side over the other. Using the tunneling site that was marked at the beginning of the operation, a two-centimeter paramedian incision is made overlying the left rectus muscle. Dissection is carried down through the subcutaneous tissues until the anterior fascia is exposed. Starting at the most cranial aspect of the incision, a five-millimeter incision is created in the fascia to expose the underlying rectus muscle. A 7/8 mm cannula and dilator trocar access needle is advanced through the rectus abdominus

muscle in a perpendicular fashion until it is just superior to the posterior sheath (Fig. 8.6). This portion of the procedure is performed under direct visualization with the laparoscope. The trocar is then tunneled on the surface of the posterior rectus sheath toward the pelvis for a distance of four to six centimeters, depending on the size of the patient. The extent of the tunnel is identified by injecting 0.25% Marcaine through the abdominal wall at the point which had been marked out at the beginning of the procedure. Once the trocar has reached the end of the dissected tunnel, downward pressure is maintained in order to gain entry through the peritoneum and into the pelvis.

As previously mentioned, we use a Tenckhoff-type double-cuffed catheter. Several studies have found no statistically significant difference in rates of technical failure between straight versus curled catheters. In our practice, we have used coiled-tip catheters exclusively [10–12]. The PD catheter is placed over a lubricated stylet and guided through the tunneled intramuscular tract into the peritoneal cavity under direct visualization. The catheter is advanced into the pelvis and the retrovesicular space until the distal cuff is visualized. This cuff is then pulled back until it is within the intramuscular portion of the tunnel.

A Maryland grasper or similar device is used to grasp the catheter within the peritoneal cavity while the stylet and trocar are removed. A 2-0 absorbable suture is used to reapproximate the fascia of our proximal tunnel. This stitch should be placed with great care to ensure that the fascial closure does not incorporate the PD catheter or put undue pressure on the catheter lumen causing partial occlusion. Using a Faller stylet, our proximal catheter is then tunneled through the abdominal wall just above the fascia and brought out through the planned exit site. During this aspect of the procedure, it is again best to grasp the distal catheter with a laparoscopic instrument in order to make sure that the catheter is taut through our subcutaneous tunnel and is not pulled out of the pelvis. The proximal cuff should then be at least several centimeters away from our exit site to prevent eventual irritation of the skin by extrusion of the cuff itself. The catheter is then secured to a titanium adaptor.

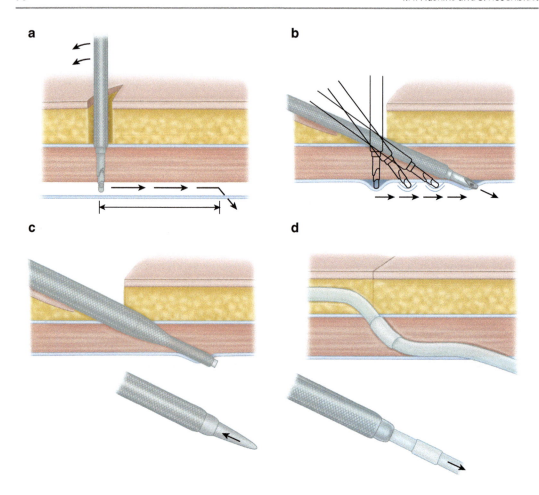

Fig. 8.6 Preperitoneal, rectus sheath tunneling. A cannula and dilator system is inserted perpendicular to the rectus muscle at the site of the transverse incision (**a**). This system is advanced towards the pelvis through the space between the rectus muscle and the peritoneum (**b**). The needle dilator is withdrawn (**c**) and the peritoneal dialysis catheter is advanced through the cannula into the peritoneal cavity (**d**) (This image was published in Kidney International Supplemental, John Crabtree, MD, "Selected Best Demonstrated Practices in Peritoneal Dialysis Access" pages 527-37. Copyright Elsevier 2006).

Confirmation of PD Catheter Function

The catheter should be tested to ensure that it is working properly prior to completion of the case. The patient is placed back into the reverse steep Trendelenburg position and CO_2 insufflation is released. Using sterile IV tubing, a 500 mL bag of sterile saline is placed to gravity and infused through the PD catheter and into the peritoneal cavity. Flushing through the catheter should be easy due to gravity. If the flow is weak, this usually indicates that there is kinking of the catheter within either the intramuscular, or more commonly, the subcutaneous tunnel. After verification of excel-

lent flow into the peritoneal cavity, the saline is then drained from the abdomen, using simple gravity drainage into a sterile basin. Again the flow should be brisk and without resistance.

If there are concerns regarding either flow into or drainage out of the peritoneal cavity, then the catheter should be carefully re-evaluated as poor flow in the operating room is indicative of catheter malfunction and non-function postoperatively. The patient is returned to the supine position, insufflation is resumed, and trouble shooting of potential causes of PD catheter malfunction is performed. As previously discussed in this chapter, the potential sources of catheter malfunction include insufficient omentopexy, catheter tip migration out of the pelvis, large epiploic appendages not previously addressed, or kinking or leakage of the catheter within the intramuscular tunnel. The source of PD catheter malfunction should be identified and addressed followed by repeat testing of PD catheter function until there is free return of the injected sterile saline.

Securing the PD Catheter in Place

Upon completion of the operation, the patient is flattened out and the CO_2 insufflation is begun once again. The abdomen should be carefully inspected to ensure that there is adequate hemostasis. Appropriate positioning of the catheter is verified. The insufflation is once again released and all trocars removed. The subcutaneous incisions should be closed according to surgeon preference for skin closure. The catheter should be connected to a transfer set, injected with approximately 50 mL of heparinized saline (5000 units of Heparin in 50 mL) to prevent fibrin clot formation, followed by a Betadine cap. The catheter exit site is secured with a sterile non-occlusive dressing. A catheter anchoring stitch predisposes the patient to early exit site and tunnel infection and should never be used. The catheter can be adequately immobilized on the abdominal wall with sterile adhesive strips and protected by an appropriately applied dressing.

If the patient is not anticipated to begin PD for several months, the catheter may be embedded into the subcutaneous tissue with interval externalization when dialysis access is required. The embedding technique has been proposed to help decrease the risk of PD-related peritonitis events by allowing the PD catheter to heal in a sterile environment [4, 13–16].

Patients Outcomes Following Laparoscopic PD Placement

PD has been shown to be an effective mode of dialysis over both the short- and long-term [4, 17–21]. In fact, PD is preferred to HD for the preservation of residual kidney function which has been shown to lead to a short-term survival advantage [5, 22, 23]. Patients who undergo PD are also offered self-autonomy through a home renal replacement modality with an improved quality of life compared to patients who undergo HD [2, 4]. Furthermore, the most common reasons for PD catheter malfunction, mainly catheter tip migration and omental occlusion, have been successfully addressed by proactive laparoscopic techniques of rectus sheath tunneling and selective omentopexy [2]. In a study published by our institution in 2010 that details the adoption of lysis of adhesions, selective omentopexy, and rectus sheath tunneling proposed by Dr. Crabtree, no patient experienced catheter outflow occlusion due to omental blockage or catheter tip migration out of the pelvis. Furthermore, the rate of PD catheter malfunction decreased from 36.7% to 4.6% [22]. Subsequently, reasons for transfer from PD to HD, including catheter related peritonitis and inadequate filtration, have received great attention in the recent years, leading to improvement in PD techniques [2].

Nevertheless, PD is not for every patient. The advantages offered with an independent mode of renal replacement therapy also come with increased patient responsibility for treating their disease. Although previously we preferred to place PD catheters mainly in younger, healthier patients as a bridge to renal transplantation at our institution, we have found that this modality can be just as successful and satisfying for those patients who are not or never will be on the transplant list. Indeed, we do not consider previous operations, size and age as contraindications to peritoneal dialysis.

Conclusion

Peritoneal dialysis is an underutilized option for renal replacement therapy. Proactive techniques enabled by a laparoscopic approach, such as adhesiolysis, omentopexy and rectus sheath tunnel leads to a decreased incidence of catheter malfunction with subsequent improvement in the long-term durability of this dialysis option. The success of peritoneal dialysis relies on the adoption of these techniques along with the collaboration and early referral of patients with chronic kidney disease to the general surgeon.

References

1. Kidney Disease Statistics for the United States. http://www.niddk.nih.gov/health-information/health-statistics/Pages/kidney-disease-statistics-united-states.aspx. Published June 2012. Accessed 22 Mar 2016.
2. Chauhary K, Sangha H, Khanna R. Peritoneal dialysis first: rationale. Clin J Am Soc Nephrol. 2011;6:447–56.
3. Jain AK, Blake P, Cordy P, Garg AX. Global trends in rates of peritoneal dialysis. J Am Soc Nephrol. 2012;23:533–44.
4. Crabtree JH. Selected best demonstrated practices in pertioneal dialysis access. Kidney Int. 2006;70:S27–36.
5. Crabtree JH. Implantation techniques for peritoneal dialysis catheters: an instructional program for healthcare providers. Viewed April 20, 2016.
6. Crabtree JH, Burchette RJ. Effect of prior abdominal surgery, peritonitis, and adhesions on catheter function and long-term outcome on peritoneal dialysis. Am Surg. 2009;75(2):140–7.
7. Keshavri A, Fazeli MS, Meyasmie A, et al. The effects of previous abdominal operations and intraperitoneal adhesions on the outcomes of peritoneal dialysis catheters. Perit Dial Int. 2010;30(1):41–5.
8. Swarnalatha G, Rapur R, Pai S, Dakshinamurty KV. Strangulated umbilical hernia in a peritoneal dialysis patient. Indian J Nephrol. 2012;22(5):381–4.
9. Imvrios G, Tsakris D, Gakis D, Takoudas D, et al. Prosthetic mesh repair of multiple recurrent and large abdominal hernias in continuous ambulatory peritoneal dialysis patients. Perit Dial Int. 1994;14:338–43.
10. Lye WC, Kour NW, van der Straaten JC, et al. A prospective randomized comparison of the Swan neck, coiled, and straight Tenckhoff catheters in patients on CAPD. Perit Dial Int. 1996;16:S333–5.
11. Eklund BH, Honkanen EO, Kala AR, et al. Peritoneal dialysis access: prospective randomized comparison of the Swan neck and Tenckhoff catheters. Perit Dial Int. 1995;15(8):353–6.
12. Eklund BH, Honkanen EO, Kala AR, et al. Catheter configuration and outcome in patients on continuous ambulatory peritoneal dialysis: a prospective comparison of two catheters. Perit Dial Int. 1994;14(1):70–4.
13. Moncrief JW, Popovich RP, Broadrick JL, He ZZ, et al. The Moncrief-Popovich catheter. A new peritoneal access technique for patients on peritoneal dialysis. ASAIO J. 1993;39(1):62–5.
14. Moncrief JW, Popovich RP, Dasgusta M, Costeron JW, et al. Reduction in peritonitis incidence in continuous ambulatory peritoneal dialysis with a new catheter and implantation technique. Perit Dial Int. 1993;13:S329–31.
15. Elhassan E, McNair B, Quinn M, Teitelbaum I. Prolonged duration of peritoneal dialysis catheter embedment does not lower the catheter success rate. Perit Dial Int. 2011;31(5):558–64.
16. Han DC, Cha HK, So IN, Chung SH, et al. Subcutaneously implanted catheters reduce the incidence of peritonitis during CAPD by eliminating infection by periluminal route. Adv Perit Dial. 1992;8:298–301.
17. Davies SJ, Phillips L, Griffiths AM, Lesley H, et al. What really happens to people on long-term peritoneal dialysis? Kidney Int. 1998;54(6):2207–17.
18. Han SH, Lee JE, Kim DK, Moon SJ, et al. Long-term clinical outcomes of peritoneal dialysis patients: single experience from Korea. Perit Dial Int. 2008;28:S21–6.
19. Fenton SS, Schaubel DE, Desmeules M, Morrison HI, et al. Hemodialysis versus peritoneal dialysis: a comparison of adjusted mortality rates. Am J Kidney Dis. 1997;30(3):334–42.
20. Coles GA, Williams JD. What is the place of peritoneal dialysis in the integrated treatment of renal failure? Kidney Int. 1998;54(6):2234–40.
21. Heaf J. Underutilization of peritoneal dialysis. JAMA. 2004;291:740–2.
22. Attaluri V, Lebeis C, Brethauer S, et al. Advanced laparoscopic techniques significantly improve function of peritoneal dialysis catheters. J Am Coll Surg. 2010;211(16):699–704.
23. Heaf JG, Lokkegaard H, Madsen M. Initial survival advantage of peritoneal dialysis relative to hemodialysis. Nephrol Dial Transplant. 2002;17(1):112–7.

Pre-sternal and Extended Catheters

9

Fahad Aziz and W. Kirt Nichols

Introduction

Placement of a peritoneal dialysis catheter with minimal or no complications is the key to the success of peritoneal dialysis. Peritoneal dialysis is now a well-established dialysis modality with fewer associated cardiovascular effects as compared to hemodialysis but it continues to be an underutilized modality. USRDS 2009 reported only 7.2% of the dialysis population on peritoneal dialysis as of 2007 [1]. A part of this problem is due to catheter-associated issues. Successful peritoneal dialysis depends on the permanent and safe access to the peritoneal cavity. A well-placed peritoneal dialysis catheter not only allows adequate dialysis but has less mechanical or infectious problems. Flanigan et al. in 2005 concluded that 20% of the patients are transferred to permanent or temporary hemodialysis due to catheter related issues and infections [2]. With the improvement in the surgical techniques, frequency of catheter related infections is going down but mechanical complications of peritoneal dialysis access continue to be a major concern for this patient population.

F. Aziz, MD
Division of Nephrology, Department of Medicine,
University of Missouri-Columbia,
Columbia, MO, USA

W. Kirt Nichols, MD, MHA (✉)
Department of Surgery, University of
Missouri-Columbia, Columbia, MO, USA
e-mail: nicholsw@health.missouri.edu

This chapter will review the different PD catheters in use with a focus on the insertion of Swan-Neck Missouri Pre-sternal PD catheters.

Background of PD Catheters Development

The word "peritoneal dialysis" was used commonly in German literature in 1920s and 1930s, where it referred to the removal of toxins from the blood through peritoneal membrane. In 1923, Ganter first ever described his experience of peritoneal dialysis in animals and two patients with the help of needles used for paracentesis [3]. Later, multiple experiments were done on animals to establish successful access to the peritoneal cavity. In 1934, Balazs and Rosenak performed the first ever continuous flow peritoneal dialysis in two patients with mercury dichloride poisoning [4]. In 1938, Wear et al. reported the first patient who survived after successful peritoneal dialysis [5]. Progress, however, seemed to halt during time of Second World War. But in mid 1940s, due to increasing number of renal failure patients during the time of time of war, multiple reports came to surface.

In 1946, Seligman, Frank and Fine performed a series of experiments in nephrectomized dogs to determine suitable peritoneal access, optimal dialysis fluid and optimal flow of continuous flow peritoneal irrigation [6]. That was the first closed system that used continuous inflow and outflow through

© Springer International Publishing AG 2017
S. Haggerty (ed.), *Surgical Aspects of Peritoneal Dialysis*, DOI 10.1007/978-3-319-52821-2_9

temporary catheters. This initial closed circuit was associated with high incidence of peritonitis.

Maxwell et al. made major progress in mid-1950 when he reported successful peritoneal dialysis in a series of 76 patients [7]. They initially introduced multiple side-hole catheters, which improved the performance of the system, and then by introducing a semi-rigid nylon design, they prevented catheter kinking. They then introduced a "paired bottle" technique, which used gravity for instillation and drainage.

In 1965, Henry Tenckhoff began to treat the patients on chronic peritoneal dialysis [8]. He introduced the concept of home peritoneal dialysis by using silicon rubber tubing, which can be used multiple times. His technique was successful in his hands but was over-all cumbersome. This initial design underwent multiple revisions until the most successful design was introduced which consisted of silicone rubber tube with a coiled intra-peritoneal portion and two Dacron cuffs at the peritoneum level, promoting tissue in growth which prevents peri-catheter leaks. This catheter was named after Dr. Tenckhoff. The Tenckhoff catheter became gold standard for the peritoneal access. Even after 50 years, the Tenckhoff catheter in its original form has remained the most widely used catheter type. Over time, it has been found that the Tenckhoff catheter is associated with exit site infection, recurrent peritonitis, external cuff extrusion and obstruction due to change in the position of catheter and omental wrapping around the catheter.

In 1976, Stephen et al. introduced a subcutaneous catheter to prevent exit infections [9]. Their catheter had two tubes in the peritoneal cavity with a subcutaneous reservoir. With each dialysis, the reservoir needed to be punctured. But with recurrent access to the reservoir, peritonitis episodes became a problem. Later, Gotloib et al. introduced a prosthesis, consisting of Teflon tube [10]. The prosthesis was implanted surgically with the head located in the subcutaneous tissue and the tube penetrating through the parietal peritoneum.

Several catheters have been introduced since then with the goal of decreasing multiple complications associated the standard Tenckhoff catheter. In 1985, Twardowaski et al., introduced silicone rubber "Swan-neck" catheters [11].

These catheters are permanently bent between two cuffs. The advantage associated with these catheters was insertion without distorting the shape of the catheter. Later, in 1992, Twardowaski et al. introduced modified "Swan-neck" catheters with exit site on the chest instead of abdomen. Moncrief et al. further modified the Swan-neck catheters with an elongated external cuff [12].

Peritoneal Dialysis

Chronic dialysis is a life-sustaining treatment for the patients with end stage renal disease. Due to lack of financial and clinical resources, dialysis access continues to remains limited through out the globe. With the growing burden of end stage renal disease and better understanding of peritoneal dialysis physiology, it's important for the both developing and developed countries to place the pattern of peritoneal dialysis use in a global context. Dialysis experts now agree that if feasible, peritoneal dialysis should be the starting dialysis modality for this group of patients [13]. Besides giving more freedom to the patient, it is gentle on the cardiovascular system. But despite these facts, peritoneal dialysis continues to be an under utilized modality. As per one estimate, only 11% of the chronic dialysis patients are treated with peritoneal dialysis. This encompasses nearly 197,000 patients worldwide [14]. Considering its effect on socioeconomics, according to one global survey, the developing countries are adopting this technique at a higher rate than the developed countries. An adequate access to the peritoneal cavity will be the key to success of peritoneal dialysis globally.

Currently Used Peritoneal Catheters

Today most peritoneal catheters used for chronic dialysis consist of two parts: Intra-peritoneal and extra-peritoneal. The extra-peritoneal part of the catheters is again composed of two parts: an intramural part and an external part. There are many combinations of intra and extra – peritoneal catheters are available for use today. As per American dialysis conference (ADC) 2005, Tenckhoff catheters have remained the most used catheters worldwide [15].

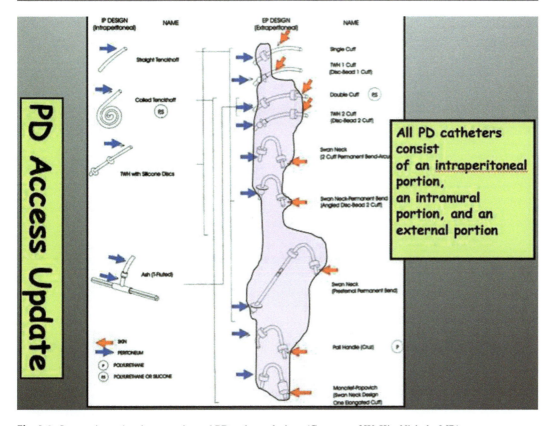

Fig. 9.1 Intraperitoneal and extraperitoneal PD catheter designs (Courtesy of W. Kirt Nichols, MD)

The Tenckhoff design has silicone rubber tubing with two polyester Dacron cuffs. The introduction of Dacron cuffs has been shown to be associated with a twofold advantage: (1) Decreasing the incidence of peritoneal fluid leaks; (2) decreasing the rates of peritoneal infections. These catheters are found with both straight and coiled intra-peritoneal portions.

Followed by Tenckhoff catheters, Swan-neck catheters were found to be the second most commonly used catheters. The permanent bend in the catheters is useful to prevent obstruction, cuff erosion and migration of these catheters. The use of Swan Neck catheters is preferentially recommended by the international society of peritoneal dialysis [16] (Fig. 9.1).

A. Tenckhoff Catheters:

Makeup: These catheters are made up of Silicone rubber with one or two polyester (Dacron) 1 cm long cuffs.

Dimensions: Internal diameter is 2.6 mm while external diameter is 5 mm. The lengths of the segments are: Intra-peritoneal 15 cm, intramural (Inter-cuff) 5–7 cm and external 16 cm.

The intra-peritoneal part has several perforations along with the distal portion of the catheter.

Coiled vs Straight Tenckhoff catheters: The coiled Tenckhoff catheters are preferred over straight ones due to decreased "jet-effect" and pressure discomfort during filling and emptying.

Both coiled and straight Tenckhoff catheters are provided with a barium-impregnated radiopaque stripe to assist in radiological visualization of the catheter.

B. Swan- neck peritoneal catheters:

Twardowaski et al. in 1993 [17], showed the complications associated with peritoneal dialysis catheters could be lowered if the double cuffed catheters were implanted

Features of Swan-Neck catheters	Advantages of specific features
1. Downwards Exit	Prevents Exit/Tunnel infections
2. Coiled intra-peritoneal tip	Prevents Infusion/pressure pain
3. Insertion through rectus muscle	Avoid peri-catheter leak due to excellent tissue ingrowth
4. Downward intraperitoneal entrance	Prevents intraperitoneal tip migration
5. Permanent bend between cuffs	Prevents external cuff extrusion

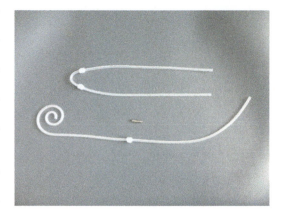

Fig. 9.2 Presternal peritoneal dilaysis catheter system including curl cath, extension piece and titanium connector (Courtesy of W. Kirt Nichols, MD)

through the belly of the rectus muscle and with both internal and skin exits of the tunnel directed downwards. But, resulting arcuate tunnel can lead to extrusion of the external cuff in straight catheters due to shape memory. Swan-neck catheters have a permanent bend between the two cuffs, which make them perfect match for the arcuate tunnel to avoid extrusion. With downward facing internal and skin exits, the rate of infections can be significantly decreased. Further, adding a coiled intra-peritoneal portion can reduce the pain and pressure discomfort with infusion. The intra-peritoneal segment in all swan neck catheters is 34 cm from the bead to the tip of the coil.

Swan-Neck Presternal Catheters

The chest is a sturdy structure with minimal motion. A catheter exit site on the chest has the advantage of: Minimal wall movement, decreasing chances of trauma and contamination due to the piston like movement of the superficial cuff in the abdominal wall. Twardowaski and Nichols in 1992 and 1993 modified Swan-neck peritoneal catheters to have an exit on the chest with preservation of all the advantages of the Swan-neck peritoneal coiled catheters [12]. The Swan-neck pre-sternal catheter is composed of two silicone rubber tubes, which are cut to an appropriate length and connected end to end at the time of implantation: (Figs. 9.2 and 9.3). The

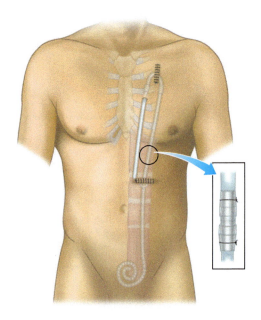

Fig. 9.3 Pre-sternal -Missouri Swan Neck Catheter insertion into peritoneal cavity with close-up of titanium connector joining the two portions of catheter (Courtesy of W. Kirt Nichols, MD)

great flexibility permitted by cutting the upper portion to length in the operating room means that the catheter exit site can actually be tailored to come out anywhere on the upper abdomen or lower chest as the patient and surgeon determine to be the best.

A. Abdominal Tube (Lower Portion):

The abdominal tube constitutes the intra-peritoneal catheter segment and a part of the intramural segment. This portion is identical to the Swan-neck abdominal catheter with exception of no bend and absence of the second cuff. The proximal end of the lower tube is straight with a redundant length, to be trimmed to the patient's size at the time of implantation. The two components are connected with a titanium connector.

B. Chest tube (Upper Portion):

The chest portion of the tube constitutes the remaining part of the intramural segment and the external catheter segment. This portion has two porous Dacron cuffs, a superficial and middle cuff, spread 5 cm apart. The tube between the cuffs has a permanent bent section defining an arc angle of 180°. The distal lumen of the upper tube communicates with the proximal lumen of the lower tube through the titanium connector. The tubing grip of the connector is strong enough to avoid spontaneous separation of the tubes.

Advantages of Swan-Neck Pre-sternal Catheters

More than 20 years after the introduction of pre-sternal catheters, they tend to perform better as compared to the abdominal catheters with respect to removal due to exit and tunnel infections, peritonitis and overall survival [18, 19]. Patients with ostomies and obesity also do better with the chest catheters as compared to the abdominal catheters. Patient acceptance of the pre-sternal exit site is also good due to psychological and body image reasons. A chest exit location allows a tub bath without the risk of contamination. Pre-sternal catheters are also very advantageous in small children because of the greater distance from diapers and are subjected to lesser trauma during crawling and with falls.

Advantages of pre-sternal Swan-neck catheters
1. Decreased risk of exit site infection
2. Decreased risk of peritonitis
3. Decreased risk of intra-peritoneal tip migration
4. Decreased risk of peri-catheter leaks
5. Better Psychosocial acceptance of the catheter

Patient Selection

The success of the peritoneal dialysis is dependent of the correct patient selection. There are only a few absolute contraindications to the initiation of peritoneal dialysis which include: Active peritoneal infections (Diverticulitis or severe inflammatory bowel disease, etc.) or uncorrectable pleuo-peritoneal connections. A majority of the relative contraindications are usually dependent on the institutional experience with peritoneal dialysis.

A majority of nephrologists now agree that the patients, if appropriate, should be offered peritoneal dialysis at the start of the dialysis in order to better preserve the residual renal function. Over time, concerns have been expressed regarding PD-dependent negative impact on survival but it has been also shown that PD provides survival advantage at least during the first few years being on dialysis. Frequent patient evaluation is essential to allow prompt adjustments in the dialysis prescription and modality when required. Important patient-related factors while considering PD include: Diabetes, large and small body size, peritoneal membrane transport status, age group and socioeconomic status.

Once the patient has been determined to have the functional capability for performing peritoneal dialysis, the relative surgical contraindications must be considered. The preoperative evaluation of a patient also includes a thorough surgical history and physical examination. Previous open abdominal operations are not a contraindication to PD catheter placement but adhesions formed to the anterior abdominal wall can increase the risk of abdominal access.

Generally, PD catheters do not require a long time to mature as compared to primary AV-fistulas. Typically from placement to training requires 2–3 weeks to before starting peritoneal dialysis.

Advantages of peritoneal dialysis
1. Preservation of residual renal function
2. Increased Survival in first 2 years
3. Patients with Coronary artery disease
4. Patients with advance liver cirrhosis and recurrent ascites
5. More patient mobility
6. More economical
7. Decreased rate of infections

Pre-sternal catheters have an advantage over abdominal catheters as they can be used in patients with obesity, with a history of multiple abdominal operations, or ostomies. Many of our patients find the "pre-sternal" location preferable for reasons of hygiene and general care of the catheter, especially those patients with urostomies, cololostomies, and those with marked obesity.

Indications of pre-sternal dialysis catheter placement
1. Obese patients (Less Subcutaneous tissue on chest wall in obese patients)
2. Previous multiple abdominal operations
3. Patients with ostomies
4. Diapered children

Surgical Technique

Pre-sternal PD catheters may be placed using traditional open surgical placement and laparoscopic techniques. In this section we will discuss the technique as well significant merits associated with each of these insertion methods.

Open Insertion Technique

Open surgical placement of peritoneal dialysis catheters such as Tenckoff catheters or Swan-Neck catheters should begin with a standing evaluation of the patient noting the belt line as well as marking with indelible ink identification of this landmark which is not obvious when the patient is supine on the operating room table, location of abdominal scars, hernias and ostomies. We also advocate supine examination with the patient lifting their head off the table. This

maneuver, much like in preoperative marking for ostomy sites, allows easier identification of the rectus musculature. Proper identification of the rectus ensures that the incision will allow trans-rectus placement of the catheter an occasional problem in those with diastasis recti (Fig. 9.4). This has been shown to decrease not only peri-catheter site leakage, but also catheter tract infections which can predispose towards peritonitis by allowing better tissue ingrowth into the cuffs [19].

The patient is positioned supine. Arm positioning is surgeon dependent, however, we find it easier to perform the pre-sternal tunneling and chest incision with the patient's arms tucked into the side and padded. After induction of appropriate anesthesia, 3–5 centimeter (cm) incisions is marked, usually lateral to the approximate location of inferior epigastric vessels but centered over the left rectus muscle, and the presternal incision and path of the catheter is also marked (Fig. 9.5). Next, an incision is made. Electrocautery is used to deepen incision and self-retaining retractors such as Weitlaner, are used to facilitate exposure. Care should be taken to have meticulous hemostasis as post-operative hematoma potentially becomes a source of catheter infection. The incision is deepened to the anterior rectus sheath which is opened transversely.

Once encountered, rectus muscle fibers are separated in the direction of their fibers with a muscle sparing technique by spreading hemostat in a cephalad-caudad direction and this exposure is maintained by a self-retaining retractor. Once the posterior sheath is encountered, a small incision is then made through the posterior sheath/ peritoneum and a pursestring suture is placed of approximately 1.5 cm diameter is placed. Elevation of this incision with forceps grasping the edges allows air to enter the abdomen creating a pneumoperitoneum and separates the viscera from the anterior abdominal wall.

The catheter of choice is then prepared on the back table by soaking the Dacron cuffs in saline and then flushing the catheter. At this point, a stiffening stylet is placed into the catheter. This provides extra support in a straight catheter to facilitate positioning and straightens the coiled

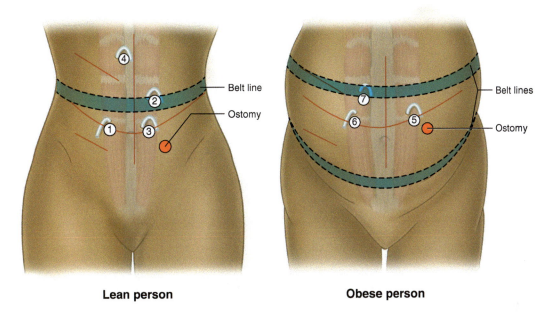

Lean person   **Obese person**

Fig. 9.4 Examination of abdomen giving consideration for old scars, location of rectus (diastasis), ostomies, belt line (Courtesy of W. Kirt Nichols, MD)

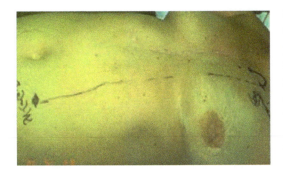

Fig. 9.5 Marking on the skin before exertion of the Pre-Sternal Missouri Swan neck Catheter (Courtesy of W. Kirt Nichols, MD)

catheter so that is may be placed in the pelvis more easily. Care should be taken in either the straight and coiled catheter to leave approximately 1 cm of soft catheter beyond the stylet to minimize trauma to the viscera during placement.

The catheter with the stiffening stylet is then used to guide the catheter carefully by feel into the pelvis. This is accomplished by elevation of the posterior sheath/peritoneum and by directing the stylet anteriorly and caudally until the area of the pubis is reached and then allowing it to fall posteriorly into the pelvis. If any resistance is felt, the catheter should be pulled back and redirected. Once placed, the catheter is held in place and the stylet carefully removed. Each catheter variation is then placed to its appropriate level (e.g. Missouri catheter placed so that purse string can be tied above the bead, or Lifecath disc folded and placed with discs beneath the peritoneum and one on the anterior sheath). Once the defect is closed in the posterior sheath and the deep cuff secured in place, a short (approximately 1.5 cm) tunnel is created in a cephalad direction through the anterior sheath and the catheter pulled through the anterior sheath into the subcutaneous space (Fig. 9.6).

To complete the pre-sternal insertion, creation of a small pocket on the chest wall is done using a vertical incision to the left of the sternum/manubrium. This pocket needs to be wide enough to allow the preformed curve to again lay flat on the chest wall. At this point, the pre-sternal catheter containing two further Dacron cuffs

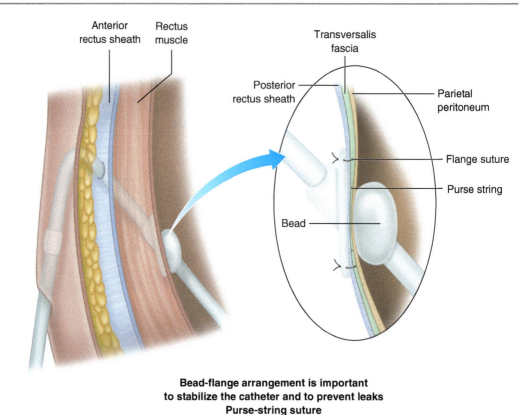

**Bead-flange arrangement is important
to stabilize the catheter and to prevent leaks
Purse-string suture**

Fig. 9.6 Missouri Swan-Neck Catheter insertion into peritoneal cavity (Courtesy of W. Kirt Nichols, MD)

is tunneled subcutaneously down to the previous incision using a vascular tunneler. These 2 catheters are then cut to appropriate length and connected using a supplied titanium connector. At this point, a 0 Ethibond suture is hand-tied around the connector on each end and then tied together. This creates a reinforced connection that is sturdy enough that we have never seen separation of the catheters in the tunnel. Once satisfied with catheter length and flow, the chest wall catheter should be externalized approximately 3 cm below the superficial cuff using a sharp trochar attached to the PD tubing. In a male the exit site is aimed laterally toward the nipple. In a woman we tunnel medially to avoid traversing the breast tissue. At this point, we recommend closing all incisions with absorbable suture in multiple layers. An infusion is done to test function and a fluoroscopic C-arm study is done to confirm placement.

Laparoscopic Technique

Presternal catheters may also be inserted using a laparoscopic technique. The ability to obtain minimally invasive access has had an increasing role in both the initial placement of peritoneal dialysis catheters as well as in revisions and repositioning. A discussion of the optimal method of abdominal entry technique is beyond the scope of this chapter and is covered in Chap. 8. For laparoscopic insertion of PD catheters, the insertion of the abdominal segment with cuff in the rectus sheath is performed using the standard best practices of preoperative marking and planning of insertion site. In addition it has been recommended that the use of rectus sheath tunnel and omentopexy may significantly reduce catheter dysfunction [20]. The parasternal incision should be planned 4–5 cm lateral to the midline but avoiding the fleshy part of the breast. As in Fig. 9.3 The swan neck presternal segment is aligned so the exit site is medial and at least 2.5–3 cm from the midline and 3–4 cm below the level of the transverse incision. Similar to open insertion a vascular tunneler is used to tunnel the presternal segment from chest to abdominal wound. The segments are then measured and the excess is trimmed. In an obese patient the catheter segments may need to be cut shorter to account for the depth of subcutaneous fat. The segments are pulled up through the abdominal wound and connected using the titanium adapter and then pulled into the tunnel [21]. Completion of the procedure is similar to the open technique described above. If one chooses to use an upper abdominal exit site the technique is the same except a small subcostal incision is used for tunneling and the exit site is 3–4 cm lateral and inferior to this.

Peritoneal Dialysis Catheter Removal

Peritoneal dialysis catheter removal is an infrequent procedure. It is typically done for one of three indications: (1) Catheter not needed after kidney transplant, (2) For patients with recurrent peritonitis, (3) Patients changing from peritoneal dialysis to hemodialysis, usually for a reason of non/malfunction.

The design of a chronic peritoneal dialysis catheter should ensure excellent tissue ingrowth into the cuffs to fix the catheter in place and prevent leak. This very design characteristic means that the catheter needs to be removed operatively and not at the bedside. This may be accomplished using conscious sedation and local or a general anesthetic. The patient's abdomen and chest are prepped and draped in a typical fashion.

In the case of an abdominal catheter the old abdominal incision is reopened and the catheter is identified by palpation. The sheath around the catheter is opened and the dissection is carried to the level of the cuffs. The cuffs are freed up with a combination electrocautery and sharp dissection. Once the cuffs and/or flange are freed up the purse string suture at the peritoneal level is divided and the catheter pulled from the abdomen. The small defect into the peritoneal cavity is closed usually with a single suture 2-0 Proline. Any additional cuffs in the subcutaneous tissue are likewise freed up using electrocautery. The catheter is divided in the subcutaneous space and the external portion of the catheter is pulled free. Any fascia defects are closed with non-absorbable suture and the subcutaneous tissue and skin are closed with absorbable suture. A gauze wick is inserted in the exit site to act as a drain for a few days.

If the patient has a pre-sternal catheter, the removal of the abdominal portion is done exactly the same as above. The pre-sternal portion of the catheter is ligated and divided through the abdominal incision, and the abdominal portion is removed. The pre-sternal incision is reopened and the catheter identified by palpation. The sheath surrounding the catheter is opened and both subcutaneous cuffs are freed up with electrocautery. The distal ligated distal portion of the catheter is pulled up into the wound and the catheter is divided just beyond the superficial cuff just beneath the exit site. The upper portion of the catheter submitted as a specimen for gross examination unless infected when specimens are sent for cultures. The wound is closed in a normal fashion using 3-0 absorbable sutures in the subcutaneous tissue and a 4-0 monofilament subcuticular suture. A piece of gauze is tucked in to the exit site to act as a wick drain.

Early Post-operative Care of the Catheters

After placement of the catheter, a plain X-ray of the abdomen, if not done in the operating room, can be done to check the position of the catheter. Catheter-tip location in the pelvis usually predicts excellent catheter function. PD catheter flushing is usually done afterwards by the dialysis nurse; exchanges are performed until the dialysate return is clear. Heparin can be added to the

Fig. 9.7 Post-operative care   Rinse until clear – discharge same day
Dressings – inspect and change weekly; Check for drainage, fever, bleeding
Flush catheter weekly
Immobilize catheter
No bath or shower till healed

dialysate to dissolve the fibrin debris. There is no consensus how frequently the catheter should be flushed after the placement of the catheter. Most of the centers prefer to perform the flushing usually once a week. Peritoneal dialysis, is usually delayed at least 2 weeks after the catheter placement, which allows better healing of the peritoneum, and helps prevents leak. Peritoneum equilibrium tests are usually performed 4 weeks after the placement of the catheter (Fig. 9.7). Within last 10 years, urgent start PD has gained considerable interest. Treatments are usually performed with low fill volumes in supine position to avoid peri-catheter leaks.

Complications

Early Complications – Peritoneal Access Related

1. **Minor Bleeding complications**:
   Blood-tinged dialysate is common post implantation but usually get resolved with post-implantation flushing. Minor bleeding occurs due to inadequate surgical hemostasis at time of implantation. Due to increased length of subcutaneous tunnel and abundant vasculature of the anterior chest wall, the risk of minor bleeding is higher with the pre-sternal catheters as compared to the abdominal catheter.

2. **Peri-catheter Leak**:
   Peri-catheter leaks are also considered an early complication. A wait of 2–4 weeks post implantation usually allows enough time for healing and tissue ingrowth and avoids peri-catheter leak. If there is an urgent need to start dialysis, low volumes should be used to avoid peri-catheter leaks.

3. **Poor Dialysate Return**:
   Poor dialysate return is usually due to catheter obstruction. Tip obstruction by bowel and/

or bladder or intra-luminal formation of clot is the most common causes of catheter obstruction. If bladder and/or bowel are the cause of poor dialysate return, emptying bladder and use of a laxative may restore catheter function. Post-implantation, catheter flushing usually prevents clot formation in the catheter. We recommended having the catheter flushed weekly to prevent intra-luminal clot formation. Use of heparin and forceful injection through the tubing into the peritoneal can dislodge the clot. If these maneuvers are unsuccessful, thrombolytics like tissue plasminogen activator or urokinase may open the obstruction in a small number of patients.

4. **Two-Way obstruction**:
   Two-way catheter obstruction is usually due to catheter kinking in the tunnel. It is recognizable on an abdominal X-ray. Surgical correction is needed as soon as the diagnosis is made. If there is no catheter kinking but there is two-way obstruction, omental wrapping or multiple adhesions are usually the reason. Omentectomy or adhesionolysis using laparoscopy may be required.

5. **Reverse One-way obstruction**:
   In reverse one-way peritoneal dialysis catheter obstruction, fluid can be drained but can't be installed for next cycle. It's extremely rare condition and is usually due to partial obstruction of the catheter with clot, which causes inflow obstruction. The clot can be removed with suction.

6. **Intra-abdominal injury**:
   The risk of intra-abdominal injury is higher in the patients with previous abdominal injuries. Injuries can occur during entry in to the abdomen or during the positioning of the catheter in the pelvis. It is usually recommended that patients with previous operations should have initial laparoscopy done to evaluate the feasibility of access into the

pelvis for placement of the catheter. Viscus perforation is extremely rare with the surgical placement of the catheter.

Outcomes

Several studies have evaluated the overall clinical outcomes of patients with end-stage renal disease. When evaluating the mortality rate, it is important to keep in mind that life expectancy of those with end-stage renal disease is only roughly 20–25% less than the general population. Despite improvements in dialysis over the years, only 54% of HD patients and 65% of PD patients are alive at 3 years after ESRD onset [22]. In studies comparing trends in dialysis patients, however, there are a number of interesting observations that have been made.

It should first be noted that overall mortality related to end-stage renal disease is significant. Many studies have been done to try to understand the reasons including those related to the modality of dialysis chosen. One fairly consistent trend that is elicited from the dialysis population data is that PD offers an early survival advantage over HD. Peritoneal dialysis patients are routinely seen to have significantly lower mortality rates in the first 2 years with dialysis dependent end-stage renal disease [23, 24]. The reasons for this are not entirely clear; however, this effect is consistently noted. We also consistently see that patients who are transferred from PD to HD suffer an increased mortality risk in the first 6 months after the changeover. This is likely due to the generally poorer health of those who suffer a peritoneal dialysis catheter complication necessitating at least temporary transfer to hemodialysis. After the initial survival advantage, rates equalize and by 5 years there appears to be a slight, but not statistically significant, increase in survival for HD patients [25].

Patient preference related to dialysis modality remains important. One of the risk factors consistently associated with increased mortality is lower overall health-related quality of life [26]. This has also been a factor in multiple studies comparing peritoneal to hemodialysis. The results of these studies have not been consistent. A recent meta-analysis was completed to help solidify the conclusions of previous studies; No statistically significant difference in health-related quality of life can be consistently found among the data confirming better quality of life using one modality of dialysis over the other [27].

Summary

Peritoneal dialysis offers an excellent alternative method for renal replacement therapy for a wide range of patients. The importance of patient selection must not be underestimated. Patients must have an adequate understanding of the lifestyle they are choosing since the patient or their care givers are the ones directly responsible for taking care of their access. Failure to properly care for the site, as well as the catheter, can result in loss of access due to infectious complications.

Surgical placement of peritoneal dialysis catheters encompasses a range of techniques which the individual surgeon can tailor to his/her practice. However, patient criteria should also be evaluated as patients will have better ability to care for their access when placed in an easily visible location (pre-sternal or upper abdominal) and this can help to prevent late infectious complications. In our present practice, virtually every patient gets a Presternal catheter. Those patients particularly benefiting by placement on the chest wall are those patients who are morbidly obese or those with an ostomy or intertrigenous skin problems which may predispose to exit site infections if catheter exit was on the abdominal wall. Likewise, extended catheter with exit in the subcostal region may offer similar benefits and not require as long of a tunnel.

Regional practice patterns will continue to play a role in the prevalence of peritoneal dialysis as an alternative method of renal replacement therapy in each community. As the vast majority of end-stage renal disease patients are controlled by nephrology referral patterns, any access surgeon performing PD catheterization procedures should make attempts to educate local nephrologists that PD access can be accommodated for any good candidates. Although no study consistently confirms an improvement in health-related quality of life, there are many patients with end-stage renal disease that find the ability to perform their own renal replacement therapy on schedule liberating.

References

1. U.S. Renal Data System: USRDS 2009 annual data report: atlas of chronic kidney disease and end-stage renal disease in the United States, Bethesda, MD, National Institute of Health, National Institute of Diabetes and Digestive and Kidney Disease; 2009.
2. Flanigan M, Gokal R. Peritoneal catheters and exit-site practices toward optimum peritoneal access: a review of current developments. Perit Dial Int. 2005;25(2):132–9.
3. Ganter G. Über die Beseitigung giftiger Stoffe aus dem Blute durch Dialyse. Münch Med Wochenschrift. 1923;50:1478–81.
4. Balázs J. Rosenak, Stephan. Zur Behandlung der Sublimatanurie durch peritoneale Dialyse. Wien klin Wchnschr. 1934;47:851.
5. Wear JB, Sisk IR, Trinkle AJ. Peritoneal lavage in the treatment of uremia, an experimental and clinical study. J Urol. 1938;39:53.
6. Seligman AM, Frank HA, Fine J. Treatment of experimental uremia by means of peritoneal irrigation. J Clin Invest. 1946;25:211.
7. Maxwell MH, Breed ES, Schwartz IL. Renal venous pressure in chronic congestive heart failure. J Clin Invest. 1950;29:342–8.
8. Tenckhoff H, Curtis FK. Experience with maintenance peritoneal dialysis in the home. Trans Am Soc Artif Intern Organs. 1970;16:90–5.
9. Stephen RL, Atkin–Thor E, Kolff WJ. Recirculating peritoneal dialysis with subcutaneous catheter. Trans Am Soc Artif Int Organs. 1976;22:575–85.
10. Gotloib L, Nisencorn I, Garmizo AL, Galili N, Servadio C, Sudarsky M. Subcutaneous intraperitoneal prosthesis for maintenance of peritoneal dialysis. Lancet. 1975;1:1318–20.
11. Twardowski ZJ, Nolph KD, Khanna R, Prowant BF, Ryan LP, Nichols WK. The need for a "swan neck" permanently bent, arcuate peritoneal dialysis catheter. Perit Dial Bull. 1985;5:219–23.
12. Twardowski ZJ, Nichols WK, Nolph KD, Khanna R. Swan neck presternal ("bath tub") catheter for peritoneal dialysis. Adv Perit Dial. 1992;8:316–24.
13. Goodlad C, Brown E. The role of peritoneal dialysis in modern renal replacement therapy. Postgrad Med J. 2013 Oct;89(1056):584–90.
14. Jain AK, Blake P, Cordy P, Garg AX. Global trends in rates of peritoneal dialysis. J Am Soc Nephrol. 2012;23(3):533–44.
15. Negoi D, Prowant BF, Twardowski ZJ. Current trends in the use of peritoneal dialysis catheters. Adv Perit Dial. 2006;22:147–52.
16. Flanigan M, Gokal R. Peritoneal catheters and exit-site practices toward optimum peritoneal access: a review of current developments. Perit Dial Int. 2005 Mar-Apr;25(2):132–9.
17. Twardowski ZJ, Van Stone JC, Jones ME, Klusmeyer ME, Haynie JD. Blood recirculation in intravenous catheters for hemodialysis. J Am Soc Nephrol. 1993;3(12):1978–81.
18. Yerram P, Gill A, Prowant B, Saab G, Misra M, Whaley-Connell A. A 9-year survival analysis of the presternal Missouri swan-neck catheter. Adv Perit Dial. 2007;23:90–3.
19. Golper TA, et al. Risk factors for peritonitis in long-term peritoneal dialysis: the Network 9 peritonitis and catheter survival studies. Academic Subcommittee of the Steering Committee of the Network 9 Peritonitis and Catheter Survival Studies. Am J Kidney Dis. 1996;28(3):428–36.
20. Haggerty S, Roth S, Walsh D, et al. Guidelines for laparoscopic peritoneal dialysis access surgery. Surg Endosc. 2014;28(11):3016–45.
21. Crabtree J, Fishman A. Laparoscopic implantation of swan neck presternal peritoneal dialysis catheters. J Laparoendosc Adv Surg Tech. 2003;13(2):131–7.
22. Guo A, Mujais S. Patient and technique survival on peritoneal dialysis in the United States: evaluation in large incident cohorts. Kidney Int Suppl. 2003;88:S3–12.
23. Heaf JG, Lokkegaard H, Madsen M. Initial survival advantage of peritoneal dialysis relative to haemodialysis. Nephrol Dial Transplant. 2002;17(1):112–7.
24. Collins AJ, et al. Mortality risks of peritoneal dialysis and hemodialysis. Am J Kidney Dis. 1999;34(6):1065–74.
25. System, U.S.R.D., 2014 USRDS annual data report: an overview of the epidemiology of kidney disease in the United States. National Institute of Health, Bethesda; 2014.
26. Moura A, et al. Predictors of health-related quality of life perceived by end-stage renal disease patients under online hemodiafiltration. Qual Life Res. 2015;24(6):1327–35.
27. Liem YS, Bosch JL, Hunink MG. Preference-based quality of life of patients on renal replacement therapy: a systematic review and meta-analysis. Value Health. 2008;11(4):733–41.

Buried Catheters: How and Why?

10

Seth B. Furgeson and Isaac Teitelbaum

Introduction

Successful peritoneal dialysis requires a well-functioning catheter that can be used long-term. For the practitioner, there are many choices that must be made regarding catheter placement. The catheter itself can have one or two cuffs and have coiled or straight intra-abdominal segments. Placement of peritoneal catheters can be performed using open or laparoscopic surgical approaches as well as percutaneous approaches. In 1993, Moncrief and Popovich described a new variation of catheter placement [1]. Instead of immediately externalizing a peritoneal catheter, the distal end was embedded in the subcutaneous fat while the catheter was allowed to heal. The distal end was exteriorized at a later point and peritoneal dialysis was begun. This chapter will highlight the benefits and disadvantages of this technique and review outcomes data regarding this procedure.

S.B. Furgeson, MD
Division of Renal Diseases and Hypertension,
University of Colorado-Anschutz Medical Campus,
Denver Health Hospital, Aurora, CO, USA

I. Teitelbaum, MD, FACP (✉)
Home Dialysis Program, University of Colorado
Hospital, AIP, 12605 E. 16th Avenue, Box F774,
Aurora, CO 80045, USA
e-mail: Isaac.Teitelbaum@ucdenver.edu

Rationale Supporting Buried Catheter

When the Moncrief-Popovich technique was first described, the proposed benefit was a reduction in infectious complications. Since the catheter is placed in a sterile subcutaneous pocket while the surgical wound heals, there is a decreased chance for periluminal or intraluminal migration of bacteria. The formation of a mature, well-healed tunnel in the absence of bacteria allows a bacteriologic barrier to develop. When the catheter is eventually exteriorized through a newly created exit site, it extends through a well-healed tunnel.

A related benefit to buried catheters is a reduction in dialysate leaks. Dialysate leaks can significantly compromise dialysis therapy and impair quality of life for patients on dialysis. In non-buried catheters, it is recommended that full volume dialysis not be performed for 2 weeks. Since buried catheters have typically been allowed to heal for many weeks, tissue ingrowth has sealed the catheter tunnel. Therefore, full volume dialysis can be initiated when dialysis is begun with a low likelihood of dialysate leaks.

As this technique has been introduced to clinical practice, it has become apparent that there are other benefits to using a buried catheter approach. Use of buried catheters may provide psychological benefits for patients and possibly improve utilization of peritoneal dialysis.

© Springer International Publishing AG 2017
S. Haggerty (ed.), *Surgical Aspects of Peritoneal Dialysis*, DOI 10.1007/978-3-319-52821-2_10

Patients with advanced chronic kidney disease (CKD) will ideally have the catheter placed before needing dialysis. In that period of time, it is easier for the patient to have an embedded catheter that requires no local care or activity limitations. For patients who may be hesitant in choosing peritoneal dialysis, this approach may increase acceptance of peritoneal dialysis. Patients may consider it similar to placing an arteriovenous fistula (AVF) months before the initiation of hemodialysis.

In many centers, there may only be one or two practitioners who specialize in the placement of peritoneal catheters. Therefore, prompt placement of peritoneal catheters may not always be feasible. Since it is difficult to predict when a patient will require dialysis, placement of buried catheters allows flexibility regarding the timing of dialysis initiation. Patients who plan to do peritoneal dialysis may develop urgent indications for dialysis. If they do not have peritoneal dialysis catheter ready to use, hemodialysis is often started through a venous catheter.

Buried catheters also require fewer resources to maintain. After a catheter is exteriorized, the exit site requires local wound care and the catheter must be flushed frequently. Non-buried catheters are more resource-intensive because dialysis staff or patients must perform these actions before the patient needs dialysis. Buried catheters also require wound care and catheter care; however, this is only necessary once the catheter is externalized and dialysis is begun.

Description of Procedure

As first described, the Moncrief-Popovich catheter was placed using a surgical approach. The catheter had two cuffs separated by a swan-neck bend configuration. The deep cuff was embedded in the rectus muscle while the superficial one was located near the skin. The external segment was completely buried in the subcutaneous tissue and the wound was closed. After a period of at least 3 weeks, the catheter was externalized through a 4 cm skin incision and dialysis was initiated.

The surgical techniques in the original technique are not completely described. Subsequent articles have detailed the catheter management and embedding techniques. After the catheter is placed, sufficient flow is ensured with saline irrigation and heparin is instilled in the lumen of the catheter [2–4] Some practitioners close the distal end of the catheter with a suture prior to embedding [2]. Embedding stylets are also commonly used to direct the catheter tip to the appropriate location [3–5]. After the tip of the catheter is placed in the correct location by the stylet, the distal end is broken off, thereby creating a plug in the distal tip of the catheter.

Since the original publications, small variations to this technique have been described. Laparoscopic implantation is commonly used [3, 4]. Coiled and straight intraperitoneal segments have been used. In addition to the swan-neck configuration, straight segment catheters have been used (Fig. 10.1) [3]. Coiled catheters and swan-neck catheters are thought to decrease risk of catheter dysfunction. However, there is limited data from well-controlled clinical trials that these catheter variants significantly impact catheter function [6].

The subcutaneous tunnels and exit sites can also be created in diverse anatomical regions (Fig. 10.1). Catheter extenders can allow to the catheters to be tunneled for longer distances to create presternal exit sites (Fig. 10.1a) [7]. Presternal exit sites may provide a lower infection rate and particularly useful in obese patients. Extenders can also be used to create exit sites in the upper abdomen (Fig. 10.1b).

At the time of externalization, an exit site is created at least 2–3 cm distal from the distal cuff. This is a routine, quick procedure that is done with local anesthesia. Under sterile technique, a small incision is made. Dissection of the subcutaneous adipose tissue is performed using a hemostat until the catheter is mobilized. Most catheters have developed a fibrin sheath along the exterior surface; careful removal of the fibrin sheath is performed with scissors and the catheter is then completely exteriorized. After removal of the distal suture and plug, an adapter set can be connected to the catheter tip in order to initiate dialysis.

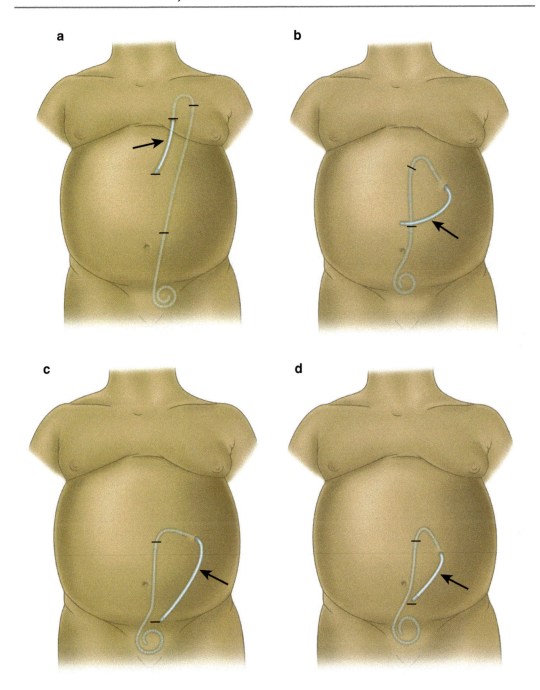

Fig. 10.1 Variations of buried catheter placement. Diagrams of different buried catheter configurations. The *arrows* point the area that is initially embedded. The different configurations are presternal exit sites (**a**), upper abdominal exit sites (**b**), straight Tenckhoff catheter (**c**), and swan-neck catheter (**d**) (Reprinted with permission Crabtree and Burchette [3])

Outcomes with Buried Catheters

Infections

Due to the above characteristics, it was predicted that subcutaneous peritoneal catheter embedding would decrease risk of infectious complications. In the initial description of the procedure, the authors performed a prospective evaluation of infections in all patients with buried catheters [1]. They found that the peritonitis rates were lower than historical controls but exit site infections appeared to occur at the same rate. The study sample included patients who performed a spike technique for exchanges and patients who used disconnect systems.

Despite that initial study, it is still unclear whether the Moncrief-Popovich technique decreases infectious complications. Two small, controlled trials have tested whether catheter burying decreases peritonitis. The first one randomized 30 patients to catheter placement with immediate externalization and 30 patients to catheters buried subcutaneously [8]. In the first group, the patients had a 6 week break-in period; in the buried catheter group, the catheters were externalized after 6 weeks. Half of the patients in each group used a Y-connector and half used the spike technique. The peritonitis-free interval was much longer in the group that received a buried catheter and used a Y-connector. This group had a peritonitis-free period of 120 patient-months while the group with a standard catheter using a Y-connector had a peritonitis-free interval of 26 patient-months. It should be noted that this study was small and had a low overall rate of peritonitis.

Another trial randomized patients at two separate hospitals to receive a buried or non-buried catheters [9]. Each center had a slightly different technique for catheter placement and catheter embedment. A total of 60 patients were included in this trial. Episodes of peritonitis were assessed at 6, 12, and 24 months. The group assigned to receive buried catheters did not have a statistically significant decrease in the time to first peritonitis episode. AS the other studies showed, there was no decrease in exit site infections. A meta-analysis pooled the results of these two studies and found that there was no reduced rate of peritonitis or exit site infections with buried catheters [10].

Catheter Damage

Since the catheter is not directly visualized during the externalization procedure, there is the risk of inadvertent damage to the catheter during the procedure. The needle used for local anesthesia can puncture the catheter as can the scalpel used for the skin incision. The rates of these complications are unclear but are likely quite low. In a retrospective review of 84 patients undergoing externalization, each complication happened in 1 patient [3]. Damage to the catheter tubing may not be a significant problem. Depending on the location of catheter tubing damage, a catheter revision can be performed without requiring further surgery.

Catheter Malfunction

One concern regarding catheter burial is a potential for catheter dysfunction after externalization. Since the catheters are typically placed before a patient requires dialysis, it is possible that the period of subcutaneous burying may last months or years. It is very difficult for practitioners to accurately predict when a patient may require dialysis. Since there is a general desire to avoid urgent dialysis, catheters are often placed well before the anticipated need for dialysis. However, it is possible that this strategy would increase risks for catheter failure since the catheter may migrate or intraluminal clots may form over the long duration.

Numerous studies have examined whether prolonged catheter burial negatively impacts catheter function. Results from a single-center study suggested that burial of single-cuff catheters was associated with increased mechanical complications [11]. The same center changed the catheter type to double-cuff catheters with a swan-neck. A retrospective analysis of outcomes with double-cuff catheters showed excellent long-term function [12].

In this study, the mean duration of catheter burial was approximately 40 days although some catheters were buried for more than 1 year. Ten percent of the catheters did not function immediately due to either fibrin plugs or omental wraps. However, all but one of these catheters were rendered functional by laparoscopic revision and ultimately 99.2% of catheters were useable. The duration of catheter embedment did not appear to predict long-term catheter function. Catheters that were embedded for longer periods had identical outcomes to catheters with short embedment duration (Fig. 10.2).

Studies from other PD centers that use buried catheters have shown similar results. In another retrospective study, Crabtree found that 99% of all externalized catheters were eventually used successfully, although only 85% functioned well immediately after externalization. Two other studies have shown similar data regarding catheter function after prolonged embedding [13, 14].

However, in contrast to other studies, Brown et al. found that prolonged catheter embedding (greater than 4 months) adversely affected catheter function.

Futile Catheters

As the Moncrief-Popovich technique has become more widely adopted, catheter burial time has increased. PD programs that aim to avoid temporary hemodialysis in prospective PD patients choose to place the buried catheter well before a patient requires dialysis. However, the risk to that strategy is that a patient will undergo a catheter placement surgery but never use the catheter (futile catheter placement). This problem is not unique to peritoneal dialysis; a number of prospective hemodialysis patients will also have futile AV fistula placement. Futile catheter placement may be due

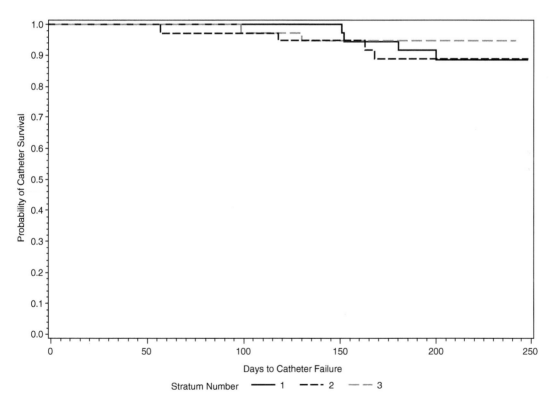

Fig. 10.2 Survival after prolonged embedding. Long-term catheter survival was analyzed as a function of embedding duration. The group with the shortest duration (*1*) had the same rate of catheter survival as the group with the longest duration (*3*) (Reprinted with permission Elhassan et al. [12])

to patient death or change in health status. The latter may preclude them from performing a home modality. It is also possible that the decrease in GFR is very slow and the patient may not need dialysis for years.

Studies have examined the risk of futile catheter placement with the buried catheter technique. In high-volume PD programs, the rate of futile catheter placement is approximately 8% [13, 15]. Clearly, there is no way to definitely predict which patients will not ever need their peritoneal catheter. Some clinical variables do help practitioners predict which patients will need dialysis sooner and, would therefore be less likely to have a futile catheter placement. Patients with lower albumin, lower GFR, and significant proteinuria are more likely to need their catheter externalized sooner [15]. A comprehensive clinical assessment using these variables may help providers identify the optimal time for catheter placement.

Summary

The use of the Moncrief-Popovich is a commonly used technique for peritoneal catheter placement that offers many potential benefits. It allows providers and patients to prepare for peritoneal dialysis and may increase utilization of peritoneal dialysis. The technique significantly reduces the probability of dialysate leaks and allows full-dose dialysis to be performed immediately after externalization. Although there are few controlled trials comparing the Moncrief-Popovich technique to standard catheter placement, data does suggest that this is an effective procedure that is associated with few complications.

References

1. Moncrief JW, Popovich RP, Broadrick LJ, He ZZ, Simmons EE, Tate RA. The Moncrief-Popovich catheter. A new peritoneal access technique for patients on peritoneal dialysis. ASAIO J. 1993;39:62–5.
2. Prischl FC, Wallner M, Kalchmair H, Povacz F, Kramar R. Initial subcutaneous embedding of the peritoneal dialysis catheter – a critical appraisal of this new implantation technique. Nephrol Dial Transplant. 1997;12:1661–7.
3. Crabtree JH, Burchette RJ. Peritoneal dialysis catheter embedment: surgical considerations, expectations, and complications. Am J Surg. 2013;206:464–71.
4. McCormick BB, Brown PA, Knoll G, et al. Use of the embedded peritoneal dialysis catheter: experience and results from a North American Center. Kidney Int Suppl. 2006;(103):S38–43.
5. Page DE, Turpin C. A simple and inexpensive method of subcutaneous implantation of catheter distal segment using a Tenckhoff curled catheter. Perit Dial Int. 2000;20:85–7.
6. Strippoli GF, Tong A, Johnson D, Schena FP, Craig JC. Catheter type, placement and insertion techniques for preventing peritonitis in peritoneal dialysis patients. Cochrane Database Syst Rev. 2004;(4):CD004680.
7. Kubota M, Kanazawa M, Takahashi Y, Io H, Ishiguro N, Tomino Y. Implantation of presternal catheter using Moncrief technique: aiming for fewer catheter-related complications. Perit Dial Int. 2001;21(Suppl 3):S205–8.
8. Park MS, Yim AS, Chung SH, et al. Effect of prolonged subcutaneous implantation of peritoneal catheter on peritonitis rate during CAPD: a prospective randomized study. Blood Purif. 1998;16:171–8.
9. Danielsson A, Blohme L, Tranaeus A, Hylander B. A prospective randomized study of the effect of a subcutaneously "buried" peritoneal dialysis catheter technique versus standard technique on the incidence of peritonitis and exit-site infection. Perit Dial Int. 2002;22:211–9.
10. Strippoli GF, Tong A, Johnson D, Schena FP, Craig JC. Catheter-related interventions to prevent peritonitis in peritoneal dialysis: a systematic review of randomized, controlled trials. J Am Soc Nephrol. 2004;15:2735–46.
11. Esson ML, Quinn MJ, Hudson EL, Teitelbaum I. Subcutaneously tunnelled peritoneal dialysis catheters with delayed externalization: long-term follow-up. Adv Perit Dial. 2000;16:123–8.
12. Elhassan E, McNair B, Quinn M, Teitelbaum I. Prolonged duration of peritoneal dialysis catheter embedment does not lower the catheter success rate. Perit Dial Int. 2011;31:558–64.
13. Brown PA, McCormick BB, Knoll G, et al. Complications and catheter survival with prolonged embedding of peritoneal dialysis catheters. Nephrol Dial Transplant. 2008;23:2299–303.
14. Brum S, Rodrigues A, Rocha S, et al. Moncrief-Popovich technique is an advantageous method of peritoneal dialysis catheter implantation. Nephrol Dial Transplant. 2010;25:3070–5.
15. Crabtree JH, Burchette RJ, Siddiqi RA. Embedded catheters: minimizing excessive embedment time and futile placement while maintaining procedure benefits. Perit Dial Int. 2015;35:545–51.

Post-operative Protocol and Maintenance of Function

11

Brendan McCormick

Background

While there have been significant clinical interest in the relative merits of different peritoneal dialysis (PD) catheter designs and different insertion methods, there is a dearth of published data on optimum post-operative care of PD catheters. The choice of post -operative dressing, frequency of dressing changes, flushing protocols, and catheter break-in protocols vary widely from center to center. In addition, the approach to leaking or obstructed catheters is typically guided by individual practitioner experience rather than published guidelines. This chapter will review the approach to post operative care of the PD catheter and highlight standard practices and, where possible, make evidence informed recommendations for practice.

Immediate Post-operative Care of the PD Catheter

Regardless of catheter placement method, the operator should confirm function of the PD catheter by flushing with either saline or dialysate prior to completion of the case. Even in the case

B. McCormick, MD, FRCPC
Division of Nephrology, Department of Medicine, University of Ottawa and the Ottawa Hospital, Ottawa, ON K1H 7W9, USA
e-mail: bmccormick@ottawahospital.on.ca

of a buried or embedded catheter, the surgeon will typically confirm catheter patency immediately prior to creation of the subcutaneous tunnel. As such, it is not necessary that PD catheters be routinely flushed in the recovery room. The major exception to this is in cases where there has been significant intraperitoneal bleeding. These cases do need immediate post-operative flushing as intraperitoneal blood may result in catheter obstruction and also give rise to intraabdominal adhesions. A retrospective cohort study has suggested that early and frequent flushing of these catheters is associated with a significantly lower subsequent rate of catheter malfunction [1]. As such, it is important that the operator inform the home dialysis team if there has been unexpected intraperitoneal bleeding as immediate post operative flushing will be required in these cases.

The International Society of Peritoneal Dialysis (ISPD) recommends that post operative dressing changes be performed using sterile technique and that the exit site be kept dry for at least 2 weeks, or until well healed [2]. More than 80% of North American centers use non occlusive gauze dressings or semi-occlusive dressings and it is recommended to avoid fully occlusive dressings due to the build up of moisture under the dressing which can delay healing [3, 4]. Dressings are typically changed once or twice weekly and care must be taken to ensure that the catheter is well immobilized as trauma to the exit site from a mobile catheter will delay healing [5]. Most PD programs also recommend that patients not

S. Haggerty (ed.), *Surgical Aspects of Peritoneal Dialysis*, DOI 10.1007/978-3-319-52821-2_11

shower or bathe for at least 1 week or do heavy lifting [3].

The time required for exit site healing is quite variable and while typically 2–6 weeks, in some cases it can be longer [6]. Risk factors for delayed exit site healing include increased body mass index, diabetes, exit site larger than 7 mm, and poor immobilization of the PD catheter [7, 8]. Delayed healing of exit sites is strongly associated with an increased risk of subsequent tunnel infection and catheter loss highlighting the importance of early exit site care [7].

The optimal solution for cleansing the new exit site is not well established. Many centers use sterile saline but some centers use antiseptics such as sodium hypochlorite, chlorhexidine or iodine based preparations. The challenge with the early use of antiseptics is that these agents are potentially cytotoxic and may delay wound healing [5]. There is a single published randomized study of povidone-iodine ointment versus saline for early exit site care. In this single center study of 117 patients, the use of povidone-iodine was associated with a decreased risk of exit site infection and peritonitis during the first 140 days [9] This are no published randomized studies of other antiseptics for early exit site care, but studies of these agents for healed exit sites have shown variable results and the author does not recommend their use on a healed exit site and suggests careful monitoring for cytotoxicity if antiseptics are used on an unhealed exit site [10, 11].

The early use of antimicrobial cream at the exit site is common but not universal. Some centers wait for the exit site to heal prior to use of antimicrobial cream, some recommend immediate use, while others reserve use of mupirocin for those who are staphylococcus aureus nasal carriers. The ISPD 2011 position statement highlights the uncertain efficacy of eradication of staphylococcus aureus nasal carriage peri-operatively but does recommend that all PD patients use topical antibiotic once the catheter exit site once healed [2]. While topical gentamicin has been shown to outperform mupirocin with respect to infectious complications in a single randomized controlled study, subsequent publications have raised concerns about the potential for fungal infection with long term use of topical gentamicin and the ISPD recommends that either gentamicin or mupirocin use is acceptable [2, 12–14].

Flushing

As discussed above, immediate post operative flushing is necessary if the insertion of the catheter was complicated by intra peritoneal bleeding. Apart from insertions complicated by intraperitoneal bleeding, the role for routine flushing of newly inserted PD catheters is unclear. At one extreme, the embedded (or buried) PD catheter cannot be flushed and the rates of initial function of these catheters exceeds 85% with a primary failure rate of less than 5% in experienced centers [15–17]. This argues that routine flushing of PD catheters is probably unnecessary. On the other hand, a recent survey of North American centers demonstrated that the practice is widespread with 76% of centers flushing catheters weekly, and only 10% reporting that they do not flush catheters at all post operatively [3].

Given the uncertainty regarding utility of catheter flushing, it is not surprising that protocols vary widely from center to center. The majority (81%) of those centers that flush catheters use dialysate to flush catheters but some do use normal saline with or without heparin [3]. Practically, the connectology of the transfer set favors the use of dialysate, and there is no published evidence to support the superiority of normal saline for flushing. The volumes used for flushing should be low, typically no more than 500 mL. Larger volumes increase the risk of an exit site leak which can result in postponement of initiation of PD. When flushing a catheter, it is also important to keep in mind that the first flush will not be completely drained as there is at least 200–300 mL of dead space in the peritoneal cavity that will not be amenable to drainage. Subsequent flushes, however, should result in return of the full flush volume. If the patient is progressively retaining fluid with each flush then the procedure should be stopped and the patient investigated for a poorly draining catheter as described further on in this chapter.

The main practical benefit to catheter flushing is to ensure patency of the catheter prior to initiation of PD training. The discovery that a PD catheter is non-functioning during the first day of PD training results in postponement of training while measures are undertaken to improve catheter function. This has logistic implications for workload and patient flow within a home dialysis program.

Bowel Routine

The use of a bowel preparation pre-operatively is not mandatory but is generally recommended to reduce the extent of fecal contamination in the case of an inadvertent bowel injury, but more importantly to ensure good early catheter function [18]. Even moderate degrees of constipation will interfere with proper drainage of the PD catheter through displacement of the catheter out of the pelvis or via extra luminal compression of the catheter. It has been reported that constipation is responsible for poor catheter drainage at least 50% of the time and any experienced PD practitioner is aware that laxatives are very effective in improving the function of a poorly draining PD catheter, even in the absence of a clinical history or radiograph supporting constipation [19].

Incident PD patients are often prescribed a combination of a stool softener (docusate) to be taken on a daily basis and a stimulant laxative such senna titrated to achieve 2 bowel movements per day. While this practice is widespread, there is no published evidence to support its utility [20]. The use of lactulose as an osmotic laxative may be preferable as it reduces intestinal pH and bacterial translocation across the colon which may result in a reduced risk of enteric peritonitis [21]. Unfortunately, lactulose is often not well tolerated due to its taste and tendency to cause bloating and flatulence. Other osmotic laxatives such as polyethylene glycol solutions are well tolerated and can be quite effective for both daily use and acute treatment of catheter dysfunction [22]. Regular or daily use of magnesium containing laxatives should be avoided due to the potential for magnesium toxicity [23]. Newer bowel preparations containing a combination of magnesium citrate and sodium picosulfate (Pico-Salax [Ferring Inc.,Toronto, Ontario] or Picolax [Nordic Pharmaceuticals,Feltham, Middlesex] should be approached with caution due to reports of increased incidence of hyponatremia with these solutions [24].

Post Operative Bleeding

Patients with stage 5 CKD have increased risk of bleeding related to disordered primary hemostasis, and in some cases secondary hemostasis [25]. Uremic platelet dysfunction, the frequent use of aspirin and other antiplatelet agents, and the use of anticoagulants for prothrombotic states are all factors which contribute to this risk. The prevalence of bleeding post PD catheter insertion has been reported between 2% and 10% [26, 27]. Significant peri-cannular, or exit site, bleeding has been defined as the need to change the exit site dressing more than twice daily during the first two post-operative weeks. Management of significant peri-cannular bleeding involves immobilization of the catheter and minimization of patient movement, and in severe cases, bed rest. The use of desmopressin 16 mcg intravenous every 12 h for three doses and the use of gauze compression with an elastic bandage are often helpful. A technique of injection of epinephrine proximal and distal to the superficial cuff has also been described as helpful in refractory cases as movement of the Dacron cuff may be responsible for bleeding due to irritation of the subcutaneous tissue [27]. The last resort for refractory bleeding is removal of the PD catheter.

Early Use of PD Catheter

Traditionally, it was recommended to allow 2 weeks for healing of a PD catheter prior to initiation of therapy due to the risk of leakage with early catheter use. Tzamaloukas and colleagues reported that 90% of early leaks occurred among patients whose catheters were inserted less than

10 days prior to usage, and a similar increased risk of early leakage with early catheter use has been shown in children [28–30]. Early use of a catheter may also be a risk factor for other mechanical complications including flow obstruction, peritonitis and need for surgical intervention for malfunctioning catheter [31]. Recently, however, there has been a resurgence in interest in early (less than 2 weeks) use of PD catheters among patients requiring urgent dialysis initiation [32–35].

Not all PD catheters are suitable for early use and two randomized controlled trials of percutaneous versus surgically inserted catheters has shown an increased risk of leakage with surgical catheters [36, 37]. Many of the centers that have reported encouraging results with urgent start PD use percutaneous catheters but some centers have reported excellent outcomes with early use of surgically inserted catheters when a purse string suture is used around the deep cuff to create a tight seal and it is generally felt that both surgical and percutaneous catheters may be used for urgent start PD [38]. Some pediatric centers have reported very low risk of early leaks among urgent start patients with surgical catheters if fibrin glue is used at the deep cuff [39].

A number of protocols for urgent start PD have been proposed [32–34].The majority of these protocols involve initiation of supine automated PD on or shortly after post operative day one. Small dwell volumes (0.5–1.2 L) and frequent exchanges over a 8–10 h period of supine positioning are started and the dwell volume progressively increased and cycle frequency decreased over a 2 week period. Patients can receive supine intermittent PD three times per week in a dialysis center while the catheter heals and after 2 weeks then start with PD training. These protocols are suitable for patients with uremic symptoms but no emergent indication for dialysis such as hyperkalemia, uremic pericarditis, severe metabolic acidosis or refractory fluid overload [32]. Suitable patients typically have some residual urine output.

The practice of urgent start PD for late presenting patients has been associated with good clinical outcomes as well as enhanced recruitment to PD among incident patients [32–34, 40]. Small studies have suggested good early technique survival, few leaks and few infections with urgent start PD when compared to patients who electively start PD. The ability to avoid placement of a central venous catheter and initiation of hemodialysis is also a less costly approach with an estimated saving of more than $3000 USD per case [41]. There is, however, requirement for an upfront investment in programmatic infrastructure so that late presenting patients can receive urgent education, timely placement of the catheter, and then outpatient intermittent automated PD with commencement of training 2 weeks post catheter insertion [42].

The Leaking PD Catheter

Leakage of dialysate can occur as a consequence of increased intra-abdominal pressure and a defect in the peritoneal membrane that allows fluid to escape. Catheter leakage may be noted following flushing of the catheter in the postoperative period, even before initiation of PD. Fluid may be observed to leak with maneuvers that increase intrabdominal pressure, such as coughing, straining, or sitting in the upright position. If the rate of leakage is slow, findings may be limited to wetness on the exit site dressing. The diagnosis of an exit site leak is based on a positive reaction for glucose on a chemical reagent strip. An exit site leak usually implies a defect in the peritoneal membrane around the catheter but may occasionally be due to fluid leakage from a hole in the catheter itself. Catheters may be damaged due to complications of insertion or exteriorization (in the case of buried catheters) or a patient may inadvertently damage the catheter.

The reported incidence of dialysate leakage varies widely based on definitions used, length of follow up, and clinical practices of the reporting center. Observational studies with long follow up periods have reported rates of dialysate leaks between 0.03 and 0.13 leaks per patient-year of follow up [43–45]. Some authors have classified leaks as early (less than 30 days after insertion), and late (greater than 30 days after insertion) [28]. Early dialysate leaks are typically exit site or incisional leaks and the reported rates vary from 3% to 5%. Late leaks are more likely to be concealed leaks and usually present as abdominal wall or genital edema, often with associated apparent ultrafiltration failure. The prevalence of late leaks is reported to vary between 3% and 18% [28, 43, 45].

There is a strong link between exit site leakage and infection. Holley and colleagues reported a retrospective series of 79 leaks among 66 prevalent PD patients [46]. In this series, 33 of the leaks (42% of total) were associated with infection, in 22 cases the infection preceded the leak, and in 11 cases the infection was diagnosed after the leak despite treatment with prophylactic antibiotics. This suggests that infection of the deep cuff may present with dialysate leak, and also that leaking dialysate is a major risk factor for catheter infection and peritonitis. Prophylactic treatment with antibiotics is indicated in patients with exit site leak. Our center typically treats patients with oral cephalexin until the leakage has ceased.

Management of early exit site leak involves discontinuing peritoneal dialysis (or flushing) for a period of 1–2 weeks if possible as the leak will seal in many cases if the abdomen is left dry [47]. This may entail temporary transfer to HD if residual renal function is not adequate [44]. Recurrent leakage after a period of rest should prompt further evaluation. A CT scan with intraperitoneal dye can confirm leakage along the tunnel and localized the site of the defect. An ultrasound of the catheter tunnel may be useful in excluding a fluid collection. Laparoscopic examination of the abdomen may allow for diagnosis and treatment of the cause of the leak. If no cause is apparent, or if infection of the deep cuff is suspected, then the catheter should be removed and a new one inserted. If early exit site leakage is a frequent problem then it is important that the surgeon be made aware to ensure that the optimal surgical technique is being employed. The deep cuff must be placed within the rectus muscle and it should be secured with a purse string suture if possible [48].

The Obstructed PD Catheter

Flow obstruction in a newly placed PD catheter is a common and vexing problem. It may be noted during post-operative flushing, prior to initiation of PD, but more commonly is first noted at the commencement of PD training. It can result in delayed training and if not adequately managed will result in early technique failure. Catheter related problems are well described to be a leading cause of early technique failure [49].

The incidence of PD catheter obstruction varies widely in the literature likely related to significant differences in insertion techniques, patient selection and differing definitions of what constitutes outflow obstruction. Some degree of outflow obstruction is reported to be present in 6–32% of catheters [34–38, 50–54]. Refractory outflow obstruction which leads to primary catheter failure is much lower, typically below 10% in most case series. Outflow obstruction with normal inflow is referred to as *one-way* obstruction and is related to a degree of malposition of the catheter in the abdomen and may be associated with catheter migration. Inflow obstruction is less common and related to obstruction of the catheter lumen with resulting bidirectional obstruction to flow, referred to *as two-way* obstruction. *Two-way* obstruction is often noted early during post- operative flushing and is typically related to obstruction of the catheter lumen from a blood clot, fibrin or sometimes a kink in the catheter tubing or transfer set.

The presence of poor drainage, or one-way obstruction, should be considered as evidence of PD catheter malposition, though not necessarily migration. Well placed catheters can be compressed by distended bowel due to constipation, or a distended bladder and this will result in poor drainage due to creation of a one way valve allowing inflow but impairing outflow of dialysate. Compartmentalization of the PD catheter by pelvic adhesions can similarly impair drainage of an apparently well placed catheter [55]. A low lying omentum can descend into the pelvis and encase a catheter without necessarily causing apparent migration of the catheter.

Catheter tip migration is a common cause of poor drainage but it is important to note that not all migrated catheters will be problematic. Three dimensional CT reconstructions show that in a supine patient, dialysate mostly pools in the pelvis though there is substantial fluid also present in the paracolic gutters and sub-phrenic space [56]. The presence of dialysate, especially in the paracolic gutters, likely explains the observation by Ersoy and colleagues that only 20% of migrated catheters had issues with poor drainage [57]. Nevertheless, upper abdominal catheter migration is a significant risk factor for poor drainage due to the potential movement of the catheter tip into the lesser sac of the peritoneal cavity or into compartments defined by the liver or spleen where there is very little free fluid present [55].

Obstruction to catheter flow should be approached in an organized manner as shown in Fig. 11.1. The initial determination is whether isolated outflow obstruction is present or if there is also inflow obstruction. As stated above, inflow obstruction suggests intraluminal obstruction and after careful examination of the catheter for kinking, the next step is to attempt vigorous irrigation of the catheter using a large (30 cc or larger) syringe filled with heparinized saline. This will often be sufficient to dislodge a fibrin or blood clot and resume PD. Some patients are prone to formation of fibrin and require chronic addition of heparin (500–1000 U/L) to their dialysate to prevent recurrent obstruction. Failure to clear an inflow obstruction with irrigation is an indication to use tissue plasminogen activator (tpa). There are a number of published protocols which typically involve filling the lumen of the catheter with concentrated heparin (1000 U/mL) with a subsequent dwell of 1 h to overnight. The success rates with this approach in appropriately selected patients is in the range of 57–83% [58, 59].

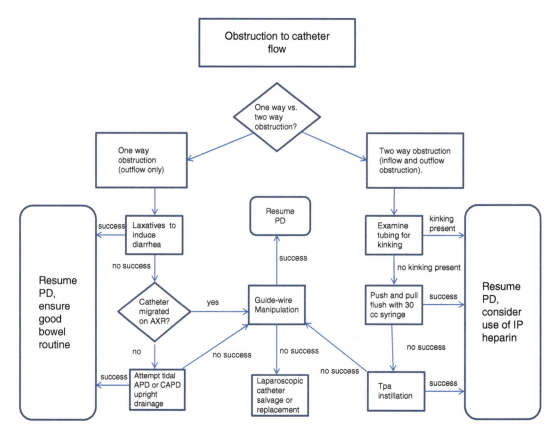

Fig. 11.1 Algorhythm for the diagnosis and management of PD catheter dysfunction

Isolated outflow obstruction often improves with use of laxatives to induce diarrhea as the vigorous peristalsis can move the catheter and reduce extrinsic compression of the catheter lumen. Patients are often reluctant to take laxatives and argue that they are not constipated so the intervention is better explained as induction of diarrhea. Appropriate bowel regimes in PD have already been discussed, but it is important to highlight that a larger dose of laxative is required for acute catheter malfunction. If catheter drainage does not improve after induction of diarrhea then an abdominal radiograph should be performed to assess for PD catheter position. A PD catheter is considered migrated if the tip of the catheter lies outside of the true pelvis. A migrated catheter may return to the true pelvis after treatment with laxatives which is why a radiograph should be performed only after the obstruction has proven refractory to laxatives. If the radiograph indicates migration then a guidewire manipulation should be performed under fluoroscopic guidance. If the catheter is not migrated on the radiograph then a trial of tidal automated PD (APD) or CAPD with upright drainage is worthwhile. Tidal APD, where a residual volume of a few hundred millilitres of fluid is left in the abdomen after each exchange, can be particularly useful for catheters that drain well initially and then slow as the residual dialysate volume contracts [60].

Fluoroscopic guide-wire manipulations are an important adjunctive procedure for salvage of poorly functioning PD catheters [52]. The radiologist inserts a stiff guide-wire through the catheter and clears out any fibrin or other intraluminal debris. The wire also serves to straighten a coiled catheter and can remedy the malposition of the catheter with respect to bowels or adhesions. The wire can also be used to reposition a migrated catheter, though this can be technically challenging and the risk of repeat migration is high and repeat malfunction is high (Table 11.1) [52, 61–67] The largest case series of fluoroscopic manipulations was reported in 2010 [66]. In this case series of 70 catheters manipulated for flow obstruction, 63% were functional at 30 days. Predictors of a successful outcome included

Table 11.1 Summary of published results of fluroscopic wire manipulation

	N subjects	Initial function	>30 day function
Moss et al. (*Am J Kidney Dis* 1990)	48	78%	25%
Kappel et al. (*Adv Perit Dial* 1995)	47		67%
Simons et al. (*Perit Dial Int* 1999)	33	85%	55%
Diax-Buxo et al. (*Clin Nephrol* 1997)	69		61%
Savader et al. (*J Vasc Interv Radiol* 1997)	12		58%
Plaza et al. (*Perit Dial Int* 2001)	14	64%	26%
Miller et al. (*Clin J Am Soc Nephrol* 2013)	70		63%
Kwon et al. (*J Vasc Interv Radiol* 2014)	68		47%

pelvic location of catheter (i.e. a non-migrated catheter) and secondary catheter malfunction (i.e. catheter became obstructed after a period of good function). Fluoroscopic manipulation can be associated with some abdominal discomfort and the patient should be aware of this prior to the procedure. There are no guidelines for the use of prophylactic antibiotics with this procedure but some centers recommend post- procedure intraperitoneal antibiotics and change of the catheter transfer set.

Obstruction that does not resolve with fluoroscopic guide wire manipulation requires surgical intervention. Traditionally, a persistently obstructed catheter would be replaced and a new one inserted, but over the past few decades there is increased interest in laparoscopic salvage for refractory drainage failure. Laparascopic salvage has a number of advantages over removal and reinsertion. It allows for direct visualization of the intra-abdominal anatomy and diagnosis as well as treatment of the precise cause of the malfunction whereas simple removal/reinsertion runs the risk of the same problem recurring with the new catheter [48]. Omental wrapping of the catheter, often due to a low lying omentum, is the most frequent cause of malfunction found at laparoscopy [68–71]. Omental wrapping of the catheter can cause migration as the omentum may pull the catheter out of the pelvis. In these cases, the catheter can be freed from the omentum and returned to the pelvis and the redundant omentum tacked up with an omentopexy. Catheter migration without omental wrapping, presumably due to excessive torque on the catheter during insertion, is also a common finding and treatment may require suturing of the catheter in the pelvis. Other frequent findings include compartmentalization of the catheter due to adhesions, wrapping of the catheter from the fimbrae of fallopian tubes, as well as intraluminal obstruction due to blood and fibrin clots [72]. Laparoscopic salvage of PD catheters is associated with a high published rate of immediate success, typically greater than 80% although there is considerable variability in the rates of recurrent obstruction [68–71]. PD can typically be restarted soon after laparoscopic manipulation in keeping with the principles described above in the section on early use of the PD catheter.

Filling and Drain Pain

Infusion pain is reported by some patients immediately after initiation of PD. The pain may be referred to the rectum or bladder, and may cause significant discomfort, especially at the beginning of the infusion. The pain is usually attributed to the jet effect of the relatively rapid infusion of dialysate into the peritoneum but may also be related to the acidity of the PD fluid [73].

The phenomenon is seen more commonly in catheters with a straight intraperitoneal segment than in coiled catheters likely due to the more diffuse nature of the spray with coiled catheters. In addition, the tip of a coiled catheter is much more flexible and less likely to abut bowel or bladder in a manner that would cause jet pain. Helpful interventions to reduce jet pain include decreasing the rate of dialysate infusion, changing the patient to tidal PD where there is always a residual pool of

dialysis fluid, and the use of laxatives to induce peristalsis and alter the position of the catheter [74]. Refractory cases of jet pain may improve with fluoroscopic guide-wire manipulation and only very rarely is removal and reinsertion of the catheter required.

Abdominal pain occurring during and after infusion may also be due to the effect of acidic PD fluid. Traditional PD solutions are lactate-buffered and acidic because the greater stability of glucose in low pH prolongs the shelf life of the dialysate. Despite the low pH, the glucose is not entirely stable in these solutions and glucose degradation products form readily. The typical pH of these solutions is 5.5 and it rises after infusion and within an hour reaches 7.2, and by 2 h is at equilibrium with the systemic pH of 7.4 [75]. The symptoms associated with acidic PD fluid are not universal and are often described more as a feeling of discomfort or unwellness rather than pain. These symptoms typically last longer than the discomfort associated with jet pain, but should subside by 1 h after the intraperitoneal pH has risen. Newer PD solutions with neutral pH and lower concentrations of GDPs are now available in the US (Balance, Fresenius, Bad Homberg, Germany) and may be helpful among those patients with acid mediated abdominal discomfort.

Pain on drainage, also referred to as dry pain, is also a frequent problem. It is usually ascribed to irritation of the peritoneal membrane by the catheter and by the negative pressure generated by the PD cycler while on drain cycle [76]. The most common solution for this problem is to avoid complete drainage of the abdomen by keeping the catheter surrounded by, or floating in, peritoneal fluid. One retrospective study reported a prevalence rate of pain on filling or draining of 13% at baseline and that the institution of tidal PD, with 25–50% tidal volume, eliminated pain in all the patients [77]. The use of tidal programs may reduce adequacy or require more frequent exchanges to maintain the clearances so this needs to be taken into account when changing to a tidal program. Alternatively, those experiencing drain pains on APD may have resolution of symptoms with CAPD as the gravity driven drainage means less negative pressure is transmitted through the catheter compared with the hydraulic suction on a cycler. Different brands of cycler also have differing amounts of negative pressure and trialing a different brand of cycler may be helpful in refractory cases.

References

1. Gadahhah MF, Torres-Rivera C, Ramdeen G, et al. Relationship between intraperitoneal bleeding, adhesions, and peritoneal dialysis catheter failure: a method of prevention. Adv Perit Dial. 2001;17:127–9.
2. Piraino B, Bernardini J, Brown E, Figueiredo A, Johnson DW, Lye WC, Price V, Ramalakshmi S, Szeto CC. ISPD position statement on reducing the risks of peritoneal dialysis–related infections. Perit Dial Int. 2011;31(6):614–30.
3. Wallace E, Fissell RB, Golper TA, Blake PG, Lewin AM, Oliver MJ, Quinn RR. Catheter insertion and perioperative practices within the ISPD North American research consortium. Perit Dial Int. 2016;36(4):382–6. pdi-2015.
4. Dombros N, Dratwa M, Gokal R, Heimbürger O, Krediet R, Plum J, Rodrigues A, Selgas R, Struijk D, Verger C. European best practice guidelines for peritoneal dialysis. 3 Peritoneal access. Nephrol Dial Transplant. 2005;20:x8–ix12.
5. Warady BA, Bakkaloglu S, Newland J, Cantwell M, Verrina E, Neu A, Chadha V, Yap HK, Schaefer F. Consensus guidelines for the prevention and treatment of catheter-related infections and peritonitis in pediatric patients receiving peritoneal dialysis: 2012 update. Perit Dial Int. 2012;32(Supplement 2):32–86.
6. Twardowski ZJ, Prowant BF. Appearance and classification of healing peritoneal catheter exit sites. Perit Dial Int. 1996;16(3):S71.
7. Twardowski ZJ, Prowant BF. Exit-site healing post catheter implantation. Perit Dial Int. 1996;16(Suppl 3):S51–70.
8. Newman LN, Tessman M, Hanslik T, Schulak J, Mayes J, Friedlander M. A retrospective view of factors that affect catheter healing: four years of experience. Adv Perit Dial. 1993;9:217.
9. Waite NM, Webster N, Laurel M, Johnson M, Fong IW. The efficacy of exit site povidone-iodine ointment in the prevention of early peritoneal dialysis-related infections. Am J Kidney Dis Off J National Kidney Foundation. 1997;29(5):763–8.
10. Luzar MA, Brown CB, Balf D, Hill L, Issad B, Monnier B, Moulart J, Sabatier JC, Wauquier JP, Peluso F. Exit-site care and exit-site infection in continuous ambulatory peritoneal dialysis (CAPD): results of a randomized multicenter trial. Perit Dial Int. 1990;10(1):25–9.
11. Findlay A, Serrano C, Punzalan S, Fan SL. Increased peritoneal dialysis exit site infections using topical antiseptic polyhexamethylene biguanide compared to

mupirocin: results of a safety interim analysis of an open-label prospective randomized study. Antimicrob Agents Chemother. 2013;57(5):2026–8.
12. Bernardini J, Bender F, Florio T, Sloand J, PalmMontalbano L, Fried L, Piraino B. Randomized, double-blind trial of antibiotic exit site cream for prevention of exit site infection in peritoneal dialysis patients. J Am Soc Nephrol. 2005;16(2):539–45.
13. Chu KH, Choy WY, Cheung CC, Fung KS, Tang HL, Lee W, Cheuk A, Yim KF, Chan WH, Tong KL. A prospective study of the efficacy of local application of gentamicin versus mupirocin in the prevention of peritoneal dialysis catheter-related infections. Perit Dial Int. 2008;28(5):505–8.
14. Mahaldar A, Weisz M, Kathuria P. Comparison of gentamicin and mupirocin in the prevention of exit-site infection and peritonitis in peritoneal dialysis. Adv Perit Dial. 2009;25:56–9.
15. Brown PA, McCormick BB, Knoll G, Su Y, Doucette S, Fergusson D, Lavoie S. Complications and catheter survival with prolonged embedding of peritoneal dialysis catheters. Nephrol Dial Transplant. 2008;23(7):2299–303.
16. Elhassan E, McNair B, Quinn M, Teitelbaum I. Prolonged duration of peritoneal dialysis catheter embedment does not lower the catheter success rate. Perit Dial Int. 2011;31(5):558–64.
17. McCormick BB, Brown PA, Knoll G, Yelle JD, Page D, Biyani M, Lavoie S. Use of the embedded peritoneal dialysis catheter: experience and results from a North American center. Kidney Int. 2006;70:S38–43.
18. Figueiredo A, Goh BL, Jenkins S, Johnson DW, Mactier R, Ramalakshmi S, Shrestha B, Struijk D, Wilkie M. Clinical practice guidelines for peritoneal access. Perit Dial Int. 2010;30(4):424–9.
19. Rodríguez-Palomares JR, Ruiz C, Granado A, Montenegro J. El acceso peritoneal. Guías de práctica clínica en diálisis peritoneal. Nefrologia. 2006;26(Suppl 4):1–184.
20. Setyapranata S, Holt SG. The gut in older patients on peritoneal dialysis. Perit Dial Int. 2015;35(6):650–4.
21. Afsar B, Elsurer R, Bilgic A, Sezer S, Ozdemir F. Regular lactulose use is associated with lower peritonitis rates: an observational study. Perit Dial Int. 2010;30(2):243–6.
22. Mimidis K, Mourvati E, Kaliontzidou M, Papadopoulos V, Thodis E, Kartalis G, Vargemezis V. Efficacy of polyethylene glycol in constipated CAPD patients. Perit Dial Int. 2005;25(6):601–3.
23. Jung GJ, Gil HW, Yang JO, Lee EY, Hong SY. Severe hypermagnesemia causing quadriparesis in a CAPD patient. Perit Dial Int. 2008;28(2):206.
24. Weir MA, Fleet JL, Vinden C, Shariff SZ, Liu K, Song H, Jain AK, Gandhi S, Clark WF, Garg AX. Hyponatremia and sodium picosulfate bowel preparations in older adults. Am J Gastroenterol. 2014;109(5):686.
25. Harman G, McCormick BB. Hemorrhage because of amyloid-related factor X deficiency after insertion of tenckhoff catheter. Perit Dial Int. 2012;32(5):567–8.

26. Mital S, Fried LF, Piraino B. Bleeding complications associated with peritoneal dialysis catheter insertion. Perit Dial Int. 2004;24(5):478–80.

27. Li JR, Chen CH, Chiu KY, Yang CR, Cheng CL, Ou YC, Ko JL, Ho HC. Management of pericannular bleeding after peritoneal dialysis catheter placement. Perit Dial Int. 2012;32(3):361–2.

28. Tzamaloukas AH, Gibel LJ, Eisenberg B, et al. Early and late peritoneal dialysate leaks in patients on CAPD. Adv Perit Dial. 1990;6:64–71.

29. Rahim KA, Seidel K, McDonald RA. Risk factors for catheter-related complications in pediatric peritoneal dialysis. Pediatr Nephrol. 2004;19:1021–8.

30. Patel UD, Mottes TA, Flynn JT. Delayed compared with immediate use of peritoneal catheter in pediatric peritoneal dialysis. Adv Perit Dial. 2001;17:253–9.

31. Liu Y, Zhang L, Lin A, Ni Z, Qian J, Fang W. Impact of break-in period on the short-term outcomes of patients started on peritoneal dialysis. Perit Dial Int. 2014;34(1):49–56.

32. Ghaffari A. Urgent-start peritoneal dialysis: a quality improvement report. Am J Kidney Dis. 2012;59(3):400–8.

33. Casaretto A, Rosario R, Kotzker WR, Pagan-Rosario Y, Groenhoff C, Guest S. Urgent-start peritoneal dialysis: report from a US private nephrology practice. Adv Perit Dial. 2011;28:102–5. Conference on Peritoneal Dialysis.

34. Povlsen JV, Ivarsen P. How to start the late referred ESRD patient urgently on chronic APD. Nephrology Dialysis Transplantation. 2006;21(Suppl 2):ii56–9.

35. Arramreddy R, Zheng S, Saxena AB, Liebman SE, Wong L. Urgent-start peritoneal dialysis: a chance for a new beginning. Am J Kidney Dis. 2014;63(3):390–5.

36. Voss D, Hawkins S, Poole G, Marshall M. Radiological versus surgical implantation of first catheter for peritoneal dialysis: a randomized non-inferiority trial. Nephrol Dial Transplant. 2012;27(11):4196–204.

37. Gadallah MF, Pervez A, El-Shahawy MA, Sorrells D, Zibari G, McDonald J, Work J. Peritoneoscopic versus surgical placement of peritoneal dialysis catheters: a prospective randomized study on outcome. Am J Kidney Dis. 1999;33(1):118–22.

38. Sharma AP, Mandhani A, Daniel SP, Filler G. Shorter break-in period is a viable option with tighter PD catheter securing during the insertion. Nephrology. 2008;13(8):672–6.

39. Sojo ET, Grosman MD, Monteverde ML, Bailez MM, Delgado N. Fibrin glue is useful in preventing early dialysate leakage in children on chronic peritoneal dialysis. Perit Dial Int. 2004;24(2):186–90.

40. Alkatheeri AM, Blake PG, Gray D, Jain AK. Success of urgent-start peritoneal dialysis in a large Canadian renal program. Perit Dial Int. 2016;36(2):171–6.

41. Liu FX, Ghaffari A, Dhatt H, Kumar V, Balsera C, Wallace E, Khairullah Q, Lesher B, Gao X, Henderson H, LaFleur P. Economic evaluation of urgent-start peritoneal dialysis versus urgent-start hemodialysis in the United States. Medicine. 2014;93(28):e293.

42. Ghaffari A, Kumar V, Guest S. Infrastructure requirements for an urgent-start peritoneal dialysis program. Perit Dial Int. 2013;33(6):611–7.

43. Balaskas EV, Ikonomopoulos D, Sioulis A, et al. Survival and complications of 225 catheters used in continuous ambulatory peritoneal dialysis: one-center experience in Northern Greece. Perit Dial Int. 1999;19(Suppl 2):S167–71.

44. Leblanc M, Ouimet D, Pichette V. Dialysate leaks in peritoneal dialysis. Semin Dial. 2001;14(1):50–4. Blackwell Science Inc.

45. Del Peso G, Bajo MA, Costero O, et al. Risk factors for abdominal wall complications in peritoneal dialysis patients. Perit Dial Int. 2003;23:249–54.

46. Holley JL, Bernardini J, Piraino B. Characteristics and outcome of peritoneal dialysate leaks and associated infections. Adv Perit Dial. 1993;9:240–3.

47. Gokal R, Alexander S, Ash S, et al. Peritoneal catheters and exit-site practices toward optimum peritoneal access: 1998 update. (Official report from the International Society for Peritoneal Dialysis). Perit Dial Int. 1998;18:11–33.

48. Crabtree JH. Selected best demonstrated practices in peritoneal dialysis access. Kidney Int. 2006;70:S27–37.

49. Kolesnyk I, Dekker FW, Boeschoten EW, Krediet RT. Time-dependent reasons for peritoneal dialysis technique failure and mortality. Perit Dial Int. 2010;30(2):170–7.

50. Ponce SP, Pierratos A, Izatt S, et al. Comparison of the survival and complications of three permanent peritoneal dialysis catheters. Perit Dial Bull. 1982; 2:82–6.

51. Diaz-Buxo JA, Geissinger WT. Single cuff versus double cuff Tenckhoff catheter. Perit Dial Bull. 1984;4:S100–2.

52. Moss JS, Minda SA, Newman GE, Dunnick NR, Vernon WB, Schwab SJ. Malpositioned peritoneal dialysis catheters: a critical reappraisal of correction by stiff-wire manipulation. Am J Kidney Dis. 1990;15(4):305–8.

53. Swartz R, Messana J, Rocher L, et al. The curled catheter: dependable device for percutaneous peritoneal access. Perit Dial Int. 1990;10:231–5.

54. Kappel JE, Ferguson GMC, Kudel RM, et al. Stiff wire manipulation of peritoneal dialysis catheters. In: Khanna R, editor. Advances in peritoneal dialysis, vol. 12. Toronto: Peritoneal Dialysis Publications; 1996. p. 223–6.

55. Diaz-Buxo JA. Peritoneal dialysis catheter malfunction due to compartmentalization. Perit Dial Int. 1997;17:209–10.

56. Hills BA, Birch S, LaMont AC. Spatial distribution of dialysate in patients and its implications to intradialysate diffusion. Perit Dial Int. 2002;22(6):698–704.

57. Ersoy FF, Twardowski ZJ, Satalowich RJ, Ketchersid T. A retrospective analysis of catheter position and function in 91 CAPD patients. Perit Dial Int. 1994;14:409–10.

58. Zorzanello MM, Fleming WJ, Prowant BE. Use of tissue plasminogen activator in peritoneal dialysis catheters: a literature review and one center's experience. Nephrol Nurs J. 2004;31:534–7.

59. Shea M, Hmiel SP, Beck AM. Use of tissue plasminogen activator for thrombolysis in occluded peritoneal dialysis catheters in children. Adv Perit Dial. 2001;17:249–52.

60. Scanziani R, Dozio B, Baragetti I, Maroni S. Intraperitoneal hydrostatic pressure and flow characteristics of peritoneal catheters in automated peritoneal dialysis. Nephrol Dial Transplant. 2003;18(11): 2391–8.

61. Kappel JE, Ferguson GM, Kudel RM, Kudel TA, Lawlor BJ, Pylypchuk GB. Stiff wire manipulation of peritoneal dialysis catheters. Adv Perit Dial. 1995; 11:202–7.

62. Simons ME, Pron G, Voros M, Vanderburgh LC, Rao PS, Oreopoulos DG. Fluoroscopically-guided manipulation of malfunctioning peritoneal dialysis catheters. Perit Dial Int. 1999;19(6):544–9.

63. Diaz-Buxo JA, Turner MW, Nelms M. Fluoroscopic manipulation of Tenckhoff catheters: outcome analysis. Clin Nephrol. 1997;47(6):384–8.

64. Savader SJ, Lund G, Scheel PJ, et al. Guide wire directed manipulation of malfunctioning peritoneal dialysis catheters: a critical analysis. J Vasc Interv Radiol. 1997;8:957–63.

65. Plaza MM, Rivas MC, Domínguez–Viguera L. Swan-neck S. Fluoroscopic manipulation is also useful for malfunctioning swan-neck peritoneal catheters. Perit Dial Int. 2001;21:193–7.

66. Miller M, McCormick B, Lavoie S, Biyani M, Zimmerman D. Fluoroscopic manipulation of peritoneal dialysis catheters: outcomes and factors associated with successful manipulation. Clin J Am Soc Nephrol. 2012;7(5):795–800.

67. Kwon YH, Kwon SH, Oh JH, Jeong KH, Lee TW. Fluoroscopic guide wire manipulation of malfunctioning peritoneal dialysis catheters initially placed by Interventional Radiologists. J Vasc Interv Radiol. 2014;25(6):904–10.

68. Santarelli S, Zeiler M, Marinelli R, Monteburini T, Federico A, Ceraudo E. Videolaparoscopy as rescue therapy and placement of peritoneal dialysis catheters: a thirty-two case single centre experience. Nephrol Dial Transplant. 2006;21(5):1348–54.

69. Yilmazlar T, Kirdak T, Bilgin S, Yavuz M, Yurtkuran M. Laparoscopic findings of peritoneal dialysis catheter malfunction and management outcomes. Perit Dial Int. 2006;26(3):374–9.

70. Skipper K, Dickerman R, Dunn E. Laparoscopic placement and revision of peritoneal dialysis catheters. JSLS. 1999;3(1):63–5.

71. Brandt CP, Ricanati ES. Use of laparoscopy in the management of malfunctioning peritoneal dialysis catheters. Adv Perit Dial. 1996;12:223–6.

72. Gudsoorkar PS, Penner T, Jassal SV, Bargman JM. The enigmatic fallopian tube: a more common cause of catheter malfunction than previously recognized. Perit Dial Int. 2016;36(4):459–61.

73. Twardowski ZJ, Prowant BF, Nichols WK, et al. Six-year experience with swan neck catheters. Perit Dial Int. 1992;12:384–9.

74. Twardowski ZJ, Nichols WK. Peritoneal dialysis access and exit-site care including surgical aspects. In: Gokal R, Khanna R, Krediet R, Nolph KD, editors. Textbook of peritoneal dialysis. 2nd ed. Dordrecht: Kluwer Academic Publishers; 2000. p. 307–61.

75. Rippe B, Simonsen O, Wieslander A, et al. Clinical and physiological effects of a new, less toxic and less acidic fluid for peritoneal dialysis. Perit Dial Int. 1997;17:27–34.

76. Blake P. Drain pain, overfill, and how they are connected. Perit Dial Int. 2014;34(4):342–4.

77. Juergensen PH, Murphy AL, Pherson KA, et al. Tidal peritoneal dialysis to achieve comfort in chronic peritoneal dialysis patients. Adv Perit Dial. 1999;15:125–6.

Diagnosis and Management of Catheter Dysfunction

12

Guner Ogunc

Introduction

Catheter malfunction, defined as mechanical failure in dialysate inflow or outflow, is not uncommon in peritoneal dialysis(PD) patient. Outflow failure occurs in 4–34.5% of PD patients [1]. Ever since the first permanent silicone catheter was introduced in 1968, a wide variety of catheters and placement techniques have been developed to attempt to eliminate catheter malfunction. However, catheter-related problems are not fully resolved [2–6].

Catheter Flow Obstruction

The most common causes of catheter malfunction are omental wrapping and catheter tip migration. Catheter obstruction due to fibrin or blood clots within the catheter lumen, kinking of the catheter, small bowel wrapping, occlusion by fimbriae and intraperitoneal adhesions are other occlusive catheter problems in CAPD patients [7–9]. Prevention of these problems during the primary insertion has been a primary goal of surgeons who insert PD catheters. Our insertion technique, which is long tunelling and routine omentopexy, is significantly effective in preventing catheter-related problems, such as omental wrapping, catheter tip migration, pericatheter leakage and drain pain [10]. Since the laparoscopic technique was introduced and used for the placement of catheters and also salvage procedures for malfunctioning CAPD catheters in the early nineties of the last century, it has proven to be superior to the open surgical technique in many medical centers [11–14]. The advantages of laparoscopy over every other techniques are the adjunctive procedures enabled by this method, principally rectus sheath tunelling, omentopexy, adhesiolysis, epiploectomy, salpigectomy, and colopexy. When these techniques are applied effectively, the laparoscopic approach can both prevent and resolve most of the common mechanical problems that complicate insertion of PD catheters [15]. Omentopexy is employed selectively since it may be unnecessary when the omentum is short or adherent to previous upper abdominal surgical site. An additional argument supporting preservation of the omentum by using omentopexy as opposed to its resection is that omental milky spots (clusters of leukocytes) appear to have a role in the peritoneal cavity immune response, especially in the pediatric age population [15].

Diagnosis and Management

In many cases, the diagnosis of outflow failure may be difficult because of a lack of noninvasive

G. Ogunc
University of Akdeniz, Faculty of Medicine, General Surgery Department, Antalya, Turkey
e-mail: ogunc@akdeniz.edu.tr

© Springer International Publishing AG 2017
S. Haggerty (ed.), *Surgical Aspects of Peritoneal Dialysis*, DOI 10.1007/978-3-319-52821-2_12

methods. Change in body position, rapid saline infusion, cathartics, enemas, the classic use of fibrinolytics, and fluoroscopic manipulation are conservative measures often used in attempting to restore drainage in patients with poorly functioning catheters. However, laparoscopy is highly accurate in its diagnosis of CAPD complications caused by obstruction and is also therapeutic. Due to the need for continuous renal replacement therapy, the rescue procedures should not be delayed beyond a few days after noticing the alfunction if concervative treatments are ineffective.

Ideally, salvage surgery should be safe, with a high success rate, ease of performance, ability to prevent recurrence, and short recovery time. Open rescue surgery can lead to new adhesion formation and, therefore, restrictions in fluid distribution in the peritoneal cavity, as well as the development of incision-related complications and the additional stress of surgery for patients. In contrast, laparoscopic rescue procedures have many advantages: they leave smaller wounds with less tissue disturbance; they allow direct examination of the catheter and whole peritoneal cavity through the scope, allowing accurate identification of the cause of catheter malfunction as well as immediate intervention to restore its function; they enable diagnosis of other intra-abdominal pathology and treatment of other surgical problems such as symptomatic cholecystolithiasis and abdominal wall/inguinal hernia in the same operation; they avoid the need to replace the catheter; they enable immediate testing for overall peritoneal catheter function; they leave the patient with diminished postoperative pain, a shorter stay in hospital, and a quicker recovery of social and professional activities; they facilitate early resumption of PD and beter functional survival; and the operation recordings can be used to share our knowledge and experience with nephrologists, our assistants, and our students. There are also a few disadvantages: the need for general anesthesia in most patients; requirement of an operating theater; the cost of equipment and instrumentation; the long duration of the operative procedure and the adverse physiologic effects of CO2 pneumoperitoneum [11]. Cosmetic problems related to port site incisions which can be eliminated with using the single port laparoscopc surgical technique by expert surgeons [1].

Technique of Laparoscopic Catheter Salvage

In our instiution, laparoscopic rescue procedures were performed under general anesthesia. The peritoneal cavity was emptied before surgery. Prophylactic antibiotic therapy (cefazolin sodium 1 g) was administired before surgery. A nasogastric tube was inserted. A 1-cm long slightly lateral subumbilical incision was made through the subcutaneous tissue, and the anterior rectus sheath. The rectus muscle fibers were then dissected bluntly down to the posterior rectus sheath. A 10-mm trocar was inserted on the opposite side of the previous catheter placement location. A pneumoperitoneum was established via this trocar, inflating to a pressure of 12 mmHg. If the patient was mobidly obese pneumoperitoneum was established through the existing PD catheter. If the catheter was completely obstructed pneumoperitoneum was established usind the Veress needle in left upper quadrant on subcostal site in morbidly obese patients with slightly reverse Trendelenburg and slightly right side position. Two 5-mm working ports were used. Once the diagnosis of catheter dysfunction was made, corrective measures were undertaken.

Omental Wrapping

Peritoneal dialysis catheter obstruction is frequently caused by omentum blocking the side holes of the catheter tubing. Omental wrapping usually develops early after catheter placement. The incidence of omental wrapping of CAPD catheters has been reported from 4.5% to 15% [16]. Clinically, the inflow of dialysate decreases slightly, and drainage is obviously blocked. Wrapping may be a result of a bulky omentum [17]. Using laparoscopic salvage, the incidence of outflow failure by omental wrapping ranged between 57% and 92% in some series [18]. Advantages of laparoscopic surgery include direct visualization of the state of obstruction and ability to lyse adhesions, and perform omental fixation after the stripping if necessary [11].

When omental wrapping is diagnosed at laparoscopy, usually only stripping is performed. This procedure can be easly done without the need for complicated laparoscopic instruments or advanced laparoscopic surgical experience. Reported series show that this simple laparoscopic stripping of the omentum from the catheter usually resolves a catheter obstruction due to omental wrapping with a high rate of success [19–21]. Some authors advocate omental fixation after the stripping procedure to prevent further omental wrapping [11, 22]. Laparoscopic partial omental resection has also been performed for recurrent catheter dysfunction due to omental wrapping [23, 24]. In our observation, the omentum was more likley to cause catheter obstruction in emaciated patients which can be related to the omentum being very thin in these individuals in contrast in obese patients. The omentum must be preserved in PD salvage procedures. The omentum possesses an inherent motility that allows it to seek out and arrest trouble that may arise within the peritoneal cavity. It has been referred to as the "police officer of the abdomen". The potent lymphatic system of the omentum can absorb enormous amounts of edema fluids and remove metabolic wastes and toxic substances. The omentum is also widely used for the treatment of some pathologies in full surgical fields if necessary [25]. To completely overcome this problem related to omental wrapping prophylactic laparoscopic omental fixation is routinely performed during CAPD catheter placement in our series [10].

Catheter Tip Migration

Catheter tip migration still accounts for a substantial number of catheter failures in blind, open and laparoscopically placed CAPD catheters [3, 17]. Mechanical obstruction usually results from either misplacement during the initial insertion or catheter migration out of the pelvis. A coiled intra-abdominal segment is generally belived to reduce catheter tip migration; however, the results of previous prospective randomized studies comparing straight and coiled catheters have been controversial [26]. Catheter tip migration is easily determined with abdominal x ray. Various noninvasive management techniques, including changing body position, enemas, and saline flushing, increase physical activity as much as possible have been described; however, the success rate is only about 25%. If such noninvasive techniques fail, before surgical revision, fluoroscopically guided manipulations using a rigid canulla, stiff metal rod, tip-deflecting wire, Lunderquist guidewire or double guidewire method may be used to reposition the catheter [7]. Different success rates of fluoroscopy-guided wire manipulation have been reported, ranging from 27% to 67% [27]. Advantages of fluoroscopy-guided wire manipulation are that it is relatively easy and safe, simple, does not require anesthesia, can be performed in radiology suite, can be attempted repeatedly, and has a relatively lower cost compared to laparoscopic surgery. Disadvantages of fluoroscopy-guided wire manipulation include a lower success rate and inapplicability of difficulty with certain special catheter design [27].

The rate of catheter misplacement has been dramatically reduced because in recent years it has been possible to place catheters more accurately under direct vision with laparoscopic insertion [10]. Surgical revision is mandatory in the treatment of peritoneal catheter malfunction due to catheter tip migration when conventional methods fail. Open repositioning of the catheter is not only more invasive, but may result in the creation of adhesions. In addition, open catheter revision inhibits immediate use of the catheter because the abdominal incision must first heal. A secondary means of dialysis is required, that is, hemodialysis (HD) which involves further cost, inconvenience, and the risks associated with HD catheters.

Catheter tip migration without adhesions, requiring only laparoscopic redirection, can be expected to be restored to normal function in a high percentage of cases. Laparoscopic surgery is also used to adhesiolysis if needed with redirection of catheter [27]. PD catheters can be safely positioned in patients with previous abdominal surgery [28].

In 1995, Julian et al. recommended the additional step of laparoscopic suturing of the catheter to the anterior abdominal wall to prevent further catheter malposition [29]. In recent years, laparoscopic repositioning and catheter fixation onto the parietal peritoneum has become an increasingly popular method of restoring the CAPD catheter due to catheter tip migration. A number of laparoscopic catheter fixation techniques have been reported. The techniques advocated for saving catheters have also been used during the initial placement for prophylaxis. Some authors have also preferred minilaparotomy and catheter fixation to the anterior abdominal wall for the treatment of malfunctioning PD catheter related to catheter tip migration [17, 30]. To prevent the catheter tip migration, rectus sheath tunellig effectively keeps the catheter oriented toward the pelvis during the PD catheter placement [15].

Fibrin or Blood Clots Within the Catheter

Catheter obstruction due to fibrin or blood clots within the catheter lumen is another problem in CAPD patients. Obstruction by blood clot or fibrin coating usually presents with blood-tinged dialysate drainage. When the catheter is blocked with fibrin/clots there is usually absent inflow and outflow. Forcibly flushing the catheter with heparinized saline, the classic use of fibrinolytics, such as urokinase, or mechanical interventions may resolve the obstruction. The channel-cleaning brush and fluoroscopy guidance can be used to restore patency with potential risks [31, 32].

Salvage surgery is required when primary noninvasive management fails. However, most of these methods are not effective in the long run. Removel of the catheter is the usual outcome [33]. Laparoscopic rescue procedure should be safe, with a high success rate, ease of performance, ability to prevent recurrence, and quick recovery time.

The obstructed catheter is examined through a laparoscope to identify the cause of obstruction. The catheter is pulled out from the abdominal cavity through the 5-mm channel in the abdominal wall with atraumatic forceps. All obstructing elements inside the lumen are removed by milking the catheter by hand. The catheter is then flushed clean with heparinized saline and pushed back into the peritoneum [19]. The fibrin and blood clots are also cleared by milking the catheter with atraumatic laparoscopic forceps and flushing intraperitoneally with heparinized saline under pressure from a 50-ml syringe [33]. This procedure is an easy task for the surgeon to perform using two ports. It does, of course, involve a longer time in the operating theater. The intraperitoneal laparoscopic cleaning minimizes the risk of catheter contamination that may occure if it is exteriorized. The reutilization of the original catheter is beneficial in that it avoids the need for additional work to remove the old catheter and reimplant a new catheter [21].

Pericatheter Leakage

Pericatheter leakage of dialysis fluid occurs in 4–36% of treated patients. Regardless of the implantation approach used, a break-in procedure for 2–4 weeks has been recommended to avoid pericatheter leakage [34]. In some reports, PD was started immediately after surgical implantation and the incidence of pericatheter leakage was less than 2% [35]. The dialysate volume which is gradually increase to allow complete wound healing, and thus promotes formation of a tight catheter passage at the begining of CAPD [36]. To treat leakage, it is recommended to have a break-in period of 7–14 days for commencement of PD [37]. Catheter replacemnt is mandatory in the treatment of dialysate leakage when conventional methods fail [38]. One method of prevention is to create the long tunelling which reduces the risk of pericatheter leaks during the PD catheter placement [10, 15].

References

1. Yamada A, Hiraiva T, Tsuji Y, Ueda N. Single-port laparoscopy for salvaging outflow failure from omental wrapping. Perit Dial Int. 2012;32(6):669–71.
2. Zhu W, Jiang J, Zheng X, Zhang M, Guo H, et al. The placement of peritoneal dialysis catheters: a

prospective randomized comparison of open surgery versus 'Mini-Perc' technique. Int Urol Nephrol. 2015;47:377–82.

3. Kang SH, Jy D, Cho KH, Park JW, Yoon KW. Blind peritoneal catheter placement with a tenckhoff trocar by nephrologists: a singlcenter experience. Nephrology. 2012;17:141–7.

4. Paolo ND, Capotondo L, Sansoni E, Romolini V, Simola M, et al. The self-locating catheter: Clinical experience and follow-up. Perit Dial Int. 2004;24:359–64.

5. Ash SR, Wolf R. Placement of the Tenckhoff peritoneal dialysis catheter under peritoneoscopic visualization. Dial Transplant. 1981;10:383–6.

6. Li JR, Chen CH, Cheng CL, Yang CK, Ou YC, et al. Five-year experience of peritoneal dialysis catheter placement. J Chin Med Assoc. 2012;75:309–13.

7. Lee CM, Ko SF, Chen HC, Leung TK. Double-guidewire method: a novel technique for correction of migrated Tenckhoff peritoneal dialysis catheter. Perit Dial Int. 2003;23:587–90.

8. Numanoglu A, McCulloch MI, Van der Pool A, Millar AJW, Rode H. Laparoscopic salvage of malfunctioning Tenckhoff Catheters. J Laparoendosc Adv Surg Tech. 2007;17:128–30.

9. Liu WJ, Hooi LS. Complications after Tenckhoff catheter insertion: a single-centre experience using multiple operators over four years. Perit Dial Int. 2010;30:509–12.

10. Ogunc G. Minilaparoscopic extraperitoneal tunelling with omentopexy: a new technique for CAPD catheter placement. Perit Dial Int. 2005;25:551–5.

11. Ogunc G. Malfunctioning peritoneal dialysis catheter and accompanying surgical pathology repaired by laparoscopic surgery. Perit Dial Int. 2002;22:454–62.

12. Kimmelstiel FM, Miller RE, Malinelli BM. Laparoscopic management of peritoneal dialysis catheters. Surg Gynecol Obstet. 1993;176:565–70.

13. Amerling R, Macic DV, Spivak H, Lo AY, White P, et al. Laparoscopic salvage of malfunctioning peritoneal catheters. Surg Endosc. 1997;11:249–52.

14. Ovnat A, Dukhno O, Pinsk I, Peiser J, Levy I. The laparoscopic option in the management of peritoneal dialysis catheter revision. Surg Endosc Other Interv Tech. 2002;16(4):698–9.

15. Crabtree JH. Development of surgical guidelines for laparoscopic peritoneal dialysis access: down a long and winding road. Perit Dial Int. 2015;35:241–4.

16. Hughes CR, Agnotti DM, Jubelirer RA. Laparoscopic repositioning of a continuous ambulatory peritoneal dialysis (CAPD) catheter. Surg Endosc. 1994;8:1108–9.

17. Li J, Cheng C, Chiu K, Cheng C, Yang C, et al. Minilaparotomy salvage of malfunctioning catheters in peritoneal dialysis. Perit Dial Int. 2011;33:46–50.

18. Goh YH. Omental folding: a novel laparoscopic technique for salvaging peritoneal dialysis catheters. Perit Dial Int. 2008;28:626–31.

19. Zadrozny D, Niemierko ML, Draczkowski T, Renke M, Liberek T. Laparoscopic approach for dysfunctional Tenckhoff catheters. Perit Dial Int. 1999;19:170–1.

20. Fukui M, Maeda K, Sakamoto K, Hamada C, Tomino Y. Laparoscopic manipulation for outflow failure of peritoneal dialysis catheter. Nephron. 1999;83:369.

21. Chao S, Tsai T. Laparoscopic rescue of dysfunctional Tenckhoff catheters in continuous ambulatory peritoneal dialysis patients. Nephron. 1993;65:157–8.

22. Crabtree JH, Fishman A. Laparoscopic epiplopexy of the greater omentum and epiploic appendices in the salvaging of dysfunctional peritoneal dialysis catheters. Surg Laparosc Endosc. 1996;6:176–80.

23. Crabtree JH, Fishman A. Laparoscopic omentectomy for peritoneal dialysis catheter flow obstruction: a case report and review of the literature. Surg Laparosc Endosc Percutan Tech. 1999;9:228–33.

24. Campisi S, Cavatorta F, Ramo E, Varano P. Videolaparoscopy with partial omentectomy in patients on peritoneal dialysis. Perit Dial Int. 1997;17:211–2.

25. Alagumuthu M, Das BB, Pattanayak SP, Rasananda M. The omentum: a unique organ of exceptional versatility. Indian J Surg. 2006;68(83):136–41.

26. Ouyang CJ, Huang FX, Yang QQ, Jiang ZP, Chen V, et al. Comparing the incidence ocatheter-related complications with straight and coiled Tenckhoff catheters in peritoneal dialysis patients- a single-center prospective randomized trial. Perit Dial Int. 2015;35:443–9.

27. Kim HJ, Lee TW, Ihm CG, Kim MJ. Use of fluoroscopy-guided wire manipulation and/or laparoscopic surgery in the repair of malfunctioning peritoneal dialysis catheters. Am J Nephrol. 2002;22:532–8.

28. Santarelli S, Zeiler M, Marinelli R, Monteburini T, Federico A, et al. Videolaparoscopy as rescue therapy and placement of peritoneal dialysis catheters: a thirty-two case single centre experience. Nephrol Dial Transplant. 2006;21:1348–54.

29. Julian TB, Ribeiro U, Bruns F, Fraley D. Malfunctioning peritonel dialysis catheter repaired by laparoscopic surgery. Perit Dial Int. 1995;15:363–6.

30. Kim SH, Lee DH, Choi HJ, Seo HJ, Jang YS, et al. Minilaparotomy with manuel correction for malfunctioning peritoneal dialysis catheters. Perit Dial Int. 2008;28:550–4.

31. Cumvenda MJ, Wright FK. The use of channel-cleaning brush for malfunctioning Tenckhoff catheters. Nephrol Dial Transplant. 1999;14:1254–7.

32. Hummeida MA, Eltahir JMA, Ali HM, Khalid SE, Mobarak AI, et al. Successful management of an obstructed Tenckhoff catheter using an endoscopic retrograde cholangiopancreatography (ERCP) cytology brush. Perit Dial Int. 2010;30:482–4.

33. Leung LC, Yiu MK, Man CW, Chan WH, Lee KW, et al. Laparoscopic management of Tenckhoff catheters in continuous ambulatoty peritoneal dialysis. A one-port technique. Surg Endosc. 1998;12:891–3.

34. Jo YI, Shin SK, Lee JH, Song JO, Park JH. Immediate initiation of CAPD following percutaneous catheter placement without break-in procedure. Perit Dial Int. 2007;22:179–83.

35. Stegmayr B. Various clinical approaches to minimise complications in peritoneal dialysis. Int J Artif Organs. 2002;25:365–72.

36. Meier CM, Poppleton A, Fliser D, Klingele M. A novel adaptation of laparoscopic Tenckhoff catheter insertion technique to enhance catheter stability and function in automated peritoneal dialysis. Langenbeck Arch Surg. 2014;399:525–32.

37. Ponce D, Banin VB, Bueloni TN, Baretti P, Caramori J, et al. Different outcomes of peritoneal catheter percutaneous placement by nephrologists using a trocar versus the Seldinger technique: the experience of two Brazilian centers. Int Urol Nephrol. 2014;46:2029–34.

38. Bergamin B, Senn O, Corsenca A, Dutkowski P, Weber M, et al. Finding the right position: A three-year, single-center experience with the "self-locating" catheter. Perit Dial Int. 2010;30:519–23.

Mechanical Complications of Peritoneal Dialysis

13

Juaquito M. Jorge, Nicolas Bonamici,
and Stephen Haggerty

Introduction

Because peritoneal dialysis relies on an intraperitoneal catheter for both inflow and outflow of dialysate, it is no wonder that mechanical complications are common and frustrating. Up to 40% of patients develop a mechanical complication of peritoneal dialysis (MCPD) at some point during their therapy [1, 2], leading to a conversion rate to hemodialysis of up to 20% [3, 4]. Examples of MCPD include inflow and outflow dysfunction, migration, hernias, peritoneal dialysate leakage, hydrothorax, superficial cuff extrusion, hydrothorax, external tubing break or leak and pain during dialysis. This chapter will focus on prevention, diagnosis and management of these common problems with the exception of catheter dysfunction and hernias which are covered in separate chapters. Most authors agree

that, like other procedure-related outcomes, equipment and operator factors are uniquely able to reduce the risk of problems before they occur. The International Society for Peritoneal Dialysis (ISPD) has published clinical practice guidelines for PD access [5] based on existing evidence, and where no evidence is available, expert consensus. These guidelines discuss having dedicated teams, surgeons, and support staff involved with each PD access case, utilizing standardized protocols for implantation (i.e. antibiotic prophylaxis, 2 week minimum between catheter insertion and PD start), and conducting regular audits of PD catheter outcomes. Notably, the ISPD guidelines do not specify recommendations on type of catheter, method of insertion, or other technical parameters. In fact, they pointedly mention that "no particular catheter type is proven to be better than another" based on grade 2C evidence.

J.M. Jorge, MD, MS
Department of Surgery, Northwestern University
Feinberg School of Medicine,
251 E. Huron, Galter 3-150, Chicago, IL 60611, USA
e-mail: juaquito.jorge@northwestern.edu

N. Bonamici, BA
Northshore University Health system,
Evanston, IL, USA
e-mail: nicolas.bonamici@northwestern.edu

S. Haggerty, MD, FACS (✉)
Department of Surgery, NorthShore University
HealthSystem, 777 Park Avenue West, Rm 3464,
Evanston, IL 60035, USA
e-mail: shaggerty@northshore.org

Technical Considerations

When it comes to discussing mechanical complications of peritoneal dialysis, prevention is key. Attention to detail, meticulous surgical technique, and following established "best practices" are paramount during PD catheter insertion surgery to reduce complications later in treatment [6]. Catheter type, length, and exit site are key considerations for surgeons involved in PD insertion. While recommendations exist on these points, no current level 1 evidence exists to

© Springer International Publishing AG 2017
S. Haggerty (ed.), *Surgical Aspects of Peritoneal Dialysis*, DOI 10.1007/978-3-319-52821-2_13

demonstrate superiority in outcome for straight vs. swan neck and single vs. double cuff catheters. No matter what catheter is used, the best way to prevent mechanical complications is a properly placed PD catheter, with curl tip under the pubis and exit site away from fat folds. Technical details for inserting catheters are found elsewhere in this book.

Peritoneal Dialysis Fluid Leaks

Introduction

Peritoneal dialysis fluid leakage is an infrequent but disruptive complication in patients on peritoneal dialysis (PD), occurring in 4–10% of this population [7–9] and can happen early (<30 days) or late (> 30 days). Although peritonitis and exit-site infections are the most frequent causes of technical failure in PD, dialysate leaks represent one of the major noninfectious complications. Causes include inguinal, umbilical, femoral or incisional hernias [10], peritoneal tears [11], leaks around the dialysis catheter, trauma, fluid overload and malignancy [12, 13]. Early leaks often overtly manifest as pericatheter leak [9] and may be related to insertion technique, timing of the start of PD after surgery, and inherent or acquired abdominal weakness. Late leaks may present more subtly with subcutaneous swelling and edema, weight gain, peripheral or genital edema, and apparent ultrafiltration failure and are predominantly due to abdominal wall hernias.

To minimize complications, particularly early in the treatment course, various options exist for PD placement location and technique, catheter type, and post-procedure CAPD management. Paramedian insertion may offer lower leak rates compared to midline insertion [14, 15]. Low leak rates have also been demonstrated after peritoneoscopic insertion [16] and laparoscopic insertion using a long peritoneal tunnel [17, 18]. While the pediatric literature tends to favor Tenckhoff catheters over other catheters as superior with respect to dialysate leakage [19, 20], similar consensus on catheter choice in adults is lacking. In addition, the International Society for Peritoneal Dialysis (ISPD) recommends a 2 week wait after PD catheter placement and prior to beginning PD in an attempt to minimize early dialysate leak [21].

Late onset PD leaks are often caused by underlying abdominal wall hernias or patent processus vaginalis, with signs and symptoms being as subtle as peripheral or genital edema. Peritoneal tears may occur from trauma or surgery and can occur at any time after the start of PD. However, hernias are the most common cause of acute genital edema (AGE), especially late-onset edema. Case studies suggest a mechanism of fluid extravasation via a tear in the hernia sac [22]. Inguinal hernias result in fluid in the hernia sac (hydrocele) and extravasation into the soft tissue causing scrotal or labial edema. Tears in ventral, incisional or umbilical hernia sacs may lead to fluid tracking down the fascial layers with gravity and entering the scrotum outside of the tunica vaginalis [22, 23]. A high index of suspicion and thorough preoperative examination prior to PD catheter placement is mandatory. Unfortunately, most dialysate leaks from hernias occur after 30 days due to de novo development of abdominal wall hernias or from a congenital patent processus vaginalis (PPV), present in about 13% of men without clinically detectable hernias [24, 25]. A number of factors predispose PD patients to hernias including obesity, chronically elevated intra-abdominal pressures, uremia, transperitoneal protein losses, and anemia [26].

Evaluation of Dialysate Leak

An evaluation for PD-related complications begins with a focused history and physical exam. Understanding how far out the patient is from PD catheter insertion, the type of catheter that was used, and how it was placed provides valuable information. Careful questioning of patient symptoms is vital. In regards to occult PPV and inguinal hernias, patients often present with the complaint of rapid, persistent swelling of the genitalia (penis, scrotum or labia). There is usually discomfort but minimal pain. There are no associated symptoms such as fever, nausea, vomiting, diarrhea or constipation. Complaints of dysuria, frequency or hesitancy are rare. On examination, bilateral scrotal or labial swelling and skin edema is often present, without redness or tenderness. During the period of severe edema, physical exam can be difficult and inaccurate. Genital swelling may be bilateral even in patients with unilateral hernias. A large hernia may be palpable, but small hernias or PPV will not be clinically apparent [7, 27–30]. While acute genital edema is not harmful to the patient, it does cause considerable distress and discomfort. It may also result in reduced dialysate outflow volumes, requiring a switch to low volume cycled peritoneal dialysis and in some cases temporary hemodialysis. Making a rapid and accurate diagnosis is therefore paramount.

Diagnostic Imaging

Evaluation for and confirmation of dialysate leakage, especially late onset, typically requires adjunctive testing and imaging. The presence of diffuse genital edema or lack of specific physical findings may make identifying overt causes of PD complications and dialysate leakage difficult. Aside from structural problems such as hernias, peritoneal tears, and pericatheter leaks, other potential causes such as salt and fluid intake /outtake imbalances may exist. Modalities such as the peritoneal equilibration test (PET) can help detect both leaks and other CAPD related complications by assessing returning volume. However, PET is best utilized in assessing patients with normal imaging since it can detect poor outflow, ultrafiltration failure and fluid overload as an alternative cause [8, 13].

Three main imaging modalities are available today which can more accurately identify the location of dialysate leak: peritoneal scintigraphy, CT peritoneography and MRI peritoneography. In the late 1970s and early 1980s, clinicians had limited options for evaluating PD leak etiology. Routine groin exploration looking for occult hernias in patients with AGE was described, but carried a success rate of only 75% [31]. Catheter peritoneography using plain roentgenograms following instillation of contrast into the peritoneal

cavity was an initial imaging mainstay. Some combination of periodic exploration along with peritoneography was also used in order to lower the incidence of unnecessary surgery [22].

Peritoneal Scintigraphy

First described in 1983, peritoneal scintigraphy was the next logical imaging advancement after catheter peritoneography. It has a higher sensitivity than either intraoperative site exploration or catheter peritoneography [32], with the success rate of picking up fluid leaks as high as 95% in some series [33].

A varying amount of radioactive isotope, usually 2–5 mCi of Tc-99m, mixed with one to two liters of dialysate is instilled into the peritoneum and imaged with a gamma camera [27, 33–35]. Standing and/or ambulating after radioisotope administration increases the sensitivity of finding a leak and shortens the duration until a positive finding can be seen. After a period of time varying from minutes to hours, imaging pictures are taken in both supine and upright positions and from different angles.

Availability of peritoneal scintigraphy is institution-specific, requiring a nuclear medicine department experienced in this technique. It is a solid diagnostic modality, especially in areas without easy availability to advanced imaging such as CT and MRI. Despite the availability of advanced technology, peritoneal scintigraphy continues to be frequently used to assess patients with suspected PD leaks [13, 36, 37]. Advantages include high diagnostic accuracy in detecting leaks and hernias, low cost, decreased radiation exposure, and low risk of contrast associated peritonitis and allergic reaction to iodine contrast. In addition, it provides whole body multi-planar images and delayed images may be taken up to 24 h later.

Computed Tomography Peritoneography

Computed tomography (CT) use in CAPD-related complications was first described circa

1984. While plain CT has been used, addition of intraperitoneal contrast has been shown to increase the diagnostic accuracy in suspected PD leak patients to between 70% and 100% [38–40].

Similar to catheter peritoneography and peritoneal scintigraphy, CT peritoneography involves instilling ~100 mL of Omnipaque or similar contrast mixed with one to two liters of dialysate into the peritoneal cavity. In order to facilitate spread of contrast, ambulatory patients are asked to walk or stand for a prescribed period of time while non-ambulatory patients may roll from side to side or sit up. Images are then taken with the patient in the supine position between 1 and 4 h later. A pre-contrast CT scan may or may not be performed. Occasionally, delayed imaging beyond 4 h may be helpful if initial imaging is negative but clinical suspicion is high.

CT peritoneography facilitates diagnosis, verifies the location of the catheter and helps in surgical planning. It allows better anatomical information regarding the etiology, location and size of fluid leak than scintigraphy. While some earlier series looking at diagnostic success demonstrated decreased sensitivity compared with peritoneal scintigraphy, advances in CT scanning technology likely will have a positive effect on this. Conversely, CT imaging generally is more expensive and subjects the patient to more radiation than other imaging modalities.

Magnetic Resonance Peritoneography

Magnetic resonance imaging (MRI) offers promising results in diagnosing etiology of PD leakage. Conducted in a manner similar to CT peritoneography, MRI peritoneography also involves imaging after intraperitoneal instillation of contrast mixed with dialysate. Single-institution case series demonstrate a sensitivity of ~65% for picking up CAPD complication etiologies [36]. In cases where contrast instillation may be contraindicated such as prior allergic reaction or sensitivity, MRI peritoneography with only dialysate medium has been described. Initial evidence seems to demonstrate equivalent sensitivity [41].

While MRI offers benefits over CT in terms of lack of radiation exposure, its diagnostic success has not been extensively studied. Additionally, its availability and cost present obvious limitations.

Other Diagnostic Modalities

Ultrasonography is often used to evaluate scrotal contents and viability of the testis. In the case of suspected PD leakage in a patient with acute genital edema and a clinically detectable hernia, some authors argue that sonographic confirmation is all that is needed prior to herniorrhaphy [42, 43]. Advantages include non-invasiveness, lack of radiation exposure and ability to be performed quickly and easily at bedside. Findings may include patent processus vaginalis containing pooling fluid and a dilated peri-testicular space of the tunica vaginalis. The presence of a communication with the peritoneal cavity may or may not be seen. However, ultrasound is highly operator dependent and lacks the sensitivity and specificity of other imaging modalities when used as a solitary diagnostic test.

Despite advances in imaging technology, there are still cases where the etiology of PD leakage is unclear, especially when differentiating unilateral from bilateral small inguinal hernias or PPV. We have previously reported the use of diagnostic laparoscopy (DL) in patients with acute genital edema and suspected PD leakage to make a definitive diagnosis and accurately differentiate bilateral and unilateral inguinal hernias [44]. This is important because the rate of PPV on the opposite side in patients with unilateral hernias approaches 25% [45, 46] and failure to identify this will result in recurrent genital edema and the need for reoperation. The accuracy of DL approaches 100% and has a less than 1% complication rate [47, 48]. Herniorrhaphy may be then undertaken during that operation.

Management

Treatment of dialysate leaks initially focuses on prevention. Delaying CAPD for 14 days after catheter insertion and initiating CAPD with low dialysate volume may prevent early leakage [5, 21]. Spending more time supine with the scrotum supported and elevated in males may help improve genital edema. Differentiating PD leaks between early and late onset is important, as etiologies are obviously managed differently. Early leaks from a peritoneal tear or catheter insertion site often respond to low volume PD in a supine position or cycled [9, 49]. If this fails, cessation of PD for a few weeks [7, 8, 10, 11] allows spontaneous closure [8, 12]. Unfortunately the latter requires temporary hemodialysis. If pericatheter leakage does not respond to conservative management, catheter replacement is an option [12, 50].

Late dialysate leaks, often manifesting as acute genital edema, usually require surgical correction. Hernias should be repaired as they generally do not respond to nonoperative measures. Open inguinal hernia repair with high ligation and excision of the hernia sac or PPV, followed by placement of onlay mesh as described by Lichtenstein [51] appears to be the best approach allowing early return to CAPD with low risk of recurrence [52–54]. In fact, if the diagnosis can be made quickly and the genital edema responds to low volume PD, hernia repair may be performed without switching to hemodialysis [55]. For ventral or incisional hernias, open anterior repair with inversion of the hernia sac without disrupting it, and placing onlay mesh has been shown to have low recurrence and leak rates in adults [56, 57]. If the peritoneum is entered, it is recommended to close the peritoneum in a watertight manner [58]. Laparoscopic inguinal and ventral hernia repair with mesh has not been adequately studied in PD patients, but may decrease the effectiveness of the peritoneal membrane and be a potential for mesh infection. Ultimately, any intraperitoneal placement of mesh, or concern for peritoneal membrane integrity after hernia repair probably should lead to cessation of PD and temporary HD for several weeks to mitigate the risk of mesh infection.

Hydrothorax

Pleural effusions and hydrothorax as a result of dialysis fluid movement from the abdominal space to the pleural space are rare but potentially life threatening complications of PD, occurring in 1–2% of patients [59, 60]. Patients with hydrothorax often present with shortness of breath and acute transudative pleural effusion, usually after dwell with dialysate and usually within the first 30 days after dialysis initiation, primarily due to catheter dysfunction or excessive peritoneal pressure due to dialysate influx [59, 60]. The primary etiology of hydrothorax in the PD patient is thought to be pleuro-peritoneal communication due to high peritoneal pressure upon dialysis in the presence of congenital or acquired defects in the diaphragm [59, 61, 62], although some cases are brought on by a malfunctioning or malpositioned catheter [63]. Notably, the presence of hydrothorax is right-sided in 90% of cases, as the left side of the diaphragm is partially supported by the heart and pericardium [64–66].

Patients often present with early onset hydrothorax within the first 30 days after catheter insertion with chest heaviness, shortness of breath, or dyspnea during dialysate indwelling, although up to 25% of patients present with no symptoms or a slight cough [67]. Like the symptoms of local edema, symptoms of hydrothorax often manifest upon dialysate influx, or directly after indwelling [68]. Because these symptoms could be misdiagnosed as congestive heart failure or inadequate dialysis, an early and accurate diagnosis is crucial to management. Many of the diagnostic tools used to detect leaks elsewhere in the body are useful in diagnosing PD-associated hydrothorax. Common methods of diagnosis are chest CT [68], X-ray imaging [70], or ultrasonography [68]. These methods can confirm the presence of fluid in the pleural space, but do not allow for appreciation of the underlying etiology of a diaphragmatic defect, which can lead to an alternate diagnosis [71]. Additionally, the presence of increased glucose levels in the pleural fluid is suggestive of a pleuro-peritoneal communication, although this does not manifest in all patients and should not be relied upon as the sole means of diagnosis [59, 70, 72]. Instead, there is increasing use of peritoneal scintigraphy [68, 69, 73–76], which allows not only for accurate diagnosis of fluid overload and transudative pleural effusion but also allows for the identification and localization of diaphragmatic defects without thoracoscopic intervention.

Management

Upon a diagnosis of PD-related hydrothorax, several management options are available. Conservative management usually involves the cessation of dialysis for 4–6 weeks, and patients are often switched to biweekly hemodialysis. This allows for the mediastinum to heal after a rupture, and is usually sufficient to prevent subsequent instances of effusion. Unfortunately, conservative management is effective in only a quarter of all PD-related hydrothorax [60]. This leaves the patient with two options, switch to hemodialysis or undertake invasive measures in attempt to remain on PD. This includes either thoracotomy or video assisted thoracoscopic surgery, usually to obliterate the pleural space via mechanical or chemical pleurodesis. Mechanical pleurodesis with an abrasive pad is performed either via open or video thoracotomy to adhere the parietal and visceral pleural via inflammation [76, 77], while chemical pleurodesis with povidone, talc, tetracycline, or other sclerosing agents can be performed by catheter infusion [76, 77]. A long term study found that pleurodesis effectively reduces the risk of hydrothorax for up to 50 months after management [77]. In cases where a large defect is identified, video-assisted thoracoscopic repair [70, 78, 79] or less commonly, thoracotomy and repair under direct vision are performed [80]. Additionally, case studies show success at closing diaphragmatic defects with automatic endoscopic staplers [81] or endoscopic suturing devices [82] combined with overlay non-absorbable mesh [79]

and fibrin glue [81]. After intervention, it is common to withhold PD for several weeks until the integrity of the diaphragm is restored [79, 82], although some advocate immediate return to PD [81]. Although the long term success of these procedures is largely unstudied, patients with hydrothorax early in their peritoneal dialysis treatment often return to PD as their preferred dialysis modality. However, if patients do not wish or are not medically fit to undergo an invasive procedure a switch to hemodialysis is needed.

Superficial Cuff Extrusion

If the external cuff of a peritoneal dialysis catheter becomes visible at the skin level, it is called extrusion (Fig. 13.1). In this case, the fibers become colonized with skin bacteria and may form a chronic exit site infection. This in turn can lead to peritonitis and even catheter loss [83]. When cuff extrusion happens it is almost always because of poor planning and technique during the surgical insertion. The exit site must be planned based on the insertion site and the shape of the catheter. If the exit site has been chosen too close to the insertion site, over time a normally straight catheter with a bend formed by the surgeon will slowly straighten and push the external cuff outward.

When the external cuff is visible, the patient is usually referred back to the surgeon for catheter replacement. Many times there is associated exit

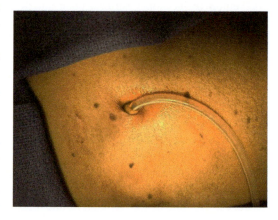

Fig. 13.1 Superficial cuff extrusion from skin (Courtesy of Dr. Stephen Haggerty)

site infection or even tunnel infection. Since maintaining a functioning catheter is of the utmost importance in renal failure patients, it is generally preferable to salvage an existing functioning catheter as opposed to replacing it and risking fluid leak, malfunction, infection and need for switch to hemodialysis. Salvage techniques such as external cuff shaving [84–89] deroofing of the exit site [90] and replacing the external segment of the catheter by splicing and repairing the catheter [91] have been reported.

Cuff-Shaving Technique

Although various techniques have been used for cuff shaving, the most standard seems to be as follows: Local anesthesia is injection into the skin around the exit site. Elliptical incision is made in the skin around exit site. Cautery is used to excise skin and soft tissue to expose the distal cuff (Fig. 13.2). Soft tissue is debrided off the distal cuff. The fibers of the cuff with a layer of silicone are then shaved off in strips using a scalpel or even a common razor [89] (Fig. 13.3). Using magnification may help the accuracy of the shaving. It should be noted that most catheters have thicker layer of silicone at the cuff to allow safe removal of all the fibers and a layer of silicone (Fig. 13.4). After all fibers are removed, the wound is packed and allowed to granulate around the catheter (Fig. 13.5).

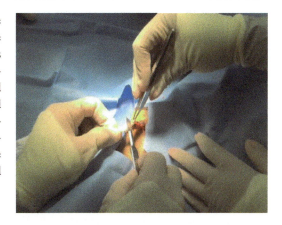

Fig. 13.3 Careful shaving of the cuff and silicone (Courtesy of Dr. Stephen Haggerty)

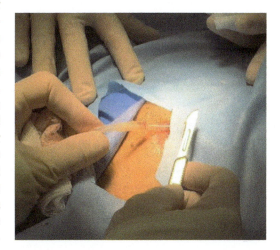

Fig. 13.4 Completed cuff shaving (Courtesy of Dr. Stephen Haggerty)

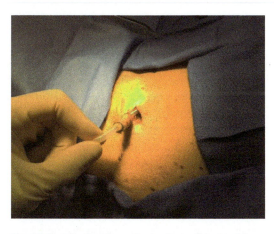

Fig. 13.2 After local anesthesia, the cuff is freed from the skin and soft tissue using knife and cautery (Courtesy of Dr. Stephen Haggerty)

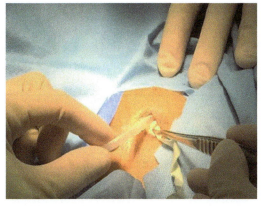

Fig. 13.5 Packing the wound around the catheter (Courtesy of Dr. Stephen Haggerty)

Results

Cuff shaving was described by Nolph and Nichols in 1983 [84] and Helfrich and Winchester were able to salvage 8 out of 12 catheters with exit site infections using this technique [85]. Piraino showed poor results from cuff shaving in 22 patients. The median catheter survival was only 1.5 months and there was high rate of dialysate leak and recurrent infection after the procedure producing a paultry 27% success rate [86]. However, in the largest series to date, Scalamogna reported a 50% 1 year survival after cuff shaving for staph aureus and staph epidermidis. Unfortunately, shortly after the procedure, 20 catheters (49%) were removed for either persistent tunnel infection or development of peritonitis [88]. In addition, Tan reported a 77% catheter survival after an average follow-up of 8.3 months using cuff shaving with a common razor [89]. Cuff shaving has also been described in children with good results. Yoshino compared 32 cuff shaving procedures with 29 catheter replacements in patients 1–20 years old. The primary outcome was time to post surgical tunnel infection and there was no significant difference between the groups. The incidence of recurrence of infection was 12.5% after the cuff shaving procedure with a 9.4% incidence of peritonitis. They concluded that compared to replacing the catheter, cuff shaving was less expensive, shortened hospital stay, and reduced the frequency of catheter replacement [92]. Another pediatric study reviewed 13 patients who underwent cuff shaving and formation of a new subcutaneous tunnel with exit site in the opposite side of the abdomen. After a mean follow-up of 31 months there were no recurrent exit site or tunnel infections. However five members of the group stopped PD due to receiving a transplant [93].

Recommendations

Based on the known literature, careful cuff shaving is a viable option to salvage a functioning PD catheter with superficial cuff extrusion or exit site infection. It may be performed under local anesthesia with minimal risk. However, if the tubing is damaged or cut during the procedure of if there is dialysate leak or persistent infection the catheter will need to be removed and a new one placed, usually on the opposite side of the abdomen.

External Tubing Damage

Peritoneal dialysis is made possible by inflow and outflow through an intraperitoneal catheter which has intraabdominal, abdominal wall and external components. Mechanical complications may occur to the external component such as cracks or leaks in the tubing which prevent adequate dialysis and predispose the patient to peritonitis. Catheter damage is an infrequent but aggravating problem that occurs most commonly from accidental damage from clamps or scissors [94, 95]. However, it can also simply weaken over time, or be damaged by disinfectants such as alcohol or iodine and even some antibiotics [96]. Mupirocin which has been used for exit site infections has been shown to cause structural damage to polyurethane catheters. Furthermore, some catheters contain barium sulfate which over time can make the catheter brittle [97]. A final reason for catheter damage may be faulty production or a "bad batch" of catheters.

If the distal end is damaged, the catheter is simply cut and the cap is replaced. If the catheter damage is less than 2–3 cm from the exit site, there is a higher risk of infection and peritonitis. In addition there is not enough length to adequately use a repair kit. Therefore, it will most likely need to be replaced [94]. However, if there is catheter damage greater than 3 cm from the exit site, it is amenable to salvage using the Argyle™ Peri-Patch peritoneal dialysis catheter repair kit (Medtronic, Inc. Mansfield, MA). This kit includes a catheter extension with double-barbed connector, glue mold, locking ring, Beta-cap and Beta-cap clamp and medical-grade adhesive silicone to "glue" the pieces together, forming an air tight, water tight, bacteria resistant connection (Fig. 13.6).

Technique for Repair

When catheter damage is reported, patients are instructed to clamp the catheter proximal to the damage and come to the outpatient clinic as soon as possible. As per the package insert, the catheter should be repaired only by a qualified, licensed physician or other health care practitioner authorized by and under the direction of such a physician. Sterile technique is observed (mask and gloves). The indwelling catheter is clamped with smooth-jawed forceps. The catheter is scrubbed with aqueous based povidone-iodine. Alcohol should be avoided. The end of the indwelling catheter is cut using sterile scissors. The barbed connector of the extension tubing is inserted all the way onto the indwelling catheter until it abuts the plastic hub of the connector (Fig. 13.7). The catheter and extension tubing is wiped to remove all iodine and any foreign matter. The empty glue mold is wrapped around the repaired segments, where the patient's existing catheter meets the extension (Fig. 13.8). Care is taken to center the glue mold over the connection and the mold is closed and secured with the locking ring. The adhesive tube is opened and the aluminum seal is broken with the piercing pin in the cap. The tube of adhesive is threaded

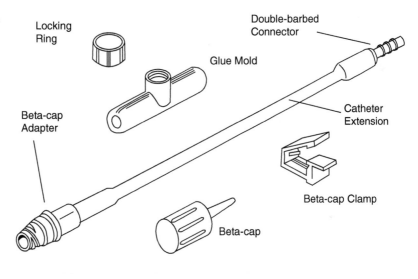

Fig. 13.6 Contents of the Peri-patch kit (Image courtesy of Medtronic. © 2016 Medtronic.)

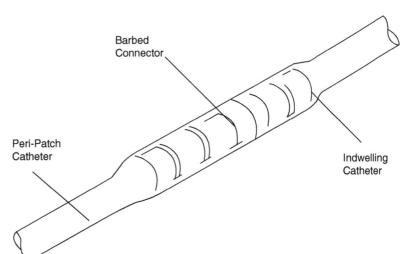

Fig. 13.7 Peri-patch catheter and connector inserted into existing catheter segment (Image courtesy of Medtronic. © 2016 Medtronic.)

Fig. 13.8 The glue mold is placed around the connected pieces and snapped shut (Image courtesy of Medtronic. © 2016 Medtronic.)

Glue Mold

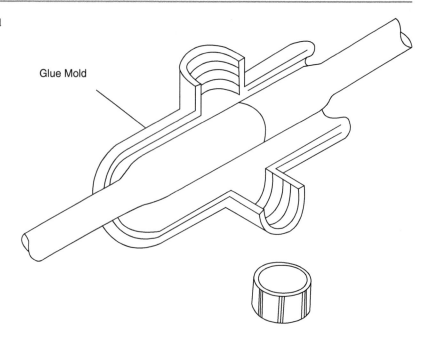

Silicone Adhesive

Catheter

Locking Ring

Glue Mold

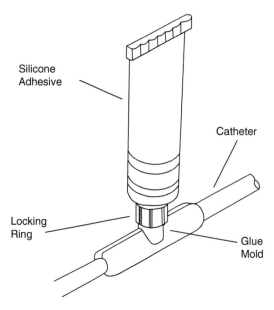

Fig. 13.9 The adhesive tube is threaded onto glue mold using the locking ring. The silicone adhesive is then squeezed into the glue mold (Image courtesy of Medtronic. © 2016 Medtronic.)

into the locking ring (Fig. 13.9). The tube of adhesive is squeezed slowly until the mold is full and excess is wiped away. The new catheter is aspirated to remove air and capped and clamped.

The mold remains for 72 h to allow the adhesive to cure. However, routine PD may be performed during this period. The mold is then opened after 72 h and if the adhesive is dry, it is removed. If it is tacky, the mold is closed for another 24 h.

Results

In a recent review of five repair procedures, Moreiras-Plaza found that none of the patients experienced dialysate leaks or peritonitis or other infectious complications after several months of follow-up [98]. A review of 11 splicing procedures by Usha in 1998 showed that the life-span of these catheters was extended by a mean of 26 months and the infection rate was not affected. Only one infection was related to trauma during the splicing resulting in chronic exit site infection requiring catheter removal [94].

Recommendations

External catheter damage can be avoided by safe handling techniques. It should be emphasized to patients not to use sharp objects to cut tape or gauze around the catheter. If there is a breakage or leak, it is important to address this immediately and also give an antibiotic to prevent peritonitis. If the break is <3 cm from the exit site, the catheter should be replaced. If it is greater than 3 cm but too close to simply divide the catheter at that spot, repair using the Peri-Patch kit is an excellent alternative to removal and should be attempted first.

Pain during Peritoneal Dialysis

Pain on instillation of PD fluid or draining (drain pain) is a known complication in patients undergoing PD occurring in 13 to 25% of patients [99–101]. It is thought to be due to shearing forces against the peritoneum or "jet" effect of dialysate emerging from the distal end of the catheter at relatively high velocity. It can also be related to the pH of the dialysate. If the pain is on outflow, it may be due to suction effect and is often positional. It is many times clinically significant, impacting the patient's quality of life. The phenomenon occurs more frequently with cycler PD where hydraulic suction rather than gravity is used to drain the dialysate. Drain pain is more likely to occur when the catheter tip is implanted too low in the pelvis, wedging it between the rectum and uterus or rectum and bladder and leaving it susceptible to early termination of dialysate outflow and abrupt contact of the catheter tip with the peritoneum. A common cause of the catheter being implanted too deep in the pelvis is when the operator uses a single catheter type for all patients, inserting it at a fixed site relative to the umbilicus without consideration of catheter dimensions or patient body habitus [102]. This is why ISPD guidelines state that the umbilicus should not be used as a reference mark for catheter insertion [103].

Treatment includes altering the pH of the fluid, slowing down the infusion, converting to non-cycler PD using gravity-only drainage or not completely draining the peritoneum at the end of dialysis (tidal dialysis) [100, 101]. The pain may resolve with time; however if it is debilitating, catheter repositioning or removal may be necessary [104, 105].

There is no satisfactory surgical salvage procedure short of replacement for a catheter implanted too deep in the pelvis. Prevention of the problem can be achieved by employing methodology during preoperative planning to select the most appropriate catheter type and using the catheter itself to determine the insertion site that produces optimal pelvic position of the catheter tip [106]. In addition, long extraperitoneal tunneling for placement of the catheter body (straight portion of the catheter) may avoid movement of the catheter which may prevent the tip of the catheter hitting the peritoneum periodically during CAPD [107].

Bibliography

1. Singh N, Davidson I, Minhajuddin A, Gieser S, Nurenberg M, Saxena R. Risk factors associated with peritoneal dialysis catheter survival: a 9-year single-center study in 315 patients. J Vasc Access. 2010;11:316–22.
2. Santarelli S, Zeiler M, Marinelli R, Monteburini T, Federico A, Ceraudo E. Videolaparoscopy as rescue therapy and placement of peritoneal dialysis catheters: a thirty-two case single centre experience. Nephrol Dial Transplant. 2006;21:1348–54.
3. Flanigan M, Gokal R. Peritoneal catheters and exit-site practices toward optimum peritoneal access: a review of current developments. Perit Dial Int. 2005;25:132–9.
4. McCormick B, Bargman J. Clinical commentary: noninfectious complications of peritoneal dialysis: implications for patient and technique survival. JASN. 2007 Dec;18:3023–5.
5. Figueiredo A, Bak-Leong G, Jenkins S, Johnson D, Mactier R, Ramalakshmi S, Shrestha B, Struijk D, Wilkie M. Clinical practice guidelines for peritoneal access. Perit Dial Int. 2010;30:424–9.
6. Crabtree JH. Selected best demonstrated practices in peritoneal dialysis access. Kidney Int Suppl. 2006 Nov;(103):S27–37.
7. Abraham G, Blake PG, Mathews RE, Bargman JM, Izatt S, Oreopoulos DG. Genital swelling as a surgical complication of continuous ambulatory peritoneal dialysis. Surg Gynecol Obstet. 1990 Apr;170(4):306–8.
8. Tzamaloukas AH. Scrotal edema in patients on CAPD: causes, differential diagnosis and management. Dial Transplant. 1992;21(9):581–90.
9. Leblanc M, Ouimet D, Pichette V. Dialysate leaks in peritoneal dialysis. Semin Dial. 2001 Jan-Feb;14(1):50–4.
10. Singal K, Segel DP, Bruns FJ, Fraley DS, Adler S, Julian TB. Genital edema in patients on continuous ambulatory peritoneal dialysis. Report of 3 cases and

review of the literature. Am J Nephrol. 1986;6(6):471–5.

11. Schroder CH, Rieu P, de Jong MC. Peritoneal laceration: a rare cause of scrotal edema in a 2-year-old boy. Adv Perit Dial. 1993;9:329–30.

12. Tzamaloukas AH, Gibel LJ, Eisenberg B, Goldman RS, Kanig SP, Zager PG, et al. Early and late peritoneal dialysate leaks in patients on CAPD. Adv Perit Dial. 1990;6:64–71.

13. Adeniyi M, Wiggins B, Sun Y, Servilla KS, Hartshorne MF, Tzamaloukas AH. Scrotal edema secondary to fluid imbalance in patients on continuous peritoneal dialysis. Adv Perit Dial. 2009;25: 68–71.

14. Helfrich GB, Pechan BW, Alifani MR. Reduction of catheter complications with lateral placement. Perit Dial Bull. 1983;2:132–3.

15. Digenis G, Khanna R, Mathews R. Abdominal wall hernias in patients undergoing continuous ambulatory peritoneal dialysis. Perit Dial Bull. 1982;(2):115.

16. Ash SR. Placement of the Tenckhoff peritoneal dialysis catheter under peritoneoscopic visualization. Dial Transplant. 1981;10:82–6.

17. Crabtree JH, Fishman A. A laparoscopic method for optimal peritoneal dialysis access. Am Surg. 2005 Feb;71(2):135–43.

18. Attaluri V, Lebeis C, Brethauer S, Rosenblatt S. Advanced laparoscopic techniques significantly improve function of peritoneal dialysis catheters. J Am Coll Surg. 2010 Dec;211(6):699–704.

19. Chadha V, Warady B, Blowey D, Simckes A, Alon U. Tenckhoff catheters prove superior to cook catheters in pediatric acute peritoneal dialysis. Am J Kidney Dis. 2000 Jun;35(6):1111–6.

20. Malcom M, Nycyk J. Practical peritoneal dialysis – the Tenckhoff catheter in acute renal failure. Pediatr Nephrol. 1992;6:470–5.

21. Gokal R, Alexander S, Ash S, Chen TW, Danielson A, Holmes C, et al. Peritoneal catheters and exit-site practices toward optimum peritoneal access: 1998 update. (Official report from the International Society for Peritoneal Dialysis). Perit Dial Int. 1998 Jan-Feb;18(1):11–33.

22. Perez FM. Rupture of hernial sac as cause of massive subcutaneous dialysate leak in CAPD: diagnostic value of peritoneography. Dial Transplant. 1986;15(2):74–7.

23. Maxwell AJ, Boggis CR, Sambrook P. Computed tomographic peritoneography in the investigation of abdominal wall and genital swelling in patients on continuous ambulatory peritoneal dialysis. Clin Radiol. 1990 Feb;41(2):100–4.

24. Paajanen H, Ojala S, Virkkunen A. Incidence of occult inguinal and Spigelian hernias during laparoscopy of other reasons. Surgery. 2006;140(1):9–12. discussion -3

25. van Wessem KJ, Simons MP, Plaisier PW, Lange JF. The etiology of indirect inguinal hernias: congenital and/or acquired? Hernia. 2003 Jun;7(2):76–9.

26. Wetherington GM, Leapman SB, Robison RJ, Filo RS. Abdominal wall and inguinal hernias in continuous ambulatory peritoneal dialysis patients. Am J Surg. 1985 Sep;150(3):357–60.

27. Orfei R, Seybold K, Blumber A. Genital edema in patients undergoing continuous ambulatory peritoneal dialysis (CAPD). Perit Dial Bull. 1984;4: 251–2.

28. Capelouto CC, DeWolf WC. Genital swelling secondary to leakage from continuous ambulatory peritoneal dialysis: computerized tomography diagnosis. J Urol. 1993 Jul;150(1):196–8.

29. Robson WL, Leung AK, Putnins RE, Boag GS. Genital edema in children on continuous ambulatory peritoneal dialysis. Child Nephrol Urol. 1990;10(4):205–10.

30. Deshmukh N, Kjellberg SI, Shaw PM. Occult inguinal hernia, a cause of rapid onset of penile and scrotal edema in patients on chronic peritoneal dialysis. Mil Med. 1995 Nov;160(11):597–8.

31. Cooper JC, Nicholls AJ, Simms JM, Platts MM, Brown CB, Johnson AG. Genital oedema in patients treated by continuous ambulatory peritoneal dialysis: an unusual presentation of inguinal hernia. Br Med J (Clin Res Ed). 1983 Jun 18;286(6382): 1923–4.

32. Davidson PG, Usal H, Fiorillo MA, Maniscalco A. The importance of peritoneal imaging in the workup of genital edema in patients on continuous ambulatory peritoneal dialysis. Mt Sinai J Med. 1999 Mar;66(2):125–7.

33. Juergensen PH, Rizvi H, Caride VJ, Kliger AS, Finkelstein FO. Value of scintigraphy in chronic peritoneal dialysis patients. Kidney Int. 1999 Mar;55(3):1111–9.

34. Ducassou D, Vuillemin L, Wone C, Ragnaud JM, Brendel AJ. Intraperitoneal injection of technetium-99m sulfur colloid in visualization of a peritoneo-vaginalis connection. J Nucl Med. 1984 Jan;25(1):68–9.

35. Schurgers ML, Boelaert JR, Daneels RF, Robbens EJ, Vandelanotte MM. Genital oedema in patients treated by continuous ambulatory peritoneal dialysis: an unusual presentation of inguinal hernia. Br Med J (Clin Res Ed). 1983 Jul 30;287(6388):358–9.

36. Bhattacharya A, Mittal BR. Peritoneo-scrotal communication: demonstration by 99mtechnetium sulphur colloid scintigraphy. Australas Radiol. 2005 Aug;49(4):335–7.

37. Tokmak H, Mudun A, Turkmen C, Sanli Y, Cantez S, Bozfakioglu S. The role of peritoneal scintigraphy in the detection of continuous ambulatory peritoneal dialysis complications. Ren Fail. 2006;28(8): 709–13.

38. Twardowski ZJ, Tully RJ, Nichols WK. Computerized tomography CT in the diagnosis of subcutaneous leak sites during continuous ambulatory peritoneal dialysis (CAPD). Perit Dial Bull. 1984;4:183–6.

39. Litherland J, Lupton EW, Ackrill PA, Venning M, Sambrook P. Computed tomographic peritoneography: CT manifestations in the investigation of leaks and abnormal collections in patients on CAPD. Nephrol Dial Transplant. 1994;9(10):1449–52.

40. Hollett MD, Marn CS, Ellis JH, Francis IR, Swartz RD. Complications of continuous ambulatory peritoneal dialysis: evaluation with CT peritoneography. AJR Am J Roentgenol. 1992 Nov;159(5):983–9.

41. Prischl FC, Muhr T, Seiringer EM, Funk S, Kronabethleitner G, Wallner M, et al. Magnetic resonance imaging of the peritoneal cavity among peritoneal dialysis patients, using the dialysate as "contrast medium". J Am Soc Nephrol. 2002 Jan; 13(1):197–203.

42. Connolly SS, Govender P, Ellanti P, Flynn R. Acute scrotal oedema complicating peritoneal dialysis. Scand J Urol Nephrol. 2008;42(6):558–9.

43. Suga K, Kaneko T, Nishigauchi K, Soejima K, Utsumi H, Yamada N. Demonstration of inguinal hernia by means of peritoneal 99mTc-MAA scintigraphy with a load produced by standing in a patient treated by continuous ambulatory peritoneal dialysis. Ann Nucl Med. 1992 Aug;6(3):203–6.

44. Haggerty SP, Jorge JM. Laparoscopy to evaluate scrotal edema during peritoneal dialysis. JSLS. 2013;17(3):429–32.

45. Schier F, Montupet P, Esposito C. Laparoscopic inguinal herniorrhaphy in children: a three-center experience with 933 repairs. J Pediatr Surg. 2002 Mar;37(3):395–7.

46. Gorsler CM, Schier F. Laparoscopic herniorrhaphy in children. Surg Endosc. 2003 Apr;17(4):571–3.

47. Orlando R, Palatini P, Lirussi F. Needle and trocar injuries in diagnostic laparoscopy under local anesthesia: what is the true incidence of these complications? J Laparoendosc Adv Surg Tech A. 2003 Jun;13(3):181–4.

48. Watson DS, Sharp KW, Vasquez JM, Richards WO. Incidence of inguinal hernias diagnosed during laparoscopy. South Med J. 1994 Jan;87(1):23–5.

49. Mobark A, Eltahir J, Mahir O. Successful conservative management of scrotal edema resulting from uncomplicated peritoneal fluid leak. Arab J Nephrol Transplant. 2009;2(2):51–4.

50. Holley JL, Bernardini J, Piraino B. Characteristics and outcome of peritoneal dialysate leaks and associated infections. Adv Perit Dial. 1993;9:240–3.

51. Lichtenstein IL, Shulman AG. Ambulatory outpatient hernia surgery. Including a new concept, introducing tension-free repair. Int Surg. 1986 Jan-Mar;71(1):1–4.

52. Pauls DG, Basinger BB, Shield 3rd CF. Inguinal herniorrhaphy in the continuous ambulatory peritoneal dialysis patient. Am J Kidney Dis. 1992 Nov;20(5): 497–9.

53. Lewis DM, Bingham C, Beaman M, Nicholls AJ, Riad HN. Polypropylene mesh hernia repair – an alternative permitting rapid return to peritoneal dialysis. Nephrol Dial Transplant. 1998 Oct;13(10):2488–9.

54. Morris-Stiff GJ, Bowrey DJ, Jurewicz WA, Lord RH. Management of inguinal herniae in patients on continuous ambulatory peritoneal dialysis: an audit of current UK practice. Postgrad Med J. 1998 Nov;74(877):669–70.

55. Shah H, Chu M, Bargman JM. Perioperative management of peritoneal dialysis patients undergoing hernia surgery without the use of interim hemodialysis. Perit Dial Int. 2006 Nov-Dec;26(6):684–7.

56. Gianetta E, Civalleri D, Serventi A, Floris F, Mariani F, Aloisi F, et al. Anterior tension-free repair under local anesthesia of abdominal wall hernias in continuous ambulatory peritoneal dialysis patients. Hernia. 2004 Dec;8(4):354–7.

57. Garcia-Urena MA, Rodriguez CR, Vega Ruiz V, Carnero Hernandez FJ, Fernandez-Ruiz E, Vazquez Gallego JM, et al. Prevalence and management of hernias in peritoneal dialysis patients. Perit Dial Int. 2006 Mar-Apr;26(2):198–202.

58. Crabtree JH. Hernia repair without delay in initiating or continuing peritoneal dialysis. Perit Dial Int. 2006 Mar-Apr;26(2):178–82.

59. Szeto CC, Chow KM. Pathogenesis and management of hydrothorax complicating peritoneal dialysis. Curr Opin Pulm Med. 2004;10:315–9.

60. Chow KM, Szeto CC, Li PKT. Management options for hydrothorax complicating peritoneal dialysis. Semin Dial. 2003;16:389–94.

61. Van Dijk CM, Ledesma SG, Teitelbaum I. Patient characteristics associated with defects of the peritoneal cavity boundary. Perit Dial Int. 2005;25:367–73.

62. Lew SQ. Hydrothorax: pleural effusion associated with peritoneal dialysis. Perit Dial Int. 2010;30:13–8.

63. Gorrin MR, et al. Hydrothorax secondary to a malpositioned peritoneal dialysis catheter. Perit Dial Int. 2015;35(3):365–6.

64. Hashimoto M, Watanabe A, Hashiguchi H, et al. Right hydrothorax found soon after introduction of continuous ambulatory peritoneal dialysis: thoracoscopic surgery for pleuroperitoneal communication. Gen Thorac Cardiovasc Surg. 2011;59:499–502.

65. Grefberg N, Danielson BG, Benson L, et al. Right-sided hydrothorax complicating peritoneal dialysis. Report of 2 cases. Nephron. 1983;34:130–4.

66. Guest S. The curious right-sided predominance of peritoneal dialysis-related hydrothorax. Clin Kidney J. 2015;8:212–4.

67. Nomoto Y, Suga T, Nakajima K, Sakai H, Osawa G, Ota K, et al. Acute hydrothorax in continuous ambulatory peritoneal dialysis—a collaborative study of 161 centers. Am J Nephrol. 1989;9:363–7.

68. Chavannes M, et al. Diagnosis by peritoneal scintigraphy of peritoneal dialysis associated hydrothorax in an infant. Perit Dial Int. 2014;34(1):140–2.

69. Kang TW, Kim CK. Pleuroperitoneal communication of peritoneal dialysis demonstrated by multidetector-row

CT peritoneography. Abdom Imaging. 2009;34: 780.

70. Wei GN, Mao JH. Hypertonic glucose pleurodesis and surgical diaphragmatic repair for tension hydrothorax complicating continuous ambulatory peritoneal dialysis. Clin Nephrol. 2016;85(5):301–4.

71. Cho Y, D'Intini V, Ranganathan D. Acute hydrothorax complicating peritoneal dialysis: a case report. J Med Case Reports. 2010;4:355.

72. Chow KM, SzetoCC WTY, Li PK. Hydrothorax complicating peritoneal dialysis: diagnostic value of glucose concentration in pleural fluid aspirate. Perit Dial Int. 2002;22:525–8.

73. Goh AS, et al. Radionuclide detection of dialysate leakage in patients on continuous ambulatory peritoneal dialysis. Ann Acad Med Singapore. 1994;23:315–8.

74. Huang JJ, et al. Hydrothorax in continuous ambulatory peritoneal dialysis: therapeutic implications of Tc-99m MAA peritoneal scintigraphy. Nephrol Dial Transplant. 1999;14:992–7.

75. Ramaema DP, Mpikashe P. Pleuroperitoneal Leak: an unusual cause of acute shortness of breath in a peritoneal dialysis patient. Case Rep Radiol. 2014;2014:614846.

76. Tsuchiya T, et al. Video assisted thoraoscopic surgery for pleuroperitoneal communications as a complication of continuous ambulatory peritoneal dialysis (CAPD). Kyobu Geka. 2014;67(11):963–6.

77. Mak SK, et al. Long-term follow-up of thoracoscopic pleurodesis for hydrothorax complicating peritoneal dialysis. Ann Thorac Surg. 2002;74(1):218–21.

78. Tsunezuka Y, Hatakeyama S, Iwase T, Watanabe G. Video-assisted thoracoscopic treatment for pleuroperitoneal communication in peritoneal dialysis. Eur J Cardiothorac Surg. 2001;20:205–7.

79. Mutter D, et al. A novel technique to treat hydrothorax in peritoneal dialysis: laparoscopic hepatodiaphragmatic adhesion. Perit Dial Int. 2011; 31(6):692–4.

80. Scheldewaert R, et al. Management of a massive hydrothorax in a CAPD patient: a case report and a review of the literature. Perit Dial Bull. 1982;2:69–72.

81. Kumagai H, Watari M, Kuratsune M. Simple surgical treatment for pleuroperitoneal communication without interruption of continuous ambulatory peritoneal dialysis. Gen Thorac Cardiovasc Surg. 2007;55:508.

82. Puri V, et al. Diaphragmatic defect complicating peritoneal dialysis. Ann Thorac Surg. 2011;92:1527.

83. Piraino B, Bernardini J, Sorkin M. The influence of peritoneal catheter exit-site infection on peritonitis, tunnel infections, and catheter loss in patients on continuous ambulatory peritoneal dialysis. Am J Kidney Dis. 1986;8:436–40.

84. Nichols WK, Nolph K. A technique for managing exit site and cuff infection in Tenckhoff catheters. Perit Dial Bull. 1983;3(4):S4–5.

85. Helfrich GB, Winchester JF. Questions and answers: 'shaving' of the subcutaneous cuff may cure persisting skin exit infection. However, in attempting this procedure one may damage the permanent catheter. Could you describe the detail of this technique? Perit Dial Bull. 1982;2:183.

86. Piraino B, Bernardini J, Peitzman A, Sorkin M. Failure of peritoneal dialysis catheter cuff shaving to eradicate infection. Perit Dial Bull. 1987;7:179–82.

87. Vas SI. What are the indications for the removal of the permanent peritoneal dialysis catheter? Perit Dial Bull. 1981;1:145–6.

88. Scalamogna A, De Vecchi A, Maccario M, Castelnovo C, Ponticelli C. Cuff-shaving procedure. A rescue treatment for exit-site infection unresponsive to medical therapy. Nephrol Dial Transplant. 1995;10:2325–7.

89. Tan SY, Thiruventhiran T. Catheter cuff shaving using a novel technique: a rescue treatment for persistent exit-site infections. Perit Dial Int. 2000;20:471–2.

90. Andreoli SP, West KW, Grosfeld JL, Bergstein JM. A technique to eradicate tunnel infection without peritoneal dialysis catheter removal. Perit Dial Bull. 1984;4:156–8.

91. Roman J, Gonzalez AR. Tenckhoff catheter repair by the splicing technique. Perit Dial Bull. 1984;4:89–91.

92. Yoshina A, Honda M, Ikeda M, Tsuchida S, Hataya H, Sakazume S, Tanaka Y, Shishido S, Nakai H. Merit of the cuff-shaving procedure in children with tunnel infection. Pediatr Nephrol. 2004;19:1267–72.

93. Macchini F, Testa S, Valade A, Torricelli M, Leva E, Ardissino G, Edefonti A. Conservative surgical management of catheter infections in children on peritoneal dialysis. Pediatr Surg Int. 2009;25:703–7.

94. Usha K, Pon Ferrada L, Prowant B, Twardowski Z. Repair of chronic peritoneal dialysis catheter. Perit Dial Int. 1998;18:419–23.

95. Golper TA, Carpenter J. Accidents with Tenchhoff catheters. Ann Intern Med. 1981;95:121–2.

96. Ward RA, Klein E, Wathen RL, editors. Peritoneal catheters. In: Investigation of the risks and hazards with devices associated with peritoneal dialysis and sorbent regenerated dialysate delivery systems. Perit Dial Bull. 1983;3(Suppl 3):S9–17.

97. Twardowski ZJ. Peritoneal catheter placement and management. In: Suki WN, Massry SG, editors. Therapy of renal diseases and related disorders. 3rd ed. Dordrecht: Kluwer Academic; 1997. p. 953–79.

98. Moreiras-Plaza M, Blanco-Garcia R, Beato-Coo L, Martin-Baez I, Fernandez-Flemming F. Repairing and recovering broken peritoneal catheters. Nefrologia. 2014;34(6):732–6.

99. Ogunc G, Tuncer M, Tekin S, Ersoy F. An unexpected complication in CAPD: severe abdominal pain. Perit Dial Int. 2001;21:84.

100. Juergensen PH, Murphy AL, Pherson KA, Chorney WS, Kliger AS, Finkelstein FO. Tidal peritoneal dialysis to achieve comfort in chronic peritoneal dialysis patients. Adv Perit Dial. 1999;15:125–6.

101. Blake PG, Sloand JA, McMurray S, Jain AK, Matthews S. A multicenter survey of why and how tidal peritoneal dialysis (TPD) is being used. Perit Dial Int. 2014;34:458–60.

102. Crabtree JH. Development of surgical guidelines for laparoscopic peritoneal dialysis access: down a long and winding road. Perit Dial Int. 2015;35:241–4.

103. Gokal R, Alexander S, Ash S, Chen TW, Danielson A, Holmes C, et al. Peritoneal catheters and exit-site practices toward optimum peritoneal access: 1998 update. Perit Dial Int. 1998;18:11–33.

104. Ash SR. Chronic peritoneal dialysis catheters: overview of design, placement, and removal procedures. Semin Dial. 2003;16:323–34.

105. Teitelbaum I, Burkart J. Peritoneal dialysis. Am J Kidney Dis. 2003;42:1082–96.

106. Crabtree JH. Selected best demonstrated practices in peritoneal dialysis access. Kidney Int. 2006;70:S27–37.

107. Ogunc G. Minilaparoscopic extraperitoneal tunelling with omentopexy: a new technique for CAPD catheter placement. Perit Dial Int. 2005;25:551–5.

Infectious Complications of Peritoneal Dialysis

L. Tammy Ho

Introduction

Infection remains the number one issue in morbidity and mortality in patients on peritoneal dialysis (PD). It remains the leading cause of technique failure and transfer to hemodialysis. Some studies estimate that peritonitis accounts for 20–25% of modality failures. In addition, exit site and tunnel infections occur in about 1 in every 24 patient months while on PD and many times lead to a disruption in dialysis. A strong home dialysis program highlights infection prevention as a main part of their quality maintenance program. In data reported by the United States Renal Data System (USRDS), collected from information received by Medicare, the incident number of all dialysis patients in 2013 was 117,162, with a prevalence of 661,638. Of this group of incident patients, only 9% initiate dialysis with PD [1]. The reported all-cause hospitalization frequency and total hospitalization days have decreased over last decade. The number of infection related hospital days per patient year in PD patients has also improved, decreasing by 24.8% compared to 2005. However, the rate for infection related hospitalization in peritoneal dialysis patients continues to exceed the rates for cardiovascular related

hospitalizations. With recognition of peritonitis as a major factor in morbidity in patients transitioning to PD, greater emphasis has been placed on finding techniques to improve rates of infection.

Presentation and Typical Organisms

Historically, the classic presentation for peritonitis among PD patients typically includes cloudy dialysate and increasing abdominal pain. The patient may or may not have accompanying fever or other symptoms of systemic infection such as rigors and hypotension. Peritonitis is frequently thought of as the result of a break in sterile technique or touch contamination. This commonly leads to dialysate contamination by gram positive skin organisms. Studies have demonstrated simple hand washing and hand drying prior to connection minimizes risk of infection [2]. Risk of infection is most when the PD system is open, during an exchange or due to leak. Use of prophylactic antibiotics following such events reduces risk of future peritonitis, although overall incidence of infection is low [3].

Touch contamination is only one of a number of ways that peritoneal fluid can be seeded. Secondary seeding of the dialysate through translocation of bacteria across bowel mucosa can also occur as a complication of elective gastrointestinal invasive procedures and through bowel related issues including gastroenteritis, diarrhea or

L.T. Ho, MD
Division of Nephrology and Hypertension,
Rm 3215 Evanston Hospital, 2650 Ridge Ave,
Evanston, IL 60201, USA
e-mail: tho@northshore.org

constipation, or bowel ischemia [4]. Resultant microbiology is reflective of the source. Peritoneal fluid cultures in these cases are typically polymicrobial or grow gram negative organisms. Secondary seeding has also been described through gynecologic procedures. Although much more rare, hematogenous spread is also a concern, through dental procedures or other systemic infections. Another major focus of attention is the relationship between catheter related infections and the progression to peritonitis. Prevention of exit site infections and tunneled infections have been associated with improved rates of peritonitis [5].

The visualization by the patient of a cloudy dialysate bag, accompanied by complaints of abdominal pain, is a standard presentation for peritonitis. The classic physical exam may show fever and abdominal rebound tendernesss. Initial workup typically includes CBC with differential, PD effluent cell count and culture. Measurement of dialysate cell count typically will demonstrate WBCs of greater than 100 cells/mm^3, 50% of which are neutrophils. However, cloudy effluent can be the result of non-infectious etiologies as well. The differential for cloudy effluent may include chemical peritonitis, allergic peritonitis, and hemoperitoneum, but both clinical presentation and dialysate cell count differential help differentiate the presence of an infectious etiology. When the percentage of eosinophils predominates, this may suggest more non-infectious etiologies or more allergic type issues. When lymphocytes are the predominant cell on cell count, fungal or mycobacterial infection need to be considered. However the cell count differential itself does not accurately predict the type of infection present.

In recent decades, the ability to rely on visual recognition of a cloudy bag has decreased due to the shift in preference by practitioners and patients from chronic ambulatory dialysis (CAPD) to automated peritoneal dialysis (APD). Patients may present with early subjective symptoms of abdominal discomfort without any history of a change in appearance of dialysis fluid. Repeated examination of dialysis fluid and collection of dialysate for cell count may become more critical in the diagnosis of peritonitis and may become abnormal later in the course of infection. Collection of cell count from the patient on APD, who does not have a last fill, may result in a WBC count below 100 cells/mm^3. In these patients, a dry abdomen during the day or much shorter contact time between dialysate and peritoneum, may result in low WBC cell count measurements. Recognition of these issues and allowing test dialysate fluid to dwell an appropriate length of time in the abdomen before collecting a cell count sample, will avoid false negative results. In APD patients, the appropriate clinical presentation, accompanied by a dialysate cell count that is mostly neutrophils, would be sufficient to support empiric antibiotic therapy for presumed peritonitis in these patients.

Prevention

Awareness of clinical risk factors that increase a peritoneal dialysis patient's likelihood of developing acute peritonitis contributes to development of interventions to lower peritonitis rates. Intervention to avoid severe constipation and education of patients regarding early notification of their home dialysis unit in the event of a break in technique, are important preventative measures. Although the incidence of secondary peritonitis is rare from invasive gastrointestinal, dental and gynecologic invasive procedures, the benefit of prophylactic antibiotics warrant their use pre-procedure [4, 6]. Typically, based upon a 1994 review by Strippoli, most centers administer intravenous aminoglycoside plus ampicillin prior to the colonoscopy. In dental procedures, typically, oral amoxacillin prophylxis is sufficient. The importance of educating patients regarding notification of their home dialysis unit prior to undergoing such elective procedures should not be overlooked.

Multiple studies have looked at a variety of catheter related characteristics and surgical techniques to assess if there may be a benefit to one type of catheter or one surgical implantation technique. Development of the double cuffed catheter, exit sit location, direction of the tip of the catheter and design of the catheter portion within the abdomen all were conceived to improve infection risk. To date, data has not strongly demonstrated a particular catheter to be superior in terms of infection prevention [7]. Laproscopic techniques with or without burying of the catheter prior to externalization and use have also not been demonstrated to lead to improved infectious outcomes, thus the International Society of Peritoneal Dialysis (ISPD) Guidelines do not recommend a specific type of peritoneal catheter as better suited to prevention of peritonitis [8]. However, data does support pre-operative administration of intravenous antibiotics prior to catheter placement. A randomized trial by Gadallah et al., showed that, in a 14 day perioperative period, single dose vancomycin pre-operatively was superior to cefazolin. A smaller benefit was also seen with the use of the first generation cephalosporin, as compared to no prophylactic antibiotic use [9]. Vancomycin use remains controversial, with ongoing concerns for development of antibiotic resistant organisms. ISPD guidelines suggest the careful consideration of cost/benefit by each center of the use of prophylactic vancomycin [8].

Identification of higher risk patients may allow for more guided surveillance and early prevention techniques in these patient groups. Kumar et al. found that neither race nor socioeconomic status predicted technique survival [10] however Nessim et al. examined data in over 4000 patients from the Baxter POET database [11]. The predictors of peritonitis in these incident patients from Canada included black race, female patients with diabetes and those who transferred from hemodialysis to peritoneal dialysis. There was no modality effect, with similar infection risk identified between CAPD and APD patients. The data is contradictory on whether CAPD increases risk of infection. There has been increased concern with the recognition that there are many more potential points/times of contact and possible contamination that result from increased frequency of connection/disconnection. Past suggestion of increased infection risk with CAPD in studies appears to be related to early connection/disconnection technology. More current studies have not found a consistent

difference in infection rates between the two PD techniques [12, 13].

Although difficult to measure and standardize, the foundation of a center's peritonitis prevention program remains the experience of the program and the effectiveness of the peritoneal dialysis nurse trainer. The years of experience of the training professional inversely correlates with the risk of peritonitis in patients trained, demonstrating the need for continuing support of the trainer nurse [14]. Ongoing reinforcement of technique and re-education of patients also appears to be important in preserving low rates of infection. The length of time spent in training is not well defined and there are no randomized trials evaluating this question. A recent Brazilian prospective cohort study of over 2000 incident PD patients found a association between greater than 15 h of training and decreased peritonitis rates. As well, centers with larger number of patients and greater length of experience had decreased peritonitis rates [15]. The ISPD Guidelines recommend that any PD training center track peritonitis episodes and maintaining ongoing continuing education for patient and staff. They recommend retraining when an acute event as hospitalization or infection occurs [16].

Exit Site and Tunnel Infections

Exit site infections are an independent risk factor for peritonitis [17]. The presence of erythema, swelling and pain on exam with purulent drainage are findings suggestive of an exit site infection. In clinical settings where there is the suggestion of active exit site infection, empiric antibiotic treatment is recommended by the ISPD guidelines [18]. Oral administration of antibiotics is generally sufficient; any empiric antibiotic therapy should provide coverage for Staphylococcal aureus organisms [19]. The presence of Staphylococcal or Pseudomonal infection is suggestive of more extensive catheter involvement and has high risk to extend into a tunnel infection. Physical exam demonstrating swelling, erythema and tenderness along the track of the catheter is supportive tunnel involvement by infection. Use of ultrasound may be helpful to define fluid collections along the track [20, 21]. Peritoneal catheter removal is recommended when there is ongoing exit site or tunnel infection which is non-responsive to therapy, or there is an exit site or tunnel infection leading to peritonitis. Some data suggests if there infection is limited to the catheter, a single surgical procedure to remove and re-implant the peritoneal catheter may be successful [22]. This may allow the patient to avoid a switch to temporary hemodialysis. Infections with pseudomonas are particularly problematic and often lead to catheter removal. Some novel techniques have been described to salvage the existing catheter in patient who have an exit site infection refractory to antibiotics. "Cuff shaving" by unroofing the subcutaneous cuff, shaving it off, and rerouting the catheter to an alternate exit site has been reported successful in 87.5% of children in one study from Japan. This technique was also successful in 13 adults with chronic tunnel infection [23]. Wu et al. described 26 catheters in 23 patients in which the entire subcutaneous tubing was replaced from just above the internal cuff with no interruption in dialysis [24].

Typical infecting organisms of the exit site include staphylococcal and streptococcal species. Identification of *staphylococcus aureus* nasal carriers and treatment of these carriers have been demonstrated to decrease infection [25]. The use of mupirocin at the exit site has also been demonstrated to effectively reduce *Staphylococcus aureus* exit site infections. There was a 72% reduction in exit site infection with use of mupirocin vs no prophylaxis in over 1200 patients and a similar reduction in peritonitis episodes, especially when considering only infections with *Staphylococcus aureus*. Mupirocin use, however, is limited due to its ineffectiveness against gram negative bacteria, especially pseudomonas infection. As well, its use has been complicated by development of mupirocin resistant organisms. Some investigators suggest that the risk of resistant bacteria is not as significant as concerns suggest [26]. However, some centers utilize gentamicin topical ointment for exit site prophylaxis, following

the demonstration of its superiority to mupirocin in a double blind, randomized trial. Bernardini et al. compared exit site use of gentamicin cream versus mupirocin [5] in 136 patients. Gentamicin has activity against both Staphyloccocal aureus and Pseudomonas aeruginosa. Patients were randomized to either mupirocin or gentamicin. Although both groups had equal catheter removal rates, the gentamicin group had fewer peritonitis rates, due to reduced rates of gram negative peritonitis. However, other investigators found, after switching from mupirocin to gentamicin topical exit site prophylaxis, that there was no difference in exit site infection and peritonitis rates [27]. It is advised that PD centers should consider including local exit site antibiotic prophylaxis as part of their peritonitis prevention program, the type of local antibiotic prophylaxis remaining an individual center choice.

Peritonitis Treatment

The most common cause of peritonitis in the PD patient is bacterial in origin and is predominantly gram positive in type. The prevalence and antibiotic sensitivities of infecting organisms are specific to the geographic location. Thus the ISPD guidelines continue to recommend center directed treatment of peritonitis. Depending on local microbial characteristics and patterns, first line empiric antibiotic regimens may include vancomycin or first generation cephalosporin plus third generation cephalosporin or aminoglycoside [8]. Prior to culture results, broad coverage for gram positive and gram negative organisms is advised. Intra-peritoneal antibiotics are preferred to intravenous agents for local concentration of drug and increased efficacy of agents used. The exception to initiation of therapy via intraperitoneal infusion is if the patient has any evidence of systemic involvement, when intravenous infusion would be appropriate. There is systemic absorption of these agents across the peritoneal membrane and levels of antibiotics should be monitored. Antibiotics can be given intermittently in a single exchange, once daily, dwelling at least for 6 h, or continuously in each exchange. Efficacy appears similar for either mode of delivery in the case of vancomycin and aminoglycosides. ISPD guidelines suggest daily intermittent dosing of aminoglycoside and vancomycin, but either continuous or intermittent dosing of cephalosporin. The supporting data for these recommendations is recognized as being of low quality. Further, tailoring of therapy can occur once cultures return. Duration of therapy depends on the aggressiveness of the infecting organism(s). Typically antibiotic duration will be 2–3 weeks, with the longer duration reserved for Enterococcus, Staphylococcus and Pseudomonas infections.

Response to antibiotics with clinical improvement in symptoms should occur in 2–3 days. Refractory peritonitis is defined as no response within 5 days and portends poor outcome. Removal of the peritoneal catheter is recommended in refractory peritonitis, recurrent or relapsing peritonitis (re-infection within 4 weeks of completion of antibiotic treatment with different or same organism, respectively), or in cases of fungal peritonitis.

In 1992, Port reported on USRDS data that included specific data collected as part of a USRDS Special Study on CAPD peritonitis [28]. He reported that positive culture results occur in approximately 60% of first time presentations of peritonitis. Culture negative results were present in about 20% of cultures. Although failure to isolate an offending microbe can occur, should culture negative results rate be greater than 15–20%, the technique of culture collection should be suspect. In a larger observational cohort study of 4675 patients on PD from the Australia and New Zealand Dialysis and Transplant Registry, patients with culture negative peritonitis tended to respond more quickly to antibiotics alone and had less catheter loss and transition to hemodialysis [29]. Prior antibiotic treatment was associated with increased frequency of culture negative peritonitis. In these patients, if there is a clinical response, treatment with empiric therapy should be continued for the recommended duration of time.

Treatment of bacterial peritonitis is complicated by increased risk for fungal peritonitis, especially in diabetic patients [30, 31]. Fungal peritonitis is a severe disease, with high rates of morbidity and mortality. The likelihood of salvage of the existing peritoneal catheter in this scenario is very small. Therefore, prevention of fungal peritonitis following treatment for a bacterial peritonitis is important. Prophylaxis with oral anti-fungal therapy during treatment with antibiotics has been effective in preventing fungal peritonitis. Restrepo et al., in a prospective, randomized trial, demonstrated that the use of fluconazole led to a statistically significant decrease in frequency of fungal peritonitis when used through the duration of antibiotics use [32]. Other anti-fungals, including Nystatin use has also been evaluated, with variable study responses. In an observational study looking at Nystatin use, Nystatin was associated with a decreased frequency of candida infection. ISPD guidelines suggest considering fungal prophylaxis in those patients on frequent or long duration anti-microbial therapy and in centers where the rates of fungal peritonitis are high.

An effective program to manage peritonitis includes regular monitoring of rates of peritonitis, type and frequency of infecting organisms and response to intervention. Any successful program includes early management of clinical risks for infection from time of catheter implantation, through training and maintenance on dialysis. Effective education of staff and patient, with periodic re-training, is essential. Ultimately, the ability to preserve the peritoneal membrane for adequate peritoneal dialysis depends on the prompt diagnosis of infection, effective treatment and recognition of when it is necessary to remove the peritoneal catheter.

References

1. Collins AJ, et al. United States renal data system public health surveillance of chronic kidney disease and end-stage renal disease. Kidney Int Suppl (2011). 2015;5(1):2–7. United States Renal Data System. 2015 USRDS annual data report: Epidemiology of Kidney Disease in the United States. National Institutes of Health, National Institute of Diabetes and Digestive and Kidney Diseases, Bethesda, MD, 2015.
2. Miller TE, Findon G. Touch contamination of connection devices in peritoneal dialysis – a quantitative

microbiologic analysis. Perit Dial Int. 1997;17(6): 560–7.

3. Yap DY, et al. Risk factors and outcome of contamination in patients on peritoneal dialysis – a single-center experience of 15 years. Perit Dial Int. 2012;32(6):612–6.

4. Yip T, et al. Risks and outcomes of peritonitis after flexible colonoscopy in CAPD patients. Perit Dial Int. 2007;27(5):560–4.

5. Bernardini J, et al. Randomized, double-blind trial of antibiotic exit site cream for prevention of exit site infection in peritoneal dialysis patients. J Am Soc Nephrol. 2005;16(2):539–45.

6. Fried L, Bernardini J, Piraino B. Iatrogenic peritonitis: the need for prophylaxis. Perit Dial Int. 2000;20(3):343–5.

7. Strippoli GF, et al. Catheter-related interventions to prevent peritonitis in peritoneal dialysis: a systematic review of randomized, controlled trials. J Am Soc Nephrol. 2004;15(10):2735–46.

8. Li PK, et al. Ispd peritonitis recommendations: 2016 update on prevention and treatment. Perit Dial Int. 2016;36:481–508.

9. Gadallah MF, et al. Role of preoperative antibiotic prophylaxis in preventing postoperative peritonitis in newly placed peritoneal dialysis catheters. Am J Kidney Dis. 2000;36(5):1014–9.

10. Kumar V. Predictors of peritonitis, hospital days and technique survival for periotneal dialysis patients in a managed care setting. Perit Dial Int. 2014;34(2): 171–8.

11. Nessim SJ, et al. Predictors of peritonitis in patients on peritoneal dialysis: results of a large, prospective Canadian database. Clin J Am Soc Nephrol. 2009; 4(7):1195–200.

12. Cnossen TT, et al. Comparison of outcomes on continuous ambulatory peritoneal dialysis versus automated peritoneal dialysis: results from a USA database. Perit Dial Int. 2011;31(6):679–84.

13. Ruger W, et al. Similar peritonitis outcome in CAPD and APD patients with dialysis modality continuation during peritonitis. Perit Dial Int. 2011;31(1):39–47.

14. Chow KM, et al. Influence of peritoneal dialysis training nurses' experience on peritonitis rates. Clin J Am Soc Nephrol. 2007;2(4):647–52.

15. Figueiredo AE, et al. Impact of patient training patterns on peritonitis rates in a large national cohort study. Nephrol Dial Transplant. 2015;30(1):137–42.

16. Bernardini J, et al. Peritoneal dialysis patient training, 2006. Perit Dial Int. 2006;26(6):625–32.

17. Lee SM, et al. Comparison of exit site infection and peritonitis incidences between povidone-iodine and normal saline use for chronic exit site care in peritoneal dialysis patients. Kidney Res Clin Pract. 2014;33(3):144–9.

18. Li PK, et al. Peritoneal dialysis-related infections recommendations: 2010 update. Perit Dial Int. 2010;30(4):393–423.

19. Strippoli GF, et al. Antimicrobial agents to prevent peritonitis in peritoneal dialysis: a systematic review of randomized controlled trials. Am J Kidney Dis. 2004;44(4):591–603.

20. Vychytil A, et al. New criteria for management of catheter infections in peritoneal dialysis patients using ultrasonography. J Am Soc Nephrol. 1998;9(2):290–6.

21. Kwan TH, et al. Ultrasonography in the management of exit site infections in peritoneal dialysis patients. Nephrology (Carlton). 2004;9(6):348–52.

22. Lui SL, et al. Simultaneous removal and reinsertion of Tenckhoff catheters for the treatment of refractory exit-site infection. Adv Perit Dial. 2000;16:195–7.

23. Crabtree JH, Burchette RJ. Surgical salvage of peritoneal dialysis catheters from chronic exit-site and tunnel infections. Am J Surg. 2005;190(1):4–8.

24. Wu YM, et al. Surgical management of refractory exit-site/tunnel infection of Tenckhoff catheter: technical innovations of partial replantation. Perit Dial Int. 1999;19(5):451–4.

25. Mahajan S, et al. Effect of local mupirocin application on exit-site infection and peritonitis in an Indian peritoneal dialysis population. Perit Dial Int. 2005;25(5):473–7.

26. Lobbedez T, et al. Routine use of mupirocin at the peritoneal catheter exit site and mupirocin resistance: still low after 7 years. Nephrol Dial Transplant. 2004;19(12):3140–3.

27. Mahaldar A, Weisz M, Kathuria P. Comparison of gentamicin and mupirocin in the prevention of exit-site infection and peritonitis in peritoneal dialysis. Adv Perit Dial. 2009;25:56–9.

28. Port FK, et al. Risk of peritonitis and technique failure by CAPD connection technique: a national study. Kidney Int. 1992;42(4):967–74.

29. Fahim M, et al. Culture-negative peritonitis in peritoneal dialysis patients in Australia: predictors, treatment, and outcomes in 435 cases. Am J Kidney Dis. 2010;55(4):690–7.

30. Wang AY, et al. Factors predicting outcome of fungal peritonitis in peritoneal dialysis: analysis of a 9-year experience of fungal peritonitis in a single center. Am J Kidney Dis. 2000;36(6):1183–92.

31. Miles R, et al. Predictors and outcomes of fungal peritonitis in peritoneal dialysis patients. Kidney Int. 2009;76(6):622–8.

32. Restrepo C, Chacon J, Manjarres G. Fungal peritonitis in peritoneal dialysis patients: successful prophylaxis with fluconazole, as demonstrated by prospective randomized control trial. Perit Dial Int. 2010;30(6): 619–25.

Management of Hernias in the Context of Peritoneal Dialysis

Pierpaolo Di Cocco, Vassilios E. Papalois,
Edwina A. Brown, and Frank J.M.F. Dor

The management of abdominal wall hernias is crucial for surgeons dedicated to peritoneal dialysis (PD). Common clinical scenarios which require different treatment algorithms, are represented by hernias diagnosed in pre-assessment (before peritoneal catheter insertion), during laparoscopic PD catheter insertion and post- operatively after dialysis starts (in the form of abdominal wall or incisional hernias).

An abdominal wall hernia is an abnormal protrusion of a peritoneal-lined sac through the musculo-aponeurotic layers of the abdomen. The prevalence of the disease in the general population, reported around 1.5–2% [1, 2] is difficult to determine, mainly due to lack of standardization in the definition, inconsistency of the data sources used (which include self-reporting by patients, audits of routine physical examinations, and insurance company databases, among others), and subjectivity of physical examination. More than 20 million hernioplasties are performed every year worldwide, the vast majority for inguinal hernias (70–75%), followed by umbilical hernias (13–24%), femoral hernias (2–14%) and rare forms (1–2%) [3–6].

The prevalence of hernias in PD patients ranges from 7% to 37%, and up to 40% in the pediatric population [7–14]. The most common type is umbilical (61.5%), followed by inguinal, both direct and indirect (27%), and incisional hernias (7%); less commonly encountered hernias include epigastric [11], cystocele or rectocele [15], Spigelian [16], paraesophageal [17] and Morgagni [18] (5%).

Traditional predisposing factors for hernia development in PD patients (Table 15.1) [7, 10] are not universally reported in the literature, suggesting that intrinsic anatomical defects in abdominal wall structure predisposing to the development of such complications are present [7–10, 19–22].

Retrospective studies reported a prevalence of abdominal wall hernias in polycystic kidney disease between 45% and 61% [7, 19]. The increased intra-abdominal pressure or the increased inside-out pressure on the abdominal wall due to large polycystic kidneys and/or primary collagen anomalies have been all postulated as being responsible for hernia formation [7, 19]. Interestingly, Modi et al. [19] showed a higher prevalence of inguinal hernias in patients with polycystic kidney disease treated with continuous ambulatory peritoneal dialysis (CAPD), compared with CAPD patients with other renal diseases. In contrast, Hadimeri et al. found no increased incidence of hernias among patients

P. Di Cocco • V.E. Papalois
E.A. Brown • F.J.M.F. Dor (✉)
West London Renal and Transplant Centre, Imperial College Healthcare NHS Trust, Hammersmith Hospital, Office 468, 4th Floor Hammersmith House, Du Cane Road, London W12 0HS, UK
e-mail: Pierpaolo.DiCocco@imperial.nhs.uk; Vassilios.Papalois@imperial.nhs.uk; Edwina.Brown@imperial.nhs.uk; Frank.dor@imperial.nhs.uk

Table 15.1 Risk factors for the development of hernia in the adult PD population

Modifiable	Non modifiable
BMI	Age
Sedentary lifestyle	Gender
Smoking	Ethnicity
Modality of PD – CAPD	Polycystic kidney disease
Comorbidities (i.e. diabetes, steroid use, BPCO)	

with polycystic kidney disease [20]. In retrospective studies, patients treated with automated peritoneal dialysis (APD) seem to have a lower prevalence of hernias compared those treated with CAPD [7, 21]. It was originally observed that patients who are at risk for hernias include those with higher body mass index, due to higher intra-abdominal pressure for a given dwell volume [22]; other studies have found the opposite result when the height and weight are adjusted for sex [8, 9]. The pathophysiological role of intra-abdominal pressure on the development of hernias has been often advocated but not been thoroughly studied in PD patients. In fact, in all the studies, the intra-abdominal pressure has been measured at rest and in a supine position and not during the patient's daily physical activities [13, 22, 23]. Since the intra-abdominal pressure varies greatly from patient to patient according to their daily physical activities, the current methodology of intra-abdominal pressure determination might be inadequate to detect patients at risk [22]. However, until the existence of a putative relation between intra-abdominal pressure and the development of hernias in PD patients has been thoroughly studied, it is prudent to continue teaching our PD patients to refrain from physical activities, which could cause straining, such as pushing, pulling and jumping. In addition, they should avoid straining with bowel movements by eating a high fiber diet or taking stool softeners to avoid constipation, without draining the peritoneal cavity first. This is particularly important postoperatively following PD catheter insertion in order to minimize the occurrence of incisional hernias.

Incisional hernia, a known complication of previous surgery, has different definitions; the most widely accepted is any abdominal wall defect, with or without a bulge, identified on clinical examination or imaging by 1 year after the index operation [24, 25]. The incidence of this complication in the literature ranges between 0% and 44%, reflecting the heterogeneity of definitions, patients, operations and follow up [26]. The discussion on the best surgical technique, type of sutures to use for which abdominal operation in order to minimize this complication is beyond the scope of this chapter [27, 28]. Incisional hernia can develop after any type of abdominal wall incision. The incidence depends upon the location and size of the incision [29–37]. Based on a recent meta-analysis on the general surgical population, midline incisions have a significantly increased risk of incisional hernia compared to transverse (relative risk [RR] 1.77, 95% CI, 1.09–2.87) and paramedian incisions (RR 3.41, 95% CI 1.02–11.45, respectively) [36]. The highest reported incidence is with midline abdominal incisions (3–20%) [31, 32]. Muscle-splitting incisions (para-median) have a cumulative incidence of incisional hernia ranging from 1% to 6% [38, 39]. Laparoscopic port sites can also develop incisional hernia, with a reported incidence between 0% and 5% [40–42]. The highest risk being 10 mm or larger ports and below the umbilicus. These findings in the general surgical population, showing the importance of the operative technique as a determinant of incisional hernia occurrence, can be applied to the PD population. We believe that in the PD population, where, unfortunately, comparative studies are missing and the incidence of all types of hernia is very high, the laparoscopic insertion technique has to be considered the gold standard since it decreases the risk of incisional hernia. The effect of hernias and their management on PD technique survival remains poorly characterized in the literature. Furthermore, the effect of hernia occurrence and treatment on residual renal function (RRF), which is known to confer significant prognostic benefit in PD, remains unknown [43].

Diagnosis

The diagnosis of hernia during the assessment for PD catheter insertion is clinical, based on the history and thorough physical examination [44–46]. The most common presentation is of a lump or a bulge (usually upon Valsalva manoeuvre); less frequently and particularly in overweight patients, the hernia may not be clinically evident with only a vague discomfort in the area. In these situations, the clinical use of ultrasonography is promising with a sensitivity and specificity of 90% and 85%, respectively [47–49]; higher resolution axial computed tomography (can be without contrast to preserve urinary output) and magnetic resonance imaging might be useful with sensitivity and specificity greater than 95% [50].

The diagnosis of hernia in patients on PD is also made on clinical ground; although rarely needed, ancillary tests used are ultrasound, CT scan or radionuclide imaging. The diagnostic accuracy of the CT scan is improved by the use of intraperitoneal dye, infused with the peritoneal fluid [51–54]. An alternative diagnostic test, described in clinical practice but rarely needed in the modern diagnostic armamentarium, is the radionuclide imaging using technetium-labelled or sulphur colloid with subsequent scanning by gamma camera to track the movement of dialysate [55, 56].

Treatment

The original technique of inguinal hernia repair, first described by Bassini more than 100 years ago, has as a major drawback the risk of recurrence [57]. Despite several modifications, introduced over the years by by Shouldice, McVay and others, the recurrence rate for primary hernia repair, according to annual statistics from various countries, is still 10–15% [58]. In the recent years, the availability of prosthetic meshes has led to an increase in the number of 'tension-free' methods of reinforcing the inguinal region to prevent recurrences [59–62]. The use of mesh is associated with a 30–50% reduction in the risk of

hernia recurrence in comparison with non-mesh methods of hernia repair [60, 61]. Open mesh methods of repair are classified as open flat mesh (i.e. the Lichtenstein method), open preperitoneal mesh (i.e. the Stoppa and Nyhus methods) and open plug and mesh repair (i.e. the Rutkow method). There are two main approaches for the laparoscopic repair of inguinal hernias. Transabdominal preperitoneal (TAPP) repair involves access to the hernia through the peritoneal cavity. Mesh is inserted through the peritoneum and placed over all potential hernia sites in the inguinal region. The peritoneum is then closed above the mesh. Totally extraperitoneal (TEP) repair is the newer laparoscopic technique, in which the hernia site is accessed via the preperitoneal plane without entering the peritoneal cavity. TEP repair is considered to be technically more difficult than the TAPP technique, but it may reduce the risk of damage to intra-abdominal organs.

The gold standard is thought to be the Lichtenstein method, although this is still a matter of debate. According to recent guidelines, laparoscopic surgery would be the preferred technique for the repair of recurrent hernias (as scar tissue from previous open repairs may be avoided) and bilateral hernias (repaired during the same operation) and should also be an option for primary repair of unilateral hernias because of the reduced incidence of long-term pain and numbness and the potential for earlier return to normal activities. [63–69]

The overall recurrence rates for primary hernia repair in the PD population range from 0% to 25%, depending upon the hernia site (direct, indirect, femoral), type of repair (mesh, no mesh, open, laparoscopic) and clinical circumstances (elective, emergent) [9, 12, 14, 70–75], which is higher than the general population (0.5–15%) [58, 61, 76]. Considering that 5–10% of PD patients undergoing surgery for recurrent hernia has to convert permanently to hemodialysis [11, 14, 73], the use of mesh in this setting is strongly advocated.

There is general agreement that all hernias should be repaired in patients considered for PD and already established on PD due to risks of bowel complications (i.e. bowel incarceration and/or strangulation) and PD failure or dialysate leak [11, 77–81].

There are a few possible scenarios for repair, depending on the residual kidney function, comorbidities and surgical technique:

– Hernia repair in patients considered for PD – before PD catheter insertion
– Hernia repair during PD catheter insertion
– Hernia repair in patients on PD – after PD catheter insertion

Hernia Repair in Patients Considered for PD – Before PD Catheter Insertion

The repair before PD catheter insertion follows the approach described above and does not differ from the treatment of the general population (Table 15.2).

Hernia Repair During PD Catheter Insertion

Special consideration is given to this approach of concomitant hernia repair and PD catheter placement. This has been described in case series with both open and laparoscopic techniques and the authors define this surgical procedure reliable and safe [78–80, 82–84]. The use of laparoscopic pre-peritoneal mesh placement in this setting has not been extensively studied but has some risk of damanging the peritoneal membrane. Further comparative trials are necessary to clarifty the best approach to concomititant laparocscopic

Table 15.2 Hernia repair before PD catheter insertion

Pros	Cons
More time for the peritoneum to heal	Two operations
More time for the mesh to grow in	Twice anaesthesia
	May delay the start of PD
	For umbilical hernia – potential interference of the mesh for optimal PD catheter insertion

Table 15.3 Hernia repair during PD catheter insertion

Pros	Cons
One operation	Potential complications (i.e. dialysate leak, recurrence) if PD treatment started early
	No guidelines on when to start PD

insertion of PD catheter and inguinal hernia repair. Given the widespread use of laparoscopy for PD catheter insertion, which allows inspection and identification of occult inguinal hernias or a patent processus vaginalis (potential site of future herniation) recent guidelines suggest fixing these defects when found (81) during the insertion. It is therefore important to counsel and consent patients for possible hernia repair prior to the laparoscopic insertion procedure (Table 15.3).

Hernia Repair in Patients on PD

The management of dialysis requirements depends on the residual function; the vast majority of patients can carry out the usual dialysis until the morning of the surgery [11, 71, 85–87]. Comparative trials of open and laparoscopic inguinal hernia repair in PD patients do not exist. Several reports have used open polypropylene mesh repair of inguinal hernias and shown very low recurrence and leak rates, despite resuming PD within a few days [74, 75, 84–88] and some authors advocate the use of mesh for a faster return to PD, thus avoiding the need for a change in dialysis modality and offering advantages both to patients and to hard-pressed haemodialysis programs [74, 75, 84, 88]. In a single centre experience, tension-free hernia repair with polypropylene mesh reinforcement allowed the patient to commence or continue PD as early as 24 h after surgery [74]. For incisional hernias, open anterior repair with inversion of the hernia sac without disrupting it, and placing a mesh has been shown to have low recurrence and leak rates in adults [11, 74]. If the peritoneum is bridged, it is recommended to close it in a watertight manner [79].

There are no guidelines as to whether PD treatment can be safely continued after hernioplasty or should be withheld postoperatively to allow proper healing, to avoid postoperative dialysate leakage from hernia repair site or early hernia recurrence. Several authors proposed different strategies [72, 75, 84]. A common strategy is to restart PD almost immediately after surgery (between 12 and 72 h) with low-volume high-frequency exchanges, avoiding temporary haemodialysis [73, 84, 88]. Shah et al. recommended continuation on standard PD therapy until the morning of the surgery, followed by no dialysis for the first 48 h and intermittent PD 3 times per week (1 L exchange for 10 h) for 2 weeks, low-volume CAPD for another 2 weeks, and resumption of the preoperative PD prescription after 4–5 weeks, with excellent results [71]. Another PD management protocol had been suggested by Crabtree et al. in which low-volume automated PD exchanges were used, with an initial fill volume of 1 L, which was gradually increased to 1.5 L the second week, and with resumption of usual dialysis regimen thereafter [79]. The above-mentioned strategies expose the patient to "underdialysis" which has to be balanced against the risk of insertion of a temporary hemodialysis line and the hemodialysis procedure itself. Dialysis is usually restarted under conditions of low abdominal pressure and small volumes after elective hernia repair; treatment is commonly withheld for several days or even weeks in case of incarcerated or strangulated hernias, which can lead to significant morbidity in this setting [89].

In our practice, we perform primary hernia repair and PD insertion during the same operation in candidates for PD. Our preferred approach in this scenario is the laparoscopic technique with sublay mesh and careful closure of the peritoneum. Following the operation peritoneal dialysis can be started as early as 12–24 hours with rapid exchange technique (low volumes, rapid frequency). For hernia repair in patients on PD our preferred approach is with open technique with mesh, reserving the laparoscopy for bilateral or recurrent hernias. Our approach to the treatment of incisional hernias, either with open or laparoscopic technique, depending on size, site and reducibility, is by applying a sublay mesh. In most cases the rapid exchange technique allows to restart PD early, avoiding temporary hemodialysis.

It is of paramount importance to adequately manage abdominal wall hernias in patients on PD since patients not successfully treated may no longer be candidates for PD. Trials are lacking to determine the best strategy towards hernia repair in PD patients, regarding timing, technique, and material. These trials should be set up nationally in multiple centers, given the relatively small numbers of PD insertions all centres are doing.

Conclusions

Abdominal wall hernias are common mechanical complications of peritoneal dialysis and their management has not been standardized. Contrary to the general population where some authors propose a strategy of watchful waiting for asymptomatic hernias [90]; in the PD setting, guidelines suggest to fix these defects to avoid complications of dialysate leak and bowel strangulation [81]. Due to the elevated recurrence rate, a mesh repair is preferred. This strategy appears to be safe, not increasing the incidence of peritonitis, and effective, reducing the recurrence rate and can be performed without temporarily converting to hemodialysis.

Bibliography

1. Rains AJH, Capper WM. Bailey & love's short practice of surgery. 15th ed. London: Lewis; 1971.
2. David C, Sabiston JR. Davis-christopher textbook of surgery. 12th ed. London: Elsevier Health Sciences; 1981.
3. Kingsworth A, LeBlanc K. Hernias: inguinal and incisional. Lancet. 2003;362:1561–71.
4. Rutkow IM. Epidemiologic, economic, and sociologic aspects of hernia surgery in the United States in the 1990s. Surg Clin North Am. 1998;78:941.
5. Dabbas N, Adams K, Pearson K, Royle GT. Frequency of abdominal wall hernias: is classical teaching out of date? JRSM Short Rep. 2011;2(1):5.
6. Burcharth J, Pedersen MS, Pommergaard HC, Bisgaard T, Pedersen CB, Rosenberg J. The prevalence of umbilical and epigastric hernia repair: a nationwide epidemiologic study. Hernia. 2015;19(5):815–9.

7. Del Peso G, Bajo MA, Costero O, et al. Risk factors for abdominal wall complications in peritoneal dialysis patients. Perit Dial Int. 2003;23:249–54.

8. Tokgoz B, Dogukan A, Guven M, Unluhizarci K, Oymak O, Utas C. Relationship between different body size indicators and hernia development in CAPD patients. Clin Nephrol. 2003;60:183–6.

9. Afthentopoulos IE, Panduranga Rao S, Mathews R, Oreopoulos DG. Hernia development in CAPD patients and the effect of 2.5l dialysate volume in selected patients. Clin Nephrol. 1998;49:251–7.

10. Van Dijk CM, Ledesma SG, Teitelbaum I. Patient characteristics associated with defects of the peritoneal cavity boundary. Perit Dial Int. 2005;25:367–73.

11. Garcia-Urena MA, Rodriguez CR, Vega Ruiz V, Carnero Hernandez FJ, Fernandez-Ruiz E, Vazquez Gallego JM, et al. Prevalence and management of hernias in peritoneal dialysis patients. Perit Dial Int. 2006;26:198–202.

12. Suh H, Wadhwa NK, Cabralda T, Sokunbi D, Pinard B. Abdominal wall hernias in ESRD patients receiving peritoneal dialysis. Adv Perit Dial. 1994;10:85–8.

13. Aranda RA, Romao Jr JE, Kakehashi E, et al. Intraperitoneal pressure and hernias in children on peritoneal dialysis. Pediatr Nephrol. 2000;14:22–4.

14. Balda S, Power A, Papalois P, Brown E. Impact of hernias on peritoneal dialysis technique survival and residual function. Perit Dial Int. 2013;33(6):629–34.

15. Nässberger L. Enterocele due to continuous ambulatory peritoneal dialysis (CAPD). Acta Obstet Gynecol Scand. 1984;63(3):283.

16. Francis DM, Schofield I, Veitch PS. Abdominal hernias in patients treated with continuous ambulatory peritoneal dialysis. Br J Surg. 1982;69(7):409.

17. Hughes GC, Ketchersid TL, Lenzen JM, Lowe JE. Thoracic complications of peritoneal dialysis. Ann Thorac Surg. 1999;67(5):1518–22.

18. Polk D, Madden RL, Lipkowitz GS, Braden GL, Germain MJ, Mulhern JG, O'Shea MH. Use of computerized tomography in the evaluation of a CAPD patient with a foramen of Morgagni hernia: a case report. Perit Dial Int. 1996;16(3):318–20.

19. Modi KB, Grant AC, Garret A, Rodger RS. Indirect inguinal hernia in CAPD patients with polycystic kidney disease. Adv Perit Dial. 1989;5:84–6.

20. Hadimeri H, Johansson A-C, Haraldsson B, Nyberg G. CAPD in patients with autosomal dominant polycystic kidney disease. Perit Dial Int. 1998;18:429–32.

21. Hussain SI, Bernardini J, Piraino B. The risk of hernia with large exchange volumes. Adv Perit Dial. 1998;14:105–7.

22. Twardowski ZJ, Khanna R, Nolph KD, et al. Intraabdominal pressures during natural activities in patients treated with continuous ambulatory peritoneal dialysis. Nephron. 1986;44:129–35.

23. Durand PY, Chanliau J, Gamberoni J, Hestin D, Kessler M. Routine measurement of hydrostatic intraperitoneal pressure. Adv Perit Dial. 1992;8:108–12.

24. Korenkov M, Paul A, Sauerland S, Neugebauer E, Arndt M, Chevrel JP, et al. Classification and surgical treatment of incisional hernia. Results of an experts' meeting. Langenbeck's Arch Surg. 2001;386:65–73.

25. Muysoms FE, Miserez M, Berrevoet F, Campanelli G, Champault GG, Chelala E, et al. Classification of primary and incisional abdominal wall hernias. Hernia. 2009;13:407–14.

26. Kössler-Ebs JB, Grummich K, Jensen K, et al. Incisional hernia rates after laparoscopic or open abdominal surgery – a systematic review and meta-analysis. World J Surg. 2016;40(10):2319–30.

27. Bosanquet DC, Ansell J, Abdelrahman T, et al. Systematic review and meta-regression of factors affecting midline incisional hernia rates: analysis of 14 618 patients. PLoS One. 2015;10(9):e0138745.

28. Harlaar JJ, Deerenberg EB, van Ramshorst GH, et al. A multicenter randomized controlled trial evaluating the effect of small stitches on the incidence of incisional hernia in midline incisions. BMC Surg. 2011;11:20.

29. Mudge M, Hughes LE. Incisional hernia: a 10 year prospective study of incidence and attitudes. Br J Surg. 1985;72(1):70.

30. Kingsnorth A, LeBlanc K. Hernias: inguinal and incisional. Lancet. 2003;362(9395):1561.

31. Bucknall TE, Cox PJ, Ellis H. Burst abdomen and incisional hernia: a prospective study of 1129 major laparotomies. Br Med J (Clin Res Ed). 1982;284(6320):931.

32. Sanders DL, Kingsnorth AN. The modern management of incisional hernias. BMJ. 2012;344:e2843.

33. Fassiadis N, Roidl M, Hennig M, South LM, Andrews SM. Randomized clinical trial of vertical or transverse laparotomy for abdominal aortic aneurysm repair. Br J Surg. 2005;92(10):1208.

34. Inaba T, Okinaga K, Fukushima R, et al. Prospective randomized study of two laparotomy incisions for gastrectomy: midline incision versus transverse incision. Gastric Cancer. 2004;7(3):167.

35. Levrant SG, Bieber E, Barnes R. Risk of anterior abdominal wall adhesions increases with number and type of previous laparotomy. J Am Assoc Gynecol Laparosc. 1994;1(4, Part 2):S19.

36. Bickenbach KA, Karanicolas PJ, Ammori JB, et al. Up and down or side to side? A systematic review and meta-analysis examining the impact of incision on outcomes after abdominal surgery. Am J Surg. 2013;206(3):400–9.

37. Brown SR, Goodfellow PB. Transverse verses midline incisions for abdominal surgery. Cochrane Database Syst Rev. 2005;4:CD005199.

38. Spence PA, Mathews RE, Khanna R, Oreopoulos DG. Improved results with a paramedian technique for the insertion of peritoneal dialysis catheters. Surg Gynecol Obstet. 1985;161(6):585–7.

39. Hughes K, Selim NM. The lateral paramedian: revisiting a forgotten incision. Am Surg. 2009;75(4):321–3.

40. Hussain A, Mahmood H, Singhal T, et al. Long-term study of port-site incisional hernia after laparoscopic procedures. JSLS. 2009;13:346–9.

41. Di Lorenzo N, Coscarella G, Lirosi F, Gaspari A. Port-site closure: a new problem, an old device. JSLS. 2002;6:181–3.

42. Klop KWJ, Hussain F, Karatepe O, Kok NFM, IJzermans JNM, Dor FJMF. Incision-related outcome after live donor nephrectomy: a single center experience. Surg Endosc. 2013;27(8):2801–6.

43. Morris-Stiff G, Coles G, Moore R, Jurewicz A, Lord R. Abdominal wall hernia in autosomal dominant polycystic disease. Br J Surg. 1997;84:615–7.

44. van den Berg JC, de Valois JC, Go PM, Rosenbusch G. Detection of groin hernia with physical examination, ultrasound, and MRI compared with laparoscopic findings. Investig Radiol. 1999;34(12): 739–43.

45. Bickley LS, Szilagyi PG, Bates B. Bates' guide to physical examination and history taking. 8th ed. Philadelphia: Lippincott Williams & Wilkins; 2003. p. 359–72.

46. Brunicardi FC, Anderson DK, Schwartz SI. Schwartz's principles of surgery. 9th ed. New York: McGraw-Hill; 2010. p. 1316–8.

47. Jamadar DA, Franz MG. Inguinal region hernias. Ultrasound Clin. 2007;2(4):711–25.

48. Jamadar DA, Jacobson JA, Morag Y, et al. Sonography of inguinal region hernias. AJR Am J Roentgenol. 2006;187(1):185–90.

49. Korenkov M, Paul A, Troidl H. Color duplex sonography: diagnostic tool in the differentiation of inguinal hernias. J Ultrasound Med. 1999;18(8):565–8.

50. Burkhardt JH, Arshanskiy Y, Munson JL, Scholz FJ. Diagnosis of inguinal region hernias with axial CT: the lateral crescent sign and other key findings. Radiographics. 2011;31(2):E1–E12.

51. Zoga AC, Mullens FE, Meyers WC. The spectrum of MR imaging in athletic pubalgia. Radiol Clin N Am. 2010;48(6):1179–97.

52. Twardowski ZJ, Tully RJ, Ersoy FF, Dedhia NM. Computerized tomography with and without intraperitoneal contrast for determination of intraabdominal fluid distribution and diagnosis of complications in peritoneal dialysis patients. ASAIO Trans. 1990;36(2):95–103.

53. Hawkins PS, Homer AJ, Murray BB, Voss MD, van der Merwe MW. Modified computed tomography peritoneography: clinical utility in continuous ambulatory peritoneal dialysis patients. Australas Radiol. 2000;44(4):398.

54. Cakir B, Kirbaş I, Cevik B, et al. Complications of continuous ambulatory peritoneal dialysis: evaluation with CT. Diagn Interv Radiol. 2008;14(4):212–20.

55. Johnson BF, Segasby CA, Holroyd AM, et al. A method for demonstrating subclinical inguinal herniae in patients undergoing peritoneal dialysis: the isotope 'peritoneoscrotogram'. Nephrol Dial Transplant. 1987;2(4):254–7.

56. Suga K, Kaneko T, Nishigauchi K, et al. Demonstration of inguinal hernia by means of peritoneal 99mTc-MAA scintigraphy with a load produced by standing in a patient treated by continuous ambulatory peritoneal dialysis. Ann Nucl Med. 1992;6(3):203–6.

57. Bassini E. Nuovo metodo operativo per la cura dell'ernia inguinale. Padua: Prosperini; 1889.

58. Bay-Nielsen M, Kehlet H, Strand L, et al. Quality assessment of 26,304 herniorrhaphies in Denmark: a prospective nationwide study. Lancet. 2001;358:1124.

59. Kald A, Anderberg B, Carlsson P, Park PO, Smedh K. Surgical outcome and cost-minimisation-analyses of laparoscopic and open hernia repair: a randomised prospective trial with one year follow up. Eur J Surg. 1997;163:505–10.

60. Scott N, Go PM, Graham P, McCormack K, Ross SJ, Grant AM. Open mesh versus non-mesh for groin hernia repair. Cochrane Database Syst Rev. 2001;4:CD002197.

61. EU Hernia Trialists Collaboration. Repair of groin hernia with synthetic mesh: meta-analysis of randomized controlled trials. Ann Surg. 2002;235:322.

62. McCormack K, Scott NW, Go PM, Ross S, Grant AM, EU Hernia Trialists Collaboration. Laparoscopic techniques versus open techniques for inguinal hernia repair. Cochrane Database Syst Rev. 2003;1:CD001785.

63. www.nice.org.uk/guidance/ta83

64. Neumayer L, Giobbie-Harder A, Jonasson O, et al. Open mesh versus laparoscopic mesh repair of inguinal hernia. N Engl J Med. 2004;350:1819.

65. Li J, Ji Z, Li Y. Comparison of laparoscopic versus open procedure in the treatment of recurrent inguinal hernia: a meta-analysis of the results. Am J Surg. 2014;207:602.

66. Alani A, Duffy F, O'Dwyer PJ. Laparoscopic or open preperitoneal repair in the management of recurrent groin hernias. Hernia. 2006;10:156.

67. Karthikesalingam A, Markar SR, Holt PJ, Praseedom RK. Meta-analysis of randomized controlled trials comparing laparoscopic with open mesh repair of recurrent inguinal hernia. Br J Surg. 2010;97:4.

68. Kuhry E, van Veen RN, Langeveld HR, Steyerberg EW, Jeekel J, Bonjer HJ. Open or endoscopic total extraperitoneal inguinal hernia repair? A systematic review. Surg Endosc. 2007;21(2):161–6.

69. Memon MA, Cooper NJ, Memon B, Memon MI, Abrams KR. Meta-analysis of randomized clinical trials comparing open and laparoscopic inguinal hernia repair. Br J Surg. 2003;90(12):1479–92.

70. Wetherington GM, Leapman SB, Robison RJ, Filo RS. Abdominal wall and inguinal hernias in continuous ambulatory peritoneal dialysis patients. Am J Surg. 1985;150:357–60.

71. Shah H, Chu M, Bargman JM. Perioperative management of peritoneal dialysis patients undergoing hernia surgery without the use of interim hemodialysis. Perit Dial Int. 2006;26:684–7.

72. Guzman-Valdivia G, Zaga I. Abdominal wall hernia repair in patients with chronic renal failure and a dialysis catheter. Hernia. 2001;5:9–11.

73. Martinez-Mier G, Garcia-Almazan E, Reyes-Devesa HE, et al. Abdominal wall hernias in end-stage renal disease patients on peritoneal dialysis. Perit Dial Int. 2008;28:391–6.

74. Gianetta E, Civalleri D, Serventi A, Floris F, Mariani F, Aloisi F, et al. Anterior tension-free repair under local anesthesia of abdominal wall hernias in continuous ambulatory peritoneal dialysis patients. Hernia. 2004;8:354–7.

75. Lewis DM, Bingham C, Beaman M, Nicholls AJ, Riad HN. Polypropylene mesh hernia repair – an alternative permitting rapid return to peritoneal dialysis. Nephrol Dial Transplant. 1998;13:2488–9.

76. Pokorny H, Klingler A, Schmid T, et al. Recurrence and complications after laparoscopic versus open inguinal hernia repair: results of a prospective randomized multicenter trial. Hernia. 2008;12(4):385–9.

77. Gokal R, Alexander S, Ash S, et al. Peritoneal catheters and exit-site practices toward optimum peritoneal access: 1998 update. (Official Report from the International Society for Peritoneal Dialysis). Perit Dial Int. 1998;18:11–33.

78. Crabtree JH. The use of the laparoscope for dialysis catheter implantation: valuable carry-on or excess baggage? Perit Dial Int. 2009;29:394–406.

79. Crabtree JH. Hernia repair without delay in initiating or continuing peritoneal dialysis. Perit Dial Int. 2006;26:178–82.

80. Nicholson ML, Madden AM, Veitch PS, Donnelly PK. Combined abdominal hernia repair and continuous ambulatory peritoneal dialysis (CAPD) catheter insertion. Perit Dial Int. 1989;9:307–8.

81. Haggerty S, Roth S, Walsh D, SAGES Guidelines Committee, et al. Guidelines for laparoscopic peritoneal dialysis access surgery. Surg Endosc. 2014;11:3016–45.

82. Li JR, Wu MJ, Chiu KY, et al. Concomitant laparoscopic peritoneal dialysis catheter placement and total extraperitoneal hernioplasty: a case report. Perit Dial Int. 2010;30(5):580–1.

83. Sodo M, Bracale U, Argentino G, et al. Simultaneous abdominal wall defect repair and Tenckhoff catheter placement in candidates for peritoneal dialysis. J Nephrol. 2016;29(5):699–702.

84. Mettang T, Stoeltzing H, Alscher DM, et al. Sustaining continuous ambulatory peritoneal dialysis after herniotomy. Adv Perit Dial. 2001;17:84–7.

85. Swarnalatha G, Rapur R, Pai S, Dakshinamurty KV. Strangulated umbilical hernia in a peritoneal dialysis patient. Indian J Nephrol. 2012;22(5):381–4.

86. Morris-Stiff GJ, Bowrey DJ, Jurewicz WA, Lord RH. Management of inguinal herniae in patients on continuous ambulatory peritoneal dialysis: an audit of current UK practice. Postgrad Med J. 1998;74:669–70.

87. Wakasugi M, Hirata T, Okamura Y, et al. Perioperative management of continuous ambulatory peritoneal dialysis patients undergoing inguinal hernia surgery. Surg Today. 2011;41:297–9.

88. Imvrios G, Tsakiris D, Gakis D, et al. Prosthetic mesh repair of multiple recurrent and large abdominal hernias in continuous ambulatory peritoneal dialysis patients. Perit Dial Int. 1994;14(4):338–43.

89. Cherney DZ, Siccion Z, Chu M, Bargman JM. Natural history and outcome of incarcerated abdominal hernias in peritoneal dialysis patients. Adv Perit Dial. 2004;20:86–9.

90. Fitzgibbons Jr RJ, Giobbie-Harder A, Gibbs JO, et al. Watchful waiting vs repair of inguinal hernia in minimally symptomatic men: a randomized clinical trial. JAMA. 2006;295(3):285–92.

Index

© Springer International Publishing AG 2017

S. Haggerty (ed.), *Surgical Aspects of Peritoneal Dialysis*, DOI 10.1007/978-3-319-52821-2

CPI Antony Rowe
Chippenham, UK
2017-12-21 21:45